X 14.86

612.04

PERSPECTIVES ON HEALTH AND EXERCISE

Perspectives on Health and Exercise

Edited by

Jim McKenna and Chris Riddoch

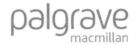

palgrave
macmillan

First published 2003 by
PALGRAVE MACMILLAN
Houndmills, Basingstoke, Hampshire RG21 6XS and
175 Fifth Avenue, New York, N.Y. 10010
Companies and representatives throughout the world

PALGRAVE MACMILLAN is the global academic imprint of the Palgrave Macmillan division of St. Martin's Press, LLC and of Palgrave Macmillan Ltd. Macmillan® is a registered trademark in the United States, United Kingdom and other countries. Palgrave is a registered trademark in the European Union and other countries.

ISBN 0–333–78700–5 paperback

This book is printed on paper suitable for recycling and made from fully managed and sustained forest sources.

A catalogue record for this book is available from the British Library.

10 9 8 7 6 5 4 3 2 1
12 11 10 09 08 07 06 05 04 03

Printed and bound in Great Britain by
Creative Print and Design (Wales), Ebbw Vale

Contents

List of Figures

List of Tables

Foreword

The 'future shock' of societal change is vividly apparent in the rapid decline of physical activity in our lives in less than a generation. In developed countries – and increasingly in developing countries – human beings have, in evolutionary terms, suddenly adopted less physically demanding work and lifestyles. Whereas this may be beneficial in some respects, in terms of human health it is an unfolding disaster, the full impact of which is only just beginning to be realised.

We are beginning to understand exactly how one's healthy life expectancy is determined by a few key health determinants and disease risks. One of the most important determinants is how physically active we are throughout our lives. The epidemic rise in avoidable chronic diseases in developed and developing countries such as cardiovascular disease, obesity, osteoporosis, diabetes and some cancers is in part caused by physical inactivity. The 'World Health Report', published in 2002 by the World Health Organisation, ranked the major contemporary health hazards and clearly demonstrated that physical inactivity is a major determinant of the global pandemic of avoidable chronic disease. The indications are that future generations may be even more afflicted as the levels of physical activity in children and young people may be declining to levels lower than that of their parents' generation.

It is therefore all the more surprising and alarming that this important area of public health has received relatively little attention from scientists, health workers and politicians given its central importance as a positive and universal solution for a broad range of public policy concerns. Professor Jerry Morris, one of the pioneers of scientific interest in physical activity, famously described physical activity as the 'best buy' in public health. There is at last a growing realisation of the importance of promoting higher levels of physical activity. The United States has recently woken up to the enormous social and economic consequences of a largely physically inactive population and is contemplating radical social change. More slowly, some European countries are also waking up to these issues.

Possibly of even more importance is that the quality of our life and well-being is greatly enriched by the quality of our experience of physical activity. In this respect physical activity can impact as much upon our mental well-being as upon our physical well-being and depends upon factors such as how we are encouraged to enjoy and experience play, sport and active recreation. How this enthusiasm and motivation might be maintained at both individual and societal levels is a key consideration of this book. The importance of a physical environment that supports individual attempts to become and remain more physically active is a major concern.

This book has not taken any short cuts but has a utilised a 'hunter-gatherer' approach to comprehensively reviewing and analysing the science and practice of physical activity promotion – from a multidisciplinary perspective. The book combines sociological, anthropological, physiological, psychological and environmental perspectives. It demonstrates the importance of physical activity throughout the lifecourse for everyone. As such, the book is a major contribution to scientific and public policy debate.

PAUL LINCOLN
Chief Executive
National Heart Forum

Acknowledgements

We would like to thank the following for their invaluable help in the preparation of this text: Houri Alavi for sowing the original seeds of the book, Magenta Lampson and Jon Reed for their helpful comments on content and design, Lucy Foster and Karen Sargent for proof reading the final text, and Margaret Thompson for administrative assistance. We would also like to thank Padma Narayanan for her thorough and professional preparation of the text.

We are also grateful to the following for their kind permission to use the material listed below:

Professor Ilkka Vuori, UKK Institute, Tampere, Finland, Figure 6.1.

Table 6.3 is reprinted with permission from the Diagnostic and Statistical Manual of Mental Disorders, Fourth Edition, Text Revision, Copyright 2000. American Psychiatric Association.

The Nutrition Society, Figure 7.1.

Human Kinetics, Figure 7.3.

Every effort has been made to contact all the copyright holders, but if any have been inadvertently omitted, the publishers will be pleased to make the necessary arrangement at the earliest opportunity.

Notes on Contributors

Colin Boreham is Professor of Sport and Exercise Science at the School of Applied Medical Sciences and Sports Studies at the University of Ulster, Northern Ireland. His main research interest is in children's physical activity and health.

David Carless works at the Department of Exercise and Health Sciences at University of Bristol. He is currently researching the mental health benefits of physical activity with a focus on clinical populations.

Douglas Carroll is Professor of Applied Psychology and Head of the School of Sport and Exercise Studies at University of Birmingham. His major research interests are in health psychology and cardiovascular psychophysiology.

Ashley Cooper is a lecturer in Exercise and Health Sciences at University of Bristol. His main research interests are physical activity in the prevention and treatment of the metabolic syndrome, and measurement of children's physical activity and associated behaviors.

Frank Eves is a lecturer in Applied Psychology at the School of Sport and Exercise Sciences at University of Birmingham. His current research interests are in psychological contributions to exercise participation and the visual regulation of locomotion.

Guy Faulkner is a lecturer in the Department of Exercise and Sport Science at the University of Exeter. His research interests lie primarily within the field of physical activity and psychological well-being.

Kenneth R. Fox is Professor in the Department of Exercise and Health Sciences at University of Bristol. His interests lie in exercise and the 'self', weight management and obesity, and exercise promotion models in primary health care.

Jo Harris is Director of the PGCE PE Teacher Education programme at Loughborough University. She is actively involved in research studying health-related policy and practice within the National Curriculum for Physical Education.

Maarike Harro and Atko Viru work in the Department of Health Promotion and Public Health at the University of Tartu in Estonia.

Rupert W. Jakes and Nicholas J. Wareham both work at the Institute of Public Health, in the Department of Community Medicine at Cambridge University. Their current research focuses on diabetes and physical activity.

Jacqueline Kerr is a researcher in the Munich Cancer Registry at the Ludwig-Maximilliams-University, Munich. Her current research addresses quality of life, doctor–patient communication and psychosocial interventions among cancer patients, and she retains an interest in promoting physical activity through environmental factors.

Jim McKenna and Chris Riddoch both are Senior Lecturers in the Department of Exercise and Health Sciences at the University of Bristol.

Nanette Mutrie is Professor of Physical Activity and Health Science at Glasgow University, Scotland. Her current research interests include physical activity and mental health (especially depression) and environmental interventions to promote active commuting.

Catherine Panter-Brick is a lecturer in the Department of Anthropology at the University of Durham. Her interests lie in human ecology and adaptation, subsistence and diet, and nutritional and medicinal anthropology.

Adrian Taylor is Professor at the School of Sport and Leisure at De Montfort University. His research interests include physical activity interventions in primary care, psychological aspects of sports injury rehabilitation, and exercise and mental health.

Allard J. van der Beek, Willem van Mechelen, Mireille N.M. van Poppel, Esther M.F. van Sluijs and Evert A.L.M. Verhagen all work in the Faculty of Medicine at the EMGO Institute in the Netherlands. Their research focuses on interventions to promote safe exercise.

Catherine Woods is a lecturer in Exercise and Sports Psychology at Dublin City University, Ireland. Her research interests include promotion of physical activity and adherence to active lifestyles across the lifespan, and public health impact of physical inactivity.

CHAPTER 1

Perspectives on Health and Exercise: an Introduction

CHRIS RIDDOCH AND JIM MCKENNA (EDITORS)

Chapter Contents

- Authors and themes
- What will the book contribute?
- Policy implications
- Working definitions

This book is obviously about physical activity and health, but the most important word in the title is 'perspectives'. 'Perspectives' means that we realise that physical activity is not just energy expenditure – something that can be quantified as 'calories burned', 'hours per week' or 'sport'. Rather, we feel that physical activity is a complex, multi-dimensional and infinitely variable behaviour that is extremely difficult to capture and explain from within a single discipline. A full understanding of physical activity, and how it affects health, can be achieved only by adopting a multi-disciplinary approach and absorbing information gleaned from a variety of perspectives. For example, many people know that an inactive lifestyle can lead to overweight and obesity, and metabolic research tells us how much physical activity we need to do to maintain normal weight. However, not everybody is active enough in this respect. Some people don't even try to become more active. Others try, but fail – they have a go at being active but soon relapse back to their sedentary ways. Therefore, on the one hand we know that we should be more active, but on the other hand we don't do it. In this simple example, the physiological perspective informs us of how much activity we need to do, and the psychological perspective tells us why we don't do it. We might also consider the environmental perspective in terms of how geographical and cultural influences impinge on the problem. And one can add other dimensions as well.

Our view is that where adverse health-related behaviours are both prevalent and resistant to change (smoking, inactivity and poor diet), the nature of the problem, and the potential answers, may be more complex than at first thought. This then is the *raison d'être* for this book – that complex problems demand complex solutions, and that both the problems and solutions can only be fully appreciated after a broad examination of the *all* available evidence. Although this might be contentious, perhaps it is only now that sufficient evidence has accumulated, from a sufficiently broad range of perspectives, to enable us to tease out the many relationships between physical activity and health that must exist.

The contributors to this book have written from defined perspectives and the resultant collection of perspectives is unique. It is precisely this *collection* of papers – constituting a broad variety of perspectives – that creates such a valuable resource. The *combined* influence of the chapters is greater than the sum of the individual chapters. Exposure to new perspectives can help to expand the thinking of professionals whose working practices are strongly defined and perhaps even entrenched. Using this idea we offer a challenge to all readers: explore how the chapters that might not ordinarily be read complement, contrast with, or challenge your own understanding (sometimes referred to as 'formalised prejudices'). An alternative perspective can often illuminate an issue that is seen as an insuperable problem from another perspective.

Authors and themes

Physical activity varies enormously in terms of its quantity, quality and type, and we have aimed to provide a range of intellectually challenging themes. Panter-Brick (University of Durham, UK – Chapter 12) questions current perspectives on levels of physical activity by considering anthropological evidence across a range of societies. Wareham and Jakes (University of Cambridge, UK – Chapter 3) provide a contemporary and critical interpretation of the epidemiological research addressing relationships between physical activity and health. Van Sluijs and colleagues (Vrei Inivesiteit Amsterdam, The Netherlands – Chapter 6) continue in this critical vein by reminding us of the risks associated with physical activity. Cooper (University of Bristol, UK – Chapter 5) shows how many of the most accepted relationships may be based on data of dubious quality, but shows how the new generation of objective measurement instruments may further enhance our current understanding of the various relationships between physical activity and health.

A well-developed perspective of biological responses to physical activity is provided by Viru and Harro (University of Tartu, Estonia – Chapter 11), and Boreham and Riddoch (University of Ulster, Northern Ireland and University of Bristol, UK – Chapter 2) show how the issues may vary across the different stages of life. Accordingly, physical activity – or rather lack of physical activity – has taken an important place on both the public health agenda (Taylor; DeMontford University, UK – Chapter 8) and education agenda (Fox & Harris; University of Bristol and Loughborough University, UK – Chapter 9).

Essentially, we have adopted the stance that no one type of evidence, no one type of researcher, and no one type of analysis or interpretation can answer all the important questions in this field. The questions are too complex, and the answers are likely to be equally complex. There are many relevant stakeholders – doctors, nurses, health-promotion specialists, politicians, exercise physiologists, exercise psychologists, epidemiologists, architects, town planners and anthropologists – the list is probably not exhaustive. Each can provide important evidence and interpretations from their own perspective. Kerr, Eves and Carroll (University of Birmingham, UK – Chapter 10) make the cogent case for physical activity promoters to work with a wider range of professionals than otherwise has been the case. They argue that this will improve the physical activity potential in our living environments. This is consistent with our (editorial) view that no individual perspective can provide a comprehensive understanding of this complex field. A clear example of this is the disappointing results of both population and individual-level interventions to promote higher levels of physical activity (Mutrie & Woods, University of Glasgow, Scotland; and Dublin City University, Ireland – Chapter 7). This 'failure' might be more easily understood after reading the chapter on the environment (Kerr *et al.*, Chapter 10). Likewise, the 'problem' of lack of vigorous activity may be more easily rationalised after absorbing the chapters on epidemiology (Chapter 3), biology (Chapter 11) and anthropology (Chapter 12).

An interesting dichotomy of perspectives that we hope you will consider is the supposed tension between the biomedical and psychosocial approaches to both physical activity and health. The biomedical approach generally encompasses the more readily quantifiable aspects of a disease, intervention or outcome. A typical example of acceptable evidence would be a randomised controlled trial, designed to reduce the incidence and/or prevalence of a disease, and assessing the potential cost savings. The alternative perspective might focus more on qualitative research approaches, examining 'man' as a complete psychosocial being, interacting in complex ways with the environment, and whose views, thoughts, feelings and desires are relevant focuses of enquiry. Appropriate research methods might be qualitative or quantitative. On-going experiences can be valued in their own right, or used to complement intervention outcomes to better understand how these outcomes are achieved. These descriptions are obviously caricatures, but serve to make the point that there is more than one way of looking at the evidence (of processes and outcomes), and perhaps even many paths to the same positive ends. Likewise, there is more than one view about what *counts* as evidence and the case for alternative perspectives has been strongly made by Carless and Faulkner (University of Exeter and University of Bristol, UK – Chapter 4) in the context of the often overlooked domain of mental health. We hope that both perspectives are substantially represented within this book, as we believe that each has an important contribution to make in furthering our understanding in this complex area.

What will the book contribute?

This book should not only broaden our understanding of physical activity and health, but it can also provide clues as to how we might best reverse the currently inexorable trend towards sedentary lifestyles. It is a mute point that 'we' might be nearing the limits of how sedentary human beings can actually become. Despite the continued popularity of physically active play (in young children), sport (in children and younger adults) and a range of physically active leisure pursuits that can be pursued by most people, it does appear that the pressures to be sedentary are now so intense that it has affected nearly everyone. The disappearance of manual work, the increasing competition from sedentary leisure activities and the plethora of labour-saving devices that surround us now dominate our existence. This milieu of social, environmental and technological pressures must be fully understood if we are to have an impact upon it through public health interventions. For example, the current policy of promoting individually focused, psychologically based interventions – however well-designed – is unlikely to succeed if social, cultural and physical environments more powerfully promote sedentary alternatives.

One of the principal aims of this book is to facilitate greater understanding of the complex interplay between individuals, groups and environments and how this affects behaviour. The pieces of this jigsaw are only just becoming clear and further editions might address the next logical question of how all of this affects individuals of differing genetic make-up. We might also explore the social world more fully, or adopt more than a First and Second World approach to further broaden the panorama of perspectives. It should be noted that there is a preponderance of studies of men in this field – especially in the more biomedical chapters – and this is undoubtedly a major limiting factor within the current evidence base. We also feel that we have been unable to do justice to how physical activity might modify the powerful demographic and socioeconomic influences on health. Potentially, these are *the* major influences on contemporary public health and they might mediate, or be mediated by, individual lifestyles, including physical activity. However, we feel that in each case the evidence base is not currently substantial enough and we must leave these important issues for a future edition of this book.

Policy implications

By drawing together all of this information we hope to guide students, policy makers and researchers towards a more complete understanding of the causes of sedentary living and a comprehensive evidence base from which to design effective 'solutions'. We have a range of authors – all acknowledged experts in their fields – offering a variety of critical perspectives on physical activity and health. We hope that within this single volume we will provide greater insight to some of the most pressing contemporary questions in this field:

- How important is physical activity in terms of physical and psychological health?
- What is the strength of the evidence?
- How easy is it to measure?
- How much activity is necessary for health?
- What happens to our bodies when we are active or inactive?
- Why are most of us inactive?
- What are the most potent barriers to being active?
- What strategies will promote increased activity in sedentary individuals?
- What strategies will promote increased activity in sedentary populations?
- Are there any risks to becoming more active?

A final point to make is that changing others' physical activity habits and patterns – such as reducing the incidence of smoking, or calories in the diet – is not easy. We suggest that those who believe it to be so either don't understand the problem, or have never tried it themselves. However, by reading and thinking about these chapters we hope you will be able to address at least one element of this problem. Each author has addressed contemporary themes that practitioners or researchers can consider in terms of improving their understanding or practice. Indeed, with so many personal, demographic and environmental influences on physical activity behaviour, it is virtually impossible to account for them all, but at least future physical activity promotion programmes can be based on a sound, multi-disciplinary evidence base. Reversing our current sedentary existence will take time, effort and resources. It will not be achieved overnight.

Unfortunately, people frequently lose sight of this fact. Equally, it is common to lose sight of the importance of sustaining the activity levels of people who have succeeded in becoming more physically active. These are important issues and are exemplified by the common negative reaction to intervention studies that aim to increase activity levels – especially when they are seen to have only a small effect. When the effects of a single intervention to promote physical activity are observed to be small, we are naturally disappointed. We tend to discount this individual contribution because it has not proved to be the 'magic bullet' that will get everyone moving. Nevertheless, this single intervention may have significantly altered – knowingly or unknowingly – an individual element in the chain of events leading to increased activity. Before population level change occurs – the essence of public health – it is quite likely that a broad range of initiatives must be in place, each constituting an important link in the chain. If you are in this chain then this book challenges you to make your particular link as strong as possible – so that the chain will hold in the worst of conditions. There are likely to be many links in the chain. For example, physical activity might be promoted by role models given frequent exposure in the media. GPs and health-promotion professionals might organise exercise-referral schemes. Physical activity specialists with high-level counselling skills might be widely available. National campaigns might promote health-related physical activity. Nutritionists and dieticians might be trained to also offer advice on physical activity. Legislation might provide incentives for activity or disincentives for sedentary activities. In addition, all of this might take place within an environment that has been designed or modified to be more conducive to physical activity. Perhaps all of these developments need to be in place before population-level shifts in physical activity take place. Perhaps some, as yet, undefined 'critical mass' of developments is needed. Perhaps there is even a 'key' element, without which the others will not 'work'.

All of this is for the future. It is our belief that large-scale improvements in physical activity behaviour will entail a well coordinated, multi-disciplinary, multi-agency approach. It will probably need a high degree of political will. It will be costly. However, substantial resources have previously been devoted to physical activity promotion, with minimal public health return. Our hope is that future strategies are more creative, more all-embracing and – most of all – more effective.

Working definitions

A range of definitions of key terms used throughout this book can be found in the literature. We have explored these and compiled the following list of 'working definitions', solely for the purposes of reading this book:

Physical activity Any force exerted by skeletal muscle that results in energy expenditure above resting level.

Exercise A subset of physical activity, which is volitional, planned, structured, repetitive and aimed at improvement or maintenance of any aspect of fitness or health.

Sport A subset of physical activity, which involves structured competitive situations governed by rules. In Europe, sport is often used in a wider context to include all exercise and leisure physical activity.

Physical fitness A set of attributes that people have or achieve that relates to the ability to perform physical activity. Some fitness components are related to sports performance, and others are also health-related. Health-related fitness components can be considered as cardio-respiratory endurance, muscular endurance, muscular strength, body composition and flexibility. These fitness components also contribute to sports performance and capacity to undertake occupational tasks. Fitness is determined by genetic inheritance, age, gender and physical activity patterns.

Dimensions of physical activity Physical activity is normally considered to vary along five basic dimensions:

- Volume: Total quantity of physical activity over a specified period. Usually expressed as kcal/day or week. Can also be expressed as MET hours/day or week (1 MET = basal metabolic rate)
- Frequency: Frequency of participation is typically expressed as number of sessions a day or week
- Intensity: Usually categorized as light, moderate, or vigorous, referring to rates of energy expenditure ($kcal\,min^{-1}$ or $kj\,h^{-1}$), multiples of resting metabolic rate (METs), oxygen consumption ($ml\,kg^{-1}\cdot min^{-1}$) or heart rate ($beats\cdot min^{-1}$)
- Duration: Time spent on a single episode of activity
- Type or mode: A qualitative descriptor, such as walking, jogging, running, swimming or rhythmic activities.

When assessing physical activity for fitness outcomes, frequency, intensity, type and duration of activity are important, whereas when assessing physical activity for health-related benefits, volume and weight-bearing modes of activity are also important. Physical activity has both physiological and behavioural dimensions. From a physiological perspective, physical activity is one component of total energy expenditure. From a behavioural perspective, physical activity can be viewed within any of several frameworks for understanding human behaviour.

SECTION I

PHYSICAL ACTIVITY: A LIFECOURSE PERSPECTIVE

The first section of this book consists of a single chapter, which establishes a 'cradle to the grave' framework for why physical activity is major contemporary health issue. The chapter also makes the point quite clearly that physical activity is a health issue for everybody – irrespective of age, gender, health status and personal circumstances. In effect, this chapter sets the 'big picture', and subsequent chapters develop and explore important sub-texts. Locating physical activity in a 'lifecourse' perspective is the first stop on any journey towards a comprehensive understanding of the full spectrum of health benefits that can be attributed to regular physical activity. It is too easy to become embroiled in debates about the nature of one specific effect of physical activity – for example how it may contribute to weight management – and to lose sight of the fact that physical activity confers substantial health benefits in a broad *range* of health outcomes. Such an approach ignores the potential summative and maybe multiplicative benefits that accrue from the full range of health effects. The nature of research and teaching often aggravates this, as researchers normally specialise in defined areas of physical activity and teaching takes place in delimited time periods during which one particular aspect of physical activity is addressed. In both cases, it is often very difficult to 'see the wood for the trees'.

Focusing on the 'big picture' is therefore an appropriate and logical starting point. In some ways the development of knowledge and understanding in this field has operated in reverse – the individual relationships with defined areas of health came first – followed by a more overarching, 'lifecourse' perspective. This may have been stimulated by the extension of the evidence-based medical climate into the field of public health, or health promotion. Just as the safety and effectiveness of a new drug needs to be ascertained, so the safety and effectiveness of new public-health interventions should also be ascertained for different population groups. A lifecourse perspective provides an appropriate framework for this exercise.

While reading this chapter it should become apparent that physical activity does not have just one effect on health – it has many. The strength of the effects varies between different diseases and conditions. The effects also vary with different dimensions of physical activity (the amount and type of activity performed) and also with age and, in some cases, gender. This variety of effects indicates that any single 'prescription' for health-related physical activity is very much a compromise message derived from a careful examination of *all* the effects of activity. Public-health professionals who work in the field of physical activity should be aware of this. While accepting that simple, singular messages about physical activity are necessary to promote physical activity on a population level, it is also crucial to retain a full understanding of the diversity of effects of physical activity.

CHAPTER 2

Physical Activity and Health through the Lifespan

COLIN BOREHAM AND CHRIS RIDDOCH

Chapter Contents

Introduction

It is now accepted that physical inactivity is a fundamental cause of several chronic diseases in adult life, including cardiovascular diseases, obesity, osteoporosis and some cancers. The majority of studies investigating these associations have, however, focused on one phase of life, usually middle-age. While such adult exposure to physical activity and other health behaviours are clearly important in the aetiology of these diseases, the 'adult lifestyle' model alone fails to explain much of the observed variation in disease between individuals and populations (Davey Smith & Hart, 1998). These explanatory limitations have given rise to recent interest in factors acting either at early stages of life ('programming'; Barker, 1992) or cumulatively throughout life ('life course epidemiology'; Kuh & Ben-Shlomo, 1997). Both models may be important to the understanding of chronic diseases, many of which, it is now acknowledged, invariably display long incubation periods (Rose, 1982). Indeed, a report from the Department of Health (GB Department of Health, 1995) concluded that '. . . it is likely that accumulative differential lifetime exposure to health-damaging or health-promoting physical and social environments is the main explanation for the observed

variations in health and life expectancy.' The purpose of this chapter will be
to examine physical activity from such a 'lifecourse' perspective, analysing
the evidence for health benefits from the foetus through to the frail elderly.
Such benefits may differ considerably in type and magnitude from one stage
of life to another, creating the need for a parallel lifecourse approach to
activity promotion and prescription.

 Chapter 3 (Epidemiology) further considers issues of lifecourse epidemiology.

Lifecourse epidemiology – background

Lifecourse epidemiology seeks to understand the biological, social and
psychological processes which influence health from conception to old age.
Health of grandparents and parents, genetic endowment, intrauterine, childhood and adult exposures, together with the interaction between these and
exposures acting in later adulthood, are all seen as influential (see Figure 2.1).
Despite large gaps in current understanding, the available evidence suggests
that there may be critical periods when preventive interventions will be most
effective. Special emphasis is given to experiences in childhood, adolescence
and early adult life, together with the interaction between these and exposures
acting in later adulthood. The lifecourse approach can also help to identify
biological mechanisms responsible for the production of later disease. Before
examining the potential interactions between physical activity, morbidity and
mortality from a lifecourse perspective, it is worth obtaining a broader
perspective of possible lifecourse influences for a specific adult disease, cardiovascular disease (CVD). CVD remains the major single cause of death among

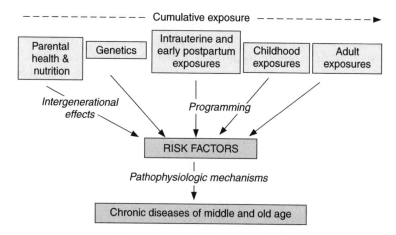

Figure 2.1   A lifecourse model of factors influencing health

men in most of the industrialised world. The aetiology of CVD is complex and several pathological processes are involved. These processes include the development of atherosclerosis, abnormalities of the haemostatic system and alterations in myocardial contractibility and function. It can be argued that CVD is the cause of death which illustrates most clearly the lifecourse perspective, since risk is associated with parental health, with intrauterine development, with growth and health in childhood and with several socio-economic and behavioural factors in adulthood. Notably, the importance of early-life exposures in the development of CVD is supported by post-mortem evidence revealing that about half of young men have evidence of atherosclerosis in their coronary vessels (McNamara *et al.*, 1971), the extent of which is related to antecedent levels of risk (Berenson *et al.*, 1998).

The importance of development *in utero* and in infancy is indicated by associations of both low birthweight and weight at one year with a high CVD risk later in life (Barker, 1992). Biological plausibility for such associations is given by the association between low birthweight and endothelial dysfunction (an indicator or early atherogenesis) in 9–11-year-olds (Leeson *et al.*, 1997). The effect of exposures acting in childhood is illustrated by relationships between adverse childhood socio-economic circumstances and CVD mortality which are independent of adult socio-economic circumstances (Davey Smith *et al.*, 1998). Poor growth in childhood – indicated by short leg length for age – is also associated with an increased risk of CVD mortality (Gunnell *et al.*, 1998a). Both low birthweight and short leg length are associated strongly with CVD if combined with obesity in adulthood, indicating biological interactions between factors at different stages of the lifecourse (Davey Smith, 1997). While childhood diet is a behaviour which may underlie links between growth and later CVD (particularly the consumption of anti-oxidants and fat; Witzum, 1994; McGill & McMahon, 1998), other behavioural factors such as smoking and physical activity may become influential only in later childhood or adolescence. Indeed, a recent study (McGill *et al.*, 2000) has indicated that the third decade of life may be particularly critical in the development of atherosclerosis. In this autopsy study of young men and women, there was a ten-fold increase in advanced lesions of left anterior descending coronary arteries between the ages of 15–19, and between 30–34 years in men. Furthermore, the extent and severity of lesions were associated with antemortem levels of risk, including non-HDL cholesterol greater than 4.14 mmol/L, smoking, HDL cholesterol less than 0.91 mmol/L, obesity (BMI greater than 30kg/m^2) and hypertension (mean arterial pressure 110 mm Hg or greater). A list of CVD risk factors is of particular interest from a lifecourse perspective is given in Table 2.1. To date, little has been written on physical activity from a lifecourse perspective, despite the growing acceptance of its myriad role in maintaining health and preventing disease (Bouchard *et al.*, 1994; Booth *et al.*, 2000). The remainder of this chapter will therefore attempt to redress this imbalance.

Table 2.1   Principal lifecourse risk factors for adult CVD

Early life	Childhood/adolescence	Adulthood
Maternal health and diet before/during pregnancy	Socio-economic deprivation	Blood pressure
Parental history of CVD	Poor growth	Serum cholesterol
Low birthweight	Obesity	Obesity
	Childhood infections	Smoking
	Diets	Diet
	Blood pressure, serum cholesterol	Fitness
	Smoking	Short stature
	Physical inactivity	Binge drinking
		Diabetes
		Physical inactivity

Modified from Davey Smith *et al.*, 1998

Physical activity and health throughout the lifecourse

It is important to emphasise at the outset that most of what can be written on this topic remains speculative. No study exists which has recorded adequate birth-to-death information relating physical activity to health. What is available can be described as a series of 'snapshots' at various stages of the lifecourse, which at best (as with the seminal Harvard Alumni study; Sesso *et al.*, 2000) covers the years of adulthood, but more commonly follows up subjects for limited time periods (typically 10–20 years), or observes relationships between activity and health at single time points. Hence there is only limited understanding of the extent to which bio-logical, social and behavioural (including physical activity) risks experienced at different life stages combine to influence adult disease. Furthermore, phys-ical activity is a complex behaviour, which varies according to type, frequency, duration and intensity. It is not, therefore, a single entity, although it is often treated as such. Although evidence is scarce, it is likely that different components of physical activity may prove more beneficial to health at different stages of life. For example, vigorous, varied and intermittent exercise may prove most beneficial to the health of young children and adolescents, while for the middle-aged, more moderate exercise stressing the cardiovascular system may be more appropriate. In old age, gentler exercise incorporating more stretching and everyday ambulatory activities might be associated with optimal health. Thus, just as the various compon-ents of blood pressure may relate differently to coronary mortality at dif-ferent stages of adulthood (Franklin *et al.*, 2001), various components of activity may prove more 'healthy' than others at different stages of the lifecourse (Table 2.2). Although exercise recommendations already exist

Table 2.2 Physical activity and health throughout the lifecourse

Stage	Gestation/childhood	Adolescence/young adulthood	Middle age	Old age
Physical activities	Maternal exercise Free play	Sport Dance Vigorous recreation Physical education	Lifestyle Gym Moderate recreation Housework Gardening DIY	Lifestyle Activities of daily living Self-paced recreation Gardening
Lifecourse influences on physical activity	Maternal circumstances Birthweight Social class Gender Siblings Garden/play area Climate Poor growth	Gender School type Social class Sports ability/self-efficacy Family influences TV watching	Educational level Car ownership Social class Job security/control Leisure time Family pressures	Health status Social class Social network Gender Spouse's influence
Health associations	Fitness Fatness CHD risk? Fundamental motor skills?	Fitness Fatness CHD risk status Bone density Other risk behaviours (smoking, diet)	Morbidity/mortality from chronic diseases (CHD, stroke, diabetes, cancer, obesity)	Functional fitness Osteoporosis Disease resistance (immune function) Independence Functional fitness Social networks

for different age groups (ACSM, 1998; Biddle *et al.*, 1998), many scientific issues relating to exercise prescription remain unresolved (Winett & Carpinelli, 2000).

Chapter 3 (Epidemiology) considers the scientific issues relating to exercise prescription.

A further complication is that physical activity behaviour varies throughout the lifecourse according to certain boundaries and 'life-events'. Free play predominates in the pre-school child, while pre-adolescents adopt more formal sporting and physical education activities. Adolescence and young adulthood may be characterised by a general decline in interest and levels of activity, as the more formal structures disappear, while recreational and household tasks may predominate in middle-age. Finally, in retirement, gentler recreational activities and so-called 'activities of daily living' become the norm. To what extent these broad boundaries are natural, biological progressions along the lifecourse and to what extent they are determined by societal norms is a moot point, and one which needs further exploration. Such abrupt changes from one stage of life to the next (for example, from school to work) will also tend to disrupt established patterns of physical activity behaviour, leading to poor or moderate 'tracking'[1] of activity between stages (Twisk *et al.*, 2000). While specific activities (and their specific health benefits) may not be carried over from one stage to the next, we need to acknowledge the importance of maintaining an overall 'background' of adequate energy expenditure in the form of moderate intensity activities (Westerterp, 2001), irrespective of the stage of life. This may be particularly important in relation to rising obesity levels (Kaplan & Dietz, 1999). Bearing the above complexities and limitations in mind, the evidence linking physical activity with health status throughout various stages of the lifecourse will now be examined.

Chapter 12 (Anthropology) explores how physical activity differs across and within cultural groups.

Early life influences

Intrauterine environment

It is now accepted that foetal under-nutrition in middle-to-late gestation, resulting in disproportionate foetal growth and low birthweight, is associated with increased CVD risk in later life (Barker, 1992). It is hypothesised that the nutrient and hormonal milieu of the foetus alters gene expression, causing developmental adaptations that lead to permanent changes in physiology and metabolism which, in turn, predispose to chronic disease in later life (Godfrey,

1998). Such 'foetal programming' of adult CVD may be mediated by a number of risk factors which have been shown to be associated with birthweight, including blood pressure (Martyn *et al.*, 1995) insulin resistance (Phillips, 1996), serum lipids (Barker *et al.*, 1993) and body-fat distribution (Barker *et al.*, 1997).

Two main questions have been addressed in relation to the intrauterine environment and exercise. Firstly, what are the effects of maternal exercise on foetal development and, secondly, what are the longer-term consequences on exercise and fitness of low birthweight? Interest in the former has stemmed from the postulated risks of exercise to foetal growth (arising from redistribution of foetal blood flow, hypothermia and reduced carbohydrate availability to the foetus) and the now well-established, independent relationships between low birthweight and adult disease (Barker, 1992; Leon & Ben Shlomo, 1997; Huxley *et al.*, 2000). However, there is almost unanimous agreement that moderate intensity exercise during pregnancy in healthy, well-nourished women is not harmful to either mother or foetus (Alderman *et al.*, 1998; Kardel & Kase, 1998; Rieman & Kanstrup Hansen, 2000). Indeed, the benefits of exercise to the foetus during pregnancy may include decreased fat mass at term, improved stress tolerance, advanced neurobehavioural maturation and greater leanness at five years of age (Clapp, 2000). Conversely, there is some evidence that more severe fitness-training regimes may result in lighter offspring (Pivarnik, 1998), although this may be partly due to reduced neonatal fat mass (Clapp & Capeless, 1990). The longer-term health consequences of maternal exercise on offspring at adulthood are unknown.

With regard to the second question – that of the possible influences of low birthweight on physical activity and or fitness, only one preliminary study (Boreham *et al.*, 1999) has indicated a positive relationship between birthweight and subsequent fitness in adolescence. Although these results require replication, they show a strength of association on a par with that which exists between birthweight and adult blood pressure. Other indirect evidence that long-term fitness, along with other established CVD risk factors which may be partly programmed by environmental influences acting at critical stages in early life, is provided by results (Phillips & Barker, 1997) showing an association between birthweight and adult resting pulse-rate (a proxy for cardiovascular fitness).

Childhood and adolescence

Although we feel instinctively that physical activity ought to be beneficial to the health of children, there is surprisingly little empirical evidence to support this notion (Riddoch, 1998). Nevertheless, a hypothetical model has been proposed (Blair *et al.*, 1989) which suggests three main health benefits arising from adequate childhood physical activity.

1. *The direct improvement of childhood health status and quality of life* Most research into this area has been carried out into relationships between physical activity and CVD risk factors (including obesity) and bone health. Beneficial relationships between physical activity and blood pressure in children have been reported (Anderson, 1994; Dwyer & Gibbons, 1994; Webber *et al.*, 1996; Boreham *et al.*, 1997), but this is not a universal finding (De Visser *et al.*, 1994). Even more equivocal is the reported association between childhood activity and blood lipids, with some studies showing benefit (Suter & Hawes, 1993; Bistritzer *et al.*, 1995; Gutin *et al.*, 1996; Twisk *et al.*, 1996; Boreham *et al.*, 1997) and others not (Dwyer & Gibbons, 1994; Harrell *et al.*, 1996; Rowland *et al.*, 1996; Webber *et al.*, 1996). In relation to obesity, a review of recent evidence (Riddoch, 1998) indicated that only two studies (Durant *et al.*, 1994, 1996) observed no association, while several others (Robinson *et al.*, 1993; Wolf *et al.*, 1993; Gutin *et al.*, 1995; Boreham *et al.*, 1997; Gutin & Owens, 1999; Epstein *et al.*, 2000) observed a beneficial association even in children as young as five years (Gutin *et al.*, 1990). It may be prudent to accept the latter consensus, given the well documented recent increase in paediatric obesity (Reilly *et al.*, 1999; Chinn & Rona, 2001) despite apparent reductions in daily energy intakes in children over recent decades (Durnin, 1992). We can suggest four reasons why an increased prevalence of childhood obesity might be a major source of concern. Firstly, obesity is a major risk factor for insulin resistance and diabetes, hypertension, dyslipidaemia, poor cardio-respiratory fitness, and atherosclerosis (Schonfeld-Warden & Warden, 1997; Berenson *et al.*, 1998; Vanhala *et al.*, 1998; Boreham *et al.*, 2001). These relationships apply throughout childhood, from 5–17 years of age (Freedman *et al.*, 1999). Secondly, obesity tends to track into adulthood (Clarke & Lauer, 1993; Sinaiko *et al.*, 1999). Thirdly, adults who had been obese in childhood have increased morbidity and mortality, irrespective of their present weight (Must *et al.*, 1992; Gunnell *et al.*, 1998b; Sinaiko *et al.*, 1999) and, fourthly, overweight adolescents may suffer long-term social and economic discrimination (Gortmaker *et al.*, 1993). For these reasons, despite the current lack of compelling evidence, childhood obesity should be a major target for intervention from both primary prevention and treatment perspectives, and physical activity should feature strongly in this intervention.

Along with CVD, osteoporosis is a major public-health burden, the latter affecting women in particular. Although it is principally a condition of old age, the optimal prevention strategy may be the attainment of a strong, dense skeleton during the growing years of childhood and adolescence (Bailey *et al.*, 1996; Vuori, 1996). Peak bone mass, which is achieved in most people by their late 20s (Theintz *et al.*, 1992; Lu *et al.*, 1994) appears to be largely under genetic control. Up to 85 per cent of the inter-individual variance in bone mass is genetically determined, with several candidate genes involved in the regulation and metabolism of collagen (COLIA 1 gene), vitamin D (VDR-gene), oestrogen (ER gene) and nitric oxide (ec NOS gene) (Ralston, 1997). However, the residual variance in bone mass appears to be under environmental influences which may be amenable to early intervention. The most important environmental factors appear to be body mass, diet – notably calcium intake (French *et al.*, 2000; Heaney *et al.*, 2000) – and the amount and type of physical activity taken throughout childhood and adolescence. Investigations examining the relationship between physical activity in childhood and bone-mineral acquisition have been reviewed in detail by Bailey *et al.* (1996). Studies of representative populations have, in the main, been conducted retrospectively (Tylavsky *et al.*, 1992; Ruiz *et al.*, 1995; Teegarden *et al.*, 1996), although longitudinal or prospective studies have been reported (Slemenda *et al.*, 1994; Gunnes & Lehmann, 1996; Morris *et al.*, 1997). These studies indicate that weight-bearing physical activity in childhood and adolescence is an important predictor of bone-mineral density, while non-weight-bearing ativity (such as swimming or cycling) is not (Grimston *et al.*, 1993). The size of the effect of physical activity (difference in BMD between the high and low fitness or activity groups) is, typically, between 5–15 per cent. In his review, Vuori (1996) estimates that physical activity, which is feasible for large numbers of young people, increases peak bone mass somewhat less than one Standard Deviation, or 7–8 per cent approximately. However, more research on the optimal type and volume of physical activity required for bone health in young people is required. From animal models (Lanyon, 1996) it is likely that activities which involve high strains, developed rapidly and distributed unevenly throughout the movement pattern, may be particularly osteogenic. Thus, activities such as aerobics, disco dancing, volleyball, basketball and racket sports may be effective, and need not necessarily be of prolonged duration, as the osteogenic response to such movement appears to saturate after only a few loading cycles (Lanyon, 1996). It is also interesting to note that the natural play activities of young children, such as skipping, chasing and climbing, provide many high-impact novel strains, and may be optimal – in type – for bone health.

 Chapter 11 (Biology) details the biological responses to different physical activity and exercise loads.

Further work also needs to be done to establish the optimal period within childhood in which to perform such activities to promote bone growth. At one end of the spectrum, adult bone seems relatively unresponsive to all but the most vigorous of exercise regimes (Friedlander *et al.*, 1995; Lohman *et al.*, 1995; Skerry, 1997) but there is some evidence (Haapasalo *et al.*, 1994; Morris *et al.*, 1997; Bradney *et al.*, 1998) that physical activity during the immediate pre-pubescent and pubescent years may be crucial for maximising peak bone mass in girls.

2. *The direct improvement of adult health status by, for example, delaying the onset of chronic disease in adulthood* It is clear from the preceding section that physical inactivity is a prime suspect in the aetiology of childhood obesity. The adverse health effects of childhood obesity may have further consequences for adult health and well-being. For example, Must and colleagues (1992) published the results of a large, prospective study with 55 years of follow-up. Overweight in adolescence predicted a wide range of adverse health effects in adulthood that were independent of adult weight. Similar findings were published by Gunnell *et al.* (1998b). It is interesting to note that risk factors for adult coronary artery disease, such as obesity, accelerate atherogenesis in the teenage years and their effects are amplified in young adulthood, some 20–30 years before coronary artery disease becomes clinically manifest (Berenson *et al.*, 1998; McGill & McMahon, 1998). Recent evidence (Boreham *et al.*, 2001) suggests that in adolescents (unlike their adult counterparts), fatness may play a central role in the atherogenic risk profile. Thus, being overweight as an adolescent may be a more significant predictor of future chronic disease than being overweight as an adult. In relation to osteoporosis, the previous section indicates that load-bearing physical activity in girls is an essential stimulus for optimal bone structure, and has the potential to increase peak bone mass. The postulated 7–8 per cent increase (Vuori, 1996) has considerable potential to reduce the risk of osteoporosis and associated fracture in later life (Rubin *et al.*, 1993), particularly if the relative increase can be maintained throughout adulthood by an appropriate lifestyle, including exercise.

 Chapter 9 (Schools) discusses issues of how physical activity might be best promoted to young people within school systems.

3. *The increased likelihood of maintaining adequate activity levels into adulthood, thus indirectly enhancing health status* The persistence of behaviour, or attribute, over time is called 'tracking' and refers to the maintenance of a rank order position over time in relation to one's peers. If being active or inactive as a child influences one's activity behaviour as an adult (good tracking), then childhood physical activity could be said to indirectly influence adult health. Given the obvious problems associated with such long-term studies, research into this question remains sparse. While tracking of activity and fitness during childhood and adolescence appears relatively good (Pate *et al.*, 1996; Janz *et al.*, 2000; Maia *et al.*, 2001), tracking of physical activity between childhood and adulthood is weak-to-moderate at best (Malina, 1996; Twisk *et al.*, 2000). This is not surprising given lack of analytical conformity in such studies (Twisk, 1997), and a growing recognition that physical activity is a relatively unstable behaviour that can vary from day to day, season to season, and stage of life to stage of life. Examples of major life events which can disturb activity patterns include

changing schools, school-to-work transition, leaving home, moving house, moving to a new neighbourhood, biological and psychological development (especially puberty and adolescence), illness, marriage and child rearing. Any one or a combination of these can significantly affect activity levels, and therefore it is to be expected that activity levels will be rather discontinuous in nature within any one individual over time. Of particular note might be the role of family and the concept of 'leaving home'. Taylor *et al.* (1994) have described three components of family influences on physical activity. The first component is 'modelling', which represents family members' current or past physical activity patterns as well as exercising with a family member. In a modelling process 'the significant others' constitute available and powerful models. Such modelling may be apparent in the play activities of very young children (Sääkslahti *et al.*, 1999). The second is 'social influence', which involves encouragement provided by the family together with persuasion, pressure, expectations and sanctions. The third is 'social support', which includes giving information about physical activity, and providing material, transport and emotional support. Upon leaving home, such parental influences are lost, and other influences predominate.

Linked with this is the fact that active individuals are likely to change the choice of activity they favour as they grow older, moving from play, through sport, to social and recreational activities. Finally, the level of 'background' or lifestyle activity we do – for example housework and walking to work – confounds the overall picture. It is, therefore, not surprising that tracking coefficients are weak or moderate at best between childhood and adulthood. However, this lack of evidence should be viewed in the context of existing methodological limitations and a relative lack of large-scale studies capable of examining tracking from childhood to young adulthood and beyond.

Adulthood

There is little doubt that a sedentary lifestyle during adulthood is an adverse health exposure. Voluminous evidence exists that a low level of activity during adulthood increases the risk of a broad range of chronic diseases in both men (Paffenbarger *et al.*, 1986; Wannamethee & Shaper, 1992) and women (Eaton *et al.*, 1995). Low cardio-respiratory fitness has been shown to be equally predictive of higher risk (Blair *et al.*, 1989; Sandvik *et al.*, 1993). Further, adults who increase activity or fitness levels during adulthood appear to reduce their risk accordingly (Paffenbarger *et al.*, 1993; Blair *et al.*, 1995). Conversely, reverting to a sedentary lifestyle after an active youth appears to negate any potential beneficial effects of that activity (Paffenbarger *et al.*, 1986). This evidence is reviewed comprehensively within this book (Chapter 3, Jakes & Wareham) and elsewhere (US Department of Health and Human Services, 1996).

Chapter 3 (Epidemiology) addresses the issues surrounding health responses to physical activity and exercise.

From a lifecourse perspective, however, a number of issues remain. Firstly, follow-up studies may *underestimate* risk reduction arising from exercise, as baseline measurements normally do not take into account subsequent changes in activity. In other words, physically active individuals will tend to become less active over time, while the inactive ones will tend to become more active. This is often referred to as 'regression to the mean' and is a well-known phenomenon in many forms of research. Any subsequent calculations of relative risk for an active lifestyle, with respect to, for example, CHD mortality, is likely to be conservative. Some studies have taken serial measurements of activity over the timecourse of the study but these studies are the exception.

Secondly, most of the larger studies of adults are monitoring mortality in cohorts – or generations – that were much more active in their early lifecourse than current younger generations. Today's 50–60-year-old adult is likely to have walked or cycled to school, played for hours outside the house, was not distracted too much by television, and eventually walked to work – which was probably a manual job. So, any baseline measurements of physical activity or fitness may be misleading, as we know there has been an inexorable decrease in activity levels in all sectors of society over the past 50 years. In effect, we are using baseline (high) measurements of activity in our analyses, but we miss the subsequent decline in activity. Studies that do not account for, or, preferably, measure, such secular changes in activity may therefore significantly underestimate the influence of activity on health.

Finally, there remains the question of whether the relationship between physical activity and health during middle-to-late adulthood is uniquely a function of adult activity. We cannot really assess to what extent the observed relationships are modified, or even determined by, the cumulative exposures that have occurred during the foetal, infant, childhood and young-adult stages of life. In other words, do low levels of exposure to adverse influences before middle age mean that inactivity as an adult is less risky? Conversely, do high levels of previous exposure mean that taking up activity during adulthood may be less effective? These are questions we cannot yet answer.

Old age

Ageing has been defined as '...a process or group of processes occurring in living organisms that, with the passage of time, lead to a loss of adaptability, functional impairment and, eventually, death' (Spirduso, 1995, p. 6). Such decline is thought to arise from a combination of inevitable biological changes associated with ageing (or 'primary' ageing) such as loss of muscle mass, balance or hearing, and the accelerated ageing that occurs as a result of disease or environmental factors ('secondary' ageing). Physical activity clearly falls into the latter environmental category, and has become the focus of much research in recent years, in relation to the preservation of function into old age. For the purposes of this chapter, old-age is characterised as the portion of the lifecourse beyond 65 years of age. It is worth noting that this age group of society in developed countries is predicted to grow by 30 and 36 per cent during 2010 and 2020 (Spirduso, 1995, p. 10).

It has often been postulated that individuals who are generally physically active live longer than their sedentary counterparts. There is some evidence to support this 'general activity' hypothesis. For example, subjects over 85 years of age – when asked for their secrets to longevity – listed 'activity' first (Hogstel & Kashka, 1989). Associations between activity levels and mortality in epidemiological studies also indicate strong relationships. For example, in the Harvard Alumni Study (Paffenbarger *et al.*, 1986), individuals in the 60+ years categories who expended at least 2000 kcals/ week in physical activity displayed a 50 per cent reduction in relative risk for all-cause mortality. More recent epidemiological studies have confirmed such associations between mortality and physical activity (Wannamethee *et al.*, 2000) and fitness (Haapanen-Niemi *et al.*, 2000) in elderly populations.

Perhaps of greatest significance is the role physical activity and the maintenance of fitness can play in the *quality* of life (as well as its quantity) in the elderly. Of particular concern is the Active Life Expectancy (Katz *et al.*, 1983) or the number of years that an individual might expect to be able to conduct the basic Activities of Daily Living (ADLs), and thus live independently. Research has shown that physical activity has the potential to maintain function and active lifespan even in the very old. Elderly muscle remains responsive to resistance training (Fiatarone *et al.*, 1990; Hagerman *et al.*, 2000), often resulting in improved functional performance (Carmeli *et al.*, 2000; Fiatarone *et al.*, 1990). There is consistent evidence that increasing physical activity in previously sedentary elderly is associated with a 20–40 per cent reduced risk of hip fracture resulting from falls (Gregg *et al.*, 2000). Even the very frail elderly may benefit from low-intensity supervised activity programmes which have been shown to significantly improve physical performance in such populations (Brown *et al.*, 2000). Furthermore, there is evidence that exercise of a duration and intensity sufficient to improve fitness may also attenuate age-related changes in the immune system (Venkatraman & Fernandes, 1997; Nieman, 2000). Finally, and perhaps not surprisingly, feelings of subjective well-being may be improved by longer term aerobic activities (McAuley *et al.*, 2000). Thus, even at the end of the lifespan, physical activity continues to make a significant contribution to the health and well being of the individual.

Chapter 4 (Mental health) addresses how physical activity is related to mental health. Chapter 7 (Inactivity) describes different approaches toward promoting physical activity with sedentary adults. Chapter 10 (Environment) describes how environmental approaches are increasingly being used to address low levels of physical activity.

Summary

In summary, it appears that there is compelling evidence linking physical activity to health and well-being at all stages of the lifecourse. Even with regard to the intrauterine environment, there is good evidence that in healthy, well-nourished pregnant women, moderate exercise is not harmful – and may be beneficial – to the foetus. More severe fitness training in pregnancy, however, may result in reduced birthweight. With regard to the influences of birthweight on subsequent fitness, evidence is slight, but indicates a positive relationship, such that heavier babies may display superior aerobic fitness at adolescence. This requires further study.

In relation to childhood, there is reasonably good evidence, both direct and circumstantial, which links higher physical activity levels in children with better health profiles in childhood. This is particularly so for certain CHD risk factors – especially obesity. As the extent of atherosclerosis in adolescents and young adults is proportional to their level of risk, there is a good rationale to start behavioural interventions at an early stage. There is also good evidence linking bone mass in young girls with the amount and type of their habitual physical activity. More research is needed to confirm putative evidence suggesting that specific exercise around puberty may be particularly osteogenic. Thus, physical activity in childhood has the potential for delivering direct health benefits to the child, as well as delaying the development of chronic diseases in adulthood.

There is strong evidence to suggest that, during middle age sedentary and less fit individuals are at increased risk of many of today's most common chronic diseases. Increasing activity and fitness levels during adulthood reduces the risk of these diseases accordingly, and reverting to a sedentary lifestyle after an active youth negates any previous benefits. We currently do not know to what extent the activity/health relationship during adulthood is influenced by exposures to risk occurring during the whole-of-life period proceeding adulthood.

In old age, regular physical activity and the maintenance of fitness continues to convey cardiovascular health benefits, but in addition is associated with a wide range of functional, social and medical benefits. From the cradle to the grave, regular physical activity appears to be an essential ingredient for human well-being.

Note

1 'Tracking', or stability of a characteristic, refers to the maintenance of relative rank or position within a group over time.

References

Alderman, B.W., Zhao, H., Holt, V.L., Walts, D.H. & Beresford, S.A. (1998) Maternal physical activity in pregnancy and infant size for gestational age, *Annals of Epidemiology*, **8**: 513–519.

American College of Sports Medicine (1998) Position Stand: The recommended quantity and quality of exercise for developing and maintaining cardiorespiratory and muscular fitness, and flexibility in healthy adults, *Medicine and Science in Sports and Exercise*, **30**: 975–999.

Anderson, L.B. (1994) Blood pressure, physical fitness and physical activity in 17-year-old Danish adolescents, *Journal of Internal Medicine*, **236**: 323–330.

Bailey, D.A., Faulkner, R.A. & McKay, H.A. (1996) Growth, physical activity and bone mineral acquisition, *Exercise and Sports Science Reviews*, **24**: 233–266.

Barker, D.J.P. (1992) *Fetal and infant origins of adult disease*. London: BMJ Publishing Group.

Barker, D.J.P., Martyn, C.N., Osmond, C. & Hales, C.N. (1993) Growth in utero and serum cholesterol concentrations in adult life, *British Medical Journal*, **307**: 1524–1527.

Barker, M., Robinson, S., Osmond, C. & Barker, D.J.P. (1997) Birthweight and body fat distribution in adolescent girls, *Archives of Disease in Childhood*, **77**: 381–383.

Berenson, G.S., Srinivasan, S.R., BAS, W., Newman, W.P., Tracy, R.E. & Wattingey, W.A. (1998) Associations between multiple cardiovascular risk factors and atherosclerosis in children and young adults, *New England Journal of Medicine*, **338**: 1650–1656.

Biddle, S., Sallis, J. & Cavill, N. (eds) (1998) *Young and Active? Young people and health-enhancing physical activity – evidence and implications*. Health Education Authority, London.

Bistritzer, T., Rosenzweig, L., Barr, J., Mayer, S., Lahat, E., Faibel, H., Schlesinger, Z. & Aladjem, M. (1995) Lipid profile with paternal history of coronary heart disease before age 40, *Archives of Disease in Childhood*, **73(1)**: 62–65.

Blair, S.N., Clark, D.G., Cureton, K.J. & Powell, K.E. (1989) Exercise and fitness in childhood: implications for a lifetime of health. In: Gisolji, C.V. & Lamb, D.R. (eds), *Perspective in Exercise Science and Sports Medicine*. New York: McGraw-Hill Companies Inc., pp. 401–430.

Blair, S.N., Kohl III, H.W., Barlow, C.E., Paffenbarger, R.S., Gibbons, L.W. & Maccra, C.A. (1995) Changes in physical fitness and all-cause mortality: a prospective study of healthy and unhealthy men. In: *Journal of the American Medical Association*, pp. 1093–1098.

Blair, S.N., Kohl, H.W., Paffenbarger, R.S.J., Clark, D.G., Cooper, K.H. & Gibbons, L.W. (1989) Physical fitness and all-cause mortality: a prospective study of healthy men and women. In: *Journal of the American Medical Association*, pp. 2395–2401.

Booth, F.W., Gordon, S.E:, Carlson, C.J. & Hamilton, M.T. (2000) Waging war on modern chronic diseases: primary prevention through exercise biology, *Journal of Applied Physiology*, **88**: 774–787.

Boreham, C., Murray, L., Dedman, D., Gray, A., Savage, M., Strain, J.J. & Davey Smith, G. (1999) Relationships between birthweight and physical fitness of adolescents: The Northern Ireland Young Hearts Project (Abstract), *Pediatric Exercise Science*, **11**: 277.

Boreham, C., Twisk, J., Murray, L., Savage, M., Strain, J.J. & Cran, G. (2001) Fitness, fatness, and coronary heart disease risk in adolescents: the Northern Ireland Young Hearts Project, *Medicine and Science in Sports and Exercise*, **33(2)**: 270–274.

Boreham, C.A., Twisk, J., Savage, M.J., Cran, G.W. & Strain, J.J. (1997) Physical activity, sports participation, and risk factors in adolescents, *Medicine and Science in Sports and Exercise*, **29(6)**: 788–793.

Bouchard, C., Shephard, R.J. & Stephens, T. (eds) (1994) *Physical Activity, Fitness and Health*. International Proceedings and Consensus Statement. Human Kinetics Publishers Inc., Champaign, Ill.

Bradney, M., Pearce, G., Naughton, G., Sullivan, C., Bass, S. & Besk, T. (1998) Moderate exercise during growth in prepubertal boys: changes in bone mass, size, volumetric density and bone strength. A controlled prospective study, *Journal of Bone Mineral Research*, **13**: 1814–1821.

Brown, M., Simacone, D.R., Ehsani, A.A., Binder, E.F., Hollozy, J.O. & Kohrt, W.M. (2000) Low intensity exercise as a modifier of physical frailty in older adults, *Archives of Physical Medicine and Rehabilitation*, **81**: 960–965.

Carmeli, E., Reznick, A.Z., Coleman, R. & Carmeli, V. (2000) Muscle strength and mass of lower extremities in relation to functional abilities in elderly adults, *Gerontology*, **46**: 249–257.

Chinn, S. & Rona, R. (2001) Prevalence and trends in overweight and obesity in three cross-sectional studies of British children 1974–94, *British Medical Journal*, **322**: 24–26.

Clapp, J.F. (2000) Exercise during pregnancy – a clinical update, *Clinics in Sports Medicine*, **19**: 273–286.

Clapp, J.F. & Capeless, E.L. (1990) Neonatal morphometrics after endurance exercise during pregnancy, *American Journal of Obstetrics and Gynaecology*, **163**: 1805–1811.

Clarke, W.R. & Lauer, R.M. (1993) Does childhood obesity track into adulthood?, *Critical Reviews in Food Science and Nutrition*, **33(4/5)**: 423–430.

Davey Smith, G. (1997) Down at heart – the meaning and implications of social inequalities in cardiovascular disease, *Journal of the Royal College of Physicians, London*, **31**: 414–424.

Davey Smith, G. & Hart, C. (1998) Socio-economic factors and determinants of mortality, *Journal of the American Medical Association*, **280**: 1744–1745.

Davey Smith, G., Hart, C., Blaire, D. & Hole, D. (1998) Adverse socio-economic conditions in childhood and cause-specific adult mortality: The Collaborative Study, *British Medical Journal*, **316**: 1631–1635.

De Visser, D.C., van Hooft, I.M., van Doornen, L.J., Hofman, A., Orlebeke, J.F. & Grobbee, D.E. (1994) Anthropometric measures, fitness and habitual physical activity in offspring of hypertensive parents. Dutch hypertension and offspring study, *American Journal of Hypertension*, **7(3)**: 242–248.

Durant, R.H., Baranowski, T., Johnson, M. & Thompson, W.O. (1994) The relationship among television watching, and body composition of young children, *Pediatrics*, **94**: 449–455.

Durant, R.H., Thompson, W.O., Johnson, M. & Baranowski, T. (1996) The relationship among television watching, physical activity, and body composition of 5- or 6-year-old children, *Pediatric Exercise Science*, **8**: 15–26.

Durnin, J.V.G.A. (1992) Physical activity and health: symposium of the Society for the Study of Human Biology. In: Norgan, N.G. (ed.), *Physical Activity Levels – Past and Present*. Cambridge: Cambridge University Press, pp. 20–27.

Dwyer, T. & Gibbons, L.E. (1994) The Australian Schools Health and Fitness Survey. Physical fitness related to blood pressure but not lipoproteins, *Circulation*, **89(4)**: 1539–1544.

Eaton, C.B., Medalie, J.H., Flocke, S.A., Zyzanski, S.J., Yaari, S. & Goldbourt, U. (1995) Self-reported physical activity predicts long-term coronary heart disease and all-cause mortalities. Twenty-one-year follow-up of the Israeli Ischemic Heart Disease Study. *Archives of Family Medicine*, **4**: 323–329.

Epstein, L.H., Paluch, R.A., Gardy, C.C. & Dorn, J. (2000) Decreasing sedentary behaviours in treating paediatric obesity, *Archives of Paediatrics and Adolescent Medicine*, **154**: 220–226.

Fiatarone, M., Marks, E., Ryan, N., Meredith, C., Lipsitz, L. & Evans, W. (1990) High intensity strength training in nonagenarians: Effects on skeletal muscle, *Journal of the American Medical Association*, **263**: 3029–3034.

Franklin, S.S., Larson, M.G., Khan, S.A., Wong, N.D., Leip, E.P., Kannel, W.B. & Levy, D. (2001) Does the relationship of blood pressure to coronary heart disease risk change with ageing? The Framingham Heart Study, *Circulation*, **103**: 1245–1249.

Freedman, D.S., Dietz, W.D., Srinivasan, S.R. & Bereson, G.S. (1999) The relation of over-weight to cardiovascular risk factors among children and adolescents: The Bogalusa Heart Study, *Paediatrics*, **103**: 1175–1182.

French, S.A., Fulkerson, J.A. & Story, M. (2000) Increasing weight-bearing physical activity and calcium intake for bone mass growth in children and adolescents: A review of intervention trials, *Preventive Medicine*, **31**: 722–731.

Friedlander, A.L., Genant, H.K., Sadowsky, S., Byl, N.N. & Gluer, C.C. (1995) A two-year program of aerobics and weight training enhances bone mineral density of young women, *Journal of Bone and Mineral Research*, **10**: 574–585.

Godfrey, J.M. (1998) Maternal regulation of foetal development and health in later life, *European Journal of Obstetrics and Gynaecology, Reproduction Biology*, **78**: 141–150.

Gortmaker *et al.* (1993) Social and economic consequences in adolescence and young adulthood, *New England Journal of Medicine*, **329**: 1008–1012.

Great Britain Department of Health (1995) *Variations in Health*. London: Department of Health.

Gregg, E.W., Pereira, M.A. & Caspersen, C.J. (2000) Physical activity, falls and fractures among older adults: A review of the epidemiologic evidence, *Journal of the American Geriatrics Society*, **48**: 883–893.

Grimston, S.K., Willows, N.D. & Hanley, D.A. (1993) Mechanical loading regime and its relationship to bone mineral density in children, *Medicine and Science in Sports and Exercise*, **25(11)**: 1203–1210.

Gunnell, D.J., Davey Smith, G., Frankel, S. *et al.* (1998a) Childhood leg length and adult mortality: follow up of the Carnegie (Boyd Orr) Survey of Diet and Health in Pre-war Britain, *Journal of Epidemiology and Community Health*, **52**: 142–152.

Gunnell, D.J., Frankel, S.J., Nanchahal, K., Peters, T.J. & Davey Smith, G. (1998b) Childhood obesity and adult cardiovascular mortality: a 57-y follow-up study based on the Boyd-Orr cohort, *American Journal of Clinical Nutrition*, **67**: 1111–1188.

Gunnes, M. & Lehmann, E.H. (1996) Physical activity and dietary constituents as predictors of forearm cortical and trabecular bone gain in healthy children and adolescents. A prospective study, *Acta Paediatrica*, **85**: 19–25.

Gutin, B. & Owens, S. (1999) Role of exercise intervention in improving body fat distribution and risk profile in children, *American Journal of Human Biology*, **11**: 237–247.

Gutin, B., Basch, C., Shea, S., Contento, I., De Lozier, M., Rips, J., Irigoyen, M. & Zypart, P. (1990) Blood pressure, fitness and fatness in five- and-six-year-old children, *Journal of the American Medical Association*, **264**: 1123–1127.

Gutin, B., Cucuzzo, N., Islam, S., Smith, C. *et al.* (1995) Physical training improves body composition of black obese 7- to 11-year-old girls, *Obesity Research*, **3(4)**: 305–312.

Gutin, B., Cucuzzo, N., Islam, S., Smith, C. & Stachura, M.E. (1996) Physical training, lifestyle education and coronary risk factors in obese girls, *Medicine and Science in Sports and Exercise*, **28(1)**: 19–23.

Haapanen-Niemi, N., Miilunpalo, S., Pasanen, M., Vuori, I., Oja, P. & Malmberg, J. (2000) Body mass index, physical inactivity and low level of physical fitness as determinants of all-cause and cardiovascular disease mortality – 16-year follow-up of middle-aged and elderly men and women, *International Journal of Obesity*, **24**: 1465–1474.

Haapasalo, H., Kannus, P., Sievanen, H., Heinonen, A., Oja, P. & Vuori, I. (1994) Long-term unilateral loading and bone mineral density and content in female squash players, *Calcified Tissue International*, **54**: 249–255.

Hagerman, F.C., Walsh, S.J., Stason, R.S., Hikida, R.S., Gilders, R.M., Murray, T.F., Toma, K. & Ragg, K. (2000) Effects of high-resistance training on untrained older men. I. Strength, cardiovascular and metabolic responses, *Journals of Gerontology*, Series A: **55(7)**, Series B: 336–346.

Harrell, J.S., McMurray, R.G., Bangdiwala, S.I., Frauman, A.C., Gansky, S.A. & Bradley, C.B. (1996) Effects of a school-based intervention to reduce cardiovascular disease risk factors in elementary-school children: The Cardiovascular Health in Children (CHIC) Study, *Journal of Pediatrics*, **128**: 797–805.

Heaney, R.P., Abrams, S., Dawson-Hughes, B., Looker, A., Marcus, R., Matkovic, V. & Weaver, C. (2000) Peak Bone Mass, *Osteoporosis International*, **11**: 985–1009.

Hogstel, M.D. & Kashka, M. (1989) Staying Healthy after 85, *Geriatric Nursing*, 16–18.

Huxley, R.R., Sheill, A.W. & Law, C.M. (2000) The role of size at birth and postnatal catch-up growth in determining systolic blood pressure – A systematic review of the literature. *Journal of Hypertension*, **18**: 815–831.

Janz, K.F., Dawson, J.D. & Mahoney, L.T. (2000) Tracking physical fitness and physical activity from childhood to adolescence: The Muscatine Study, *Medicine and Science in Sport and Exercise*, **32**: 1250–1257.

Kaplan, J.P. & Dietz, W.H. (1999) Caloric imbalance and public health policy, *Journal of the American Medical Association*, **282**: 1579–1581.

Kardel, K.R. & Kase, T. (1998) Training in pregnant women: effects on foetal development and birth, *American Journal of Obstetrics and Gynaecology*, **178**: 280–286.

Katz, S., Brauch, L.G., Branson, M.H., Papsidero, J., Beck, J.C. & Greek, D.S. (1983) Active life expectancy, *New England Journal of Medicine*, **309**: 1218–1224.

Kuh, D. & Ben-Shlomo, Y. (eds) (1997) *A lifecourse approach to chronic disease epidemiology*, Oxford: Oxford University Press.

Lanyon, L.E. (1996) Using functional loading to influence bone mass and architecture: object-ives, mechanisms and relationship with estrogen of the mechanically adaptive process in bone, *Bone Mineral*, **18**: 37S–43S.

Leeson, C.P.M., Whincup, P.H., Cook, D.G. *et al.* (1997) Flow mediated dilation in 9- to 11-year-old-children, *Circulation*, **96**: 2233–2238.

Leon, D. & Ben Shlomo, Y. (1997) *Pre-adult influences on cardiovascular disease and cancer. A life course approach to chronic disease epidemiology*, Oxford: OUP, 1997: 45–77.

Lohman, T., Going, S., Pamenter, R., Hall, M., Boyden, T., Houtkooper, L., Ritenbaugh, C., Bare, L., Hill, A. & Aickin, M. (1995) Effects of resistance training on regional and total bone mineral density in premenopausal women: a randomized prospective study, *Journal of Bone and Mineral Research*, **10**: 1015–1024.

Lu, P.W., Brody, J.N. & Ogle, G.D. (1994) Bone mineral density of total body, spine and femoral neck in children and young adults: A cross-sectional and longitudinal study, *Journal of Bone and Mineral Research*, **9**: 1451–1588.

McAuley, E., Blissmer, B., Marqurez, D.X., Jerome, D., Krames, A. & Katula, J. (2000) Social relations, physical activity and well-being in older adults, *Preventative Medicine*, **31**: 608–617.

McGill, H.C. & McMahon, C.A. (1998) Determinants of atherosclerosis in the young. Patho-biological Determinants of Atherosclerosis in Youth (PDAY) Research Group, *American Journal of Cardiology*, **82**: 30T–36T.

McGill, H.C., McMahan, A., Zieske, A.W., Tracy, R.E. *et al.* (2000) Association of coronary heart disease risk factors with microscopic qualities of coronary atherosclerosis in youth, *Circulation*, **102**: 374–379.

McNamara, J.J., Molot, M.A., Stremple, J.F. & Cutting, R.T. (1971) Coronary artery disease in combat casualties in Vietnam, *Journal of the American Medical Association*, **216**: 1185–1187.

Maia, J.A.R., Lefevre, J., Claessens, A., Renson, R., Vanreusel, B. & Beunen, G. (2001) Tracking of physical fitness during adolescence: a panel study in boys, *Medicine and Science in Sports and Exercise*, **33**: 765–771.

Malina, R.M. (1996) Tracking of physical activity and physical fitness across the life span, *Research Quarterly for Exercise and Sport*, **67**: (Suppl. to No. 3) S1–S10.

Martyn, C.N., Barker, D.J.P., Jespersen, S. *et al.* (1995) Growth in utero, adult blood pressure and arterial compliance, *British Heart Journal*, **73**: 116–121.

Morris, F., Naughton, G.A., Gibbs, J.L., Carlson, J. & Wark, J.G. (1997) Prospective ten-month exercise intervention in premenarcheal girls: positive effects on bone and lean mass, *Journal of Bone and Mineral Research*, **12**: 1453–1462.

Must A., Jacques P.F., Dallal G.E., Bajema C.J. and Dietz W.H. (1992) Long-term morbidity and mortality of overweight adolescents, *New England Journal of Medicine*, **327**: 1350–1355.

Nieman, D.C. (2000) Exercise Immunology: Future directions for research related to athletes, nutrition and the elderly, *International Journal of Sports Medicine*, **21**: (Suppl.) S61–S68.

Paffenbarger, R.S., Hyde, R.T., Wing, A.L. & Hsieh, C.C. (1986) Physical activity, all-cause mortality, and longevity of college alumni, *New England Journal of Medicine*, **314**: 605–613.

Paffenbarger R.S.J., Hyde, R.T., Wing, A.L., Lee, I.-M., Jung, D.L. & Kampert, J.B. (1993) The association of changes in physical activity level and other lifestyle characteristics with mortality among men. In: *New England Journal of Medicine*, pp. 538–545.

Pate, R.R., Baranowski, T., Dowda, M. & Trost, S. (1996) Tracking of physical activity in young children, *Medicine and Science in Sports and Exercise*, **28**: 92–96.

Phillips, D.I.W. (1996) Insulin resistance as a programmed response to fetal undernutrition, *Diabetologia*, **39**: 1119–1122.

Phillips, D.I.W. & Barker, D.J.P. (1997) Association between low birth weight and high resting pulse in adult life: is the sympathetic nervous system involved in programming the insulin resist-ance syndrome? *Diabetic Medicine*, **14**: 673–677.

Pivarnik, J.M. (1998) Potential effects of maternal physical activity on birth weight: brief review, *Medicine and Science in Sports and Exercise*, **30**: 400–406.

Ralston, S.H. (1997) Osteoporosis, *British Medical Journal*, 315: 469–472.

Reilly, J.J., Dorosty, A.R. & Emmett, P.M. (1999) Prevalence of overweight and obesity in British children: cohort study, *British Medical Journal*, 319: 1039.

Riddoch, C.J. (1998) Relationships between physical activity and physical health in young people. In: Biddle, S., Sallis, J.C.N. & Cavill, N. (eds), *Young and Active?* London Health Education Authority, pp. 17–48.

Rieman, M.K. & Kanstrup Hansen, I.L. (2000) Effects on the foetus of exercise in pregnancy, *Scandinavian Journal of Medicine and Science in Sports*, 10: 12–19.

Robinson, T.N., Hammer, L.D., Killen, J.D., Kraemer, H.C., Wilson, D.M. & Hayward, C. (1993) Does television viewing increase obesity and reduce physical activity? Cross-sectional and longitudinal analyses among adolescent girls, *Pediatrics*, 91(2): 273–280.

Rose, G. (1982) Incubation period of coronary heart disease, *British Medical Journal*, 284: 1600–1601.

Rowland, T.W., Martel, L., Vanderburgh, P., Manos, T. & Charkoudian, N. (1996) The influence of short-term aerobic training on blood lipids in healthy 10–12-year-old children, *International Journal of Sports Medicine*, 17(7): 487–492.

Rubin, K., Schirduan, V., Geudreau, P., Sarfrazi, M., Mendola, R. & Dalsky, G. (1993) Predictors of axial and peripheral bone mineral density in healthy children and adolescents, with special attention to the role of puberty, *Journal of Paediatrics*, 123: 863–870.

Ruiz, J.C., Mandel, C. & Garabedian, M. (1995) Influence of spontaneous calcium intake and physical exercise on the vertebral and femoral bone mineral density of children and adolescents, *Journal of Bone and Mineral Research*, 10: 675–682.

Sääkslahti, A.P., Numminen, P., Niinikoski, H., Rask-Nissilä, L., Viikari, J., Tuominen, J. & Välimäki, I. (1999) Is physical activity related to body size, fundamental motor skills, and CHD risk factors in early childhood?, *Pediatric Exercise Science*, 11: 327–340.

Sandvik, L., Erikssen, J., Thaulow, E., Eriksson, G., Mundal, R. & Rodahl, K. (1993) Physical fitness as a predictor of mortality among healthy, middle-aged Norwegian men. In: *New England Journal of Medicine*, pp. 533–537.

Schonfeld-Warden, N. & Warden, C.H. (1997) Pediatric obesity. An overview of etiology and treatment, *Pediatric Clinics of North America*, 44(2): 339–361.

Sesso, H.D., Paffenbarger, R.S. & Lee, I.M. (2000) Physical activity and coronary heart disease in men: The Harvard Alumni Health Study, *Circulation*, 102: 975–980.

Sinaiko, A.R., Donahue, R.P., Jacobs, D.R. & Prineas, R.J. (1999) Relation of weight and rate of increase of weight during childhood and adolescence and body size, blood pressure, fasting insulin and lipids in young adults. The Minneapolis Children's' Blood pressure Study, *Circulation*, 99: 1471–1476.

Skerry, T.M. (1997) Mechanical loading and bone: what sort of exercise is beneficial to the skeleton? *Bone Mineral*, 20: 179–181.

Slemenda, C.W., Reister, T.K., Hui, S.L., Miller, J.Z., Christian, J.C. & Johnston, C.C. (1994) Influences on skeletal mineralization in children and adolescents: Evidence for varying effects of sexual maturation and physical activity, *Journal of Pediatrics*, 125: 201–207.

Spirduso, W. (1995) *Physical dimensions of ageing*. Human Kinetics, Champaigne, Il.

Suter, E. & Hawes, M.R. (1993) Relationship of physical activity, body fat, diet and blood lipid profile in youths 10–15 Years, *Medicine and Science in Sports and Exercise*, 25(6): 748–754.

Taylor, W.C., Baranowski, T. & Sallis, J.F. (1994) Family determinants of childhood physical activity: A social-cognitive model. In: Dishman R.K. (ed.), *Advances in Exercise Adherence*. Human Kinetics: Champaigne, pp. 319–342.

Teegarden, D., Proulx, W.R., Kern, M., Sedlock, D., Weaver, C.M., Johnston, C.C. & Lyle, R.M. (1996) Previous physical activity relates to bone mineral measures in young women, *Medicine and Science in Sports and Exercise*, 28: 105–113.

Theintz, G., Buchs, B., Rizzoli, R., Slosman, D., Clavien, H., Sizonenko, P.C. & Bonjour, J.P. (1992) Longitudinal monitoring of bone mass accumulation in healthy adolescents: evidence for a marked reduction after 16 years of age at the levels of the lumbar spine and femoral neck in female subjects, *Journal of Clinical Endocrinology and Metabolism*, 75: 1060–1065.

Twisk *et al.* (1996) Relationship between the longitudinal development of lipoprotein levels and life-style parameters during adolescence and young adulthood, *Annals of Epidemiology*, 6: 246–256.

Twisk, J. (1997) Different statistical models to analyse observational longitudinal data: An example from the Amsterdam Growth and Health Study, *International Journal of Sports Medicine*, **18**: (Suppl. 3) S216–224.

Twisk, J.W., Kemper, H.C. & Van Mechelen, W. (2000) Tracking of activity and fitness and the relationships with cardiovascular disease risk factors, *Medicine and Science in Sports and Exercise*, **32**: 1455–1462.

Tylavsky, F.A., Anderson, J.J.B., Talmage, R.V. & Taft, T.N. (1992) Are calcium intakes and physical activity patterns during adolescence related to radial bone mass of white college-age females?, *Osteoporosis International*, **2**: 232–240.

US Department of Health and Human Services (1996) *Physical activity and health: a report of the surgeon general*. Pittsburgh, PA: Department of Health and Human Services, Centers for Disease Control and Prevention, National Center for Chronic Disease Prevention and Health Promotion.

Vanhala, M., Vanhala, P., Kumpusalo, E., Halonen, P. & Takala, J. (1998) Relation between obesity from childhood to adulthood and the metabolic syndrome: population based study, *British Medical Journal*, **317**: 319.

Venkatraman, J.T. & Fernandes, G. (1997) Exercise, immunity and ageing, *Ageing-Clinical and Experimental Research*, **9**: 42–56.

Vuori, I. (1996) Peak bone mass and physical activity: A short review, *Nutrition Reviews*, **54(4)**: S11–S14.

Wannamethee, G. & Shaper, A.G. (1992) Physical activity and stroke in British middle-aged men. In: *British Medical Journal*, **304**: 597–601.

Wannamethee, S.G., Shaper, A.G. & Walker, M. (2000) Physical activity and mortality in older men with diagnosed coronary heart disease, *Circulation*, **102**: 1358–1363.

Webber, L.S., Osganian, S.K., Feldman, H.A., Wu, M., McKenzie, T.L., Nichaman, M., Lytle, L.A., Edmundson, E., Cutler, J., Nader, P.R. & Luepker, R.V. (1996) Cardiovascular risk factors among children after a two and a half year intervention – The CATCH Study, *Preventive Medicine*, **25**: 432–441.

Westerterp, K.R. (2001) Pattern and intensity of physical activity. Keeping moderately active is the best way to boost total daily energy expenditure, *Nature*, **410**: 539.

Winett, R.A. & Carpinelli, R.N. (2000) Examining the validity of exercise guidelines for the prevention of morbidity and all-cause mortality, *Annals of Behavioural Medicine*, **22(3)**: 237–245.

Witzum, J.L. (1994) The oxidation hypothesis of atherosclerosis, *Lancet*, **344**: 793–795.

Wolf, A.M., Gortmaker, S.L., Cheung, L., Gray, H.M., Herzog, D.B. & Colditz, G.A. (1993) Activity, inactivity, and obesity: racial, ethnic, and age differences among schoolgirls, *American Journal of Public Health*, **83(11)**: 1625–1627.

SECTION II

PHYSICAL ACTIVITY AND HEALTH RELATIONSHIPS

Each chapter in this section explores the nature and strength of relationships between physical activity and health. Jakes and Wareham begin by reminding us of basic principles in epidemiology, and contend that that we should remain 'sceptically positive' about the contribution of physical activity to health. They highlight the fact that although we have abundant evidence suggesting that active people have a better health prognosis, we require further evidence to clarify the effects of different levels and patterns of activity. Not everybody exercises in the same way, and we need to ascertain how, for example, walking the dog for two miles every night compares with three sessions of aerobics a week. Such detailed dose–response evidence is currently sparse for many health outcomes, and in these cases it would be prudent to exercise caution in our claims for physical activity.

Carless and Faulkner argue clearly that physical activity has more than just 'bodily' or 'physiological' effects. Mental health is a major public health issue and there are indications that physical activity might have an important role to play in both prevention and treatment. Despite being relatively under-researched, the growing body of evidence confirms the hitherto unrealised potential of physical activity to positively influence mental well-being in both normal and clinical populations. As the aetiology of mental ill-health and mental well-being are better defined, and as the effects of physical activity become clearer, physical activity prescriptions for improved mental health will be more accurately characterised.

The same authors also remind us of the importance of the qualitative research paradigm in exploring both individual experiences and their associated meanings. Medical research is dominated by quantitative research and there is no question that this is important. However, qualitative evidence may be crucial in order to fully understand the health effects of physical activity with respect to mental-health outcomes such as depression or anxiety. It may also be the case that a combination of quantitative and qualitative evidence would tell us more about the true effects of physical activity interventions in terms of both physical and mental outcomes. There is little doubt that such an approach – concerned for the total 'patient experience' – is consistent with medical concerns to become more patient-centred. A good example of this is that the US National Plan for arthritis has identified a need to explore the total life experiences of arthritis patients. There may also be a need to address the experiences of doctors, nurses and other health professionals in the promotion of physical activity with different patient groups.

Cooper then makes the case for more accurate measurement of physical activity, which can be achieved by using objective monitors, rather than self-report methods. He presents a case for exercising caution in our claims for the health effects of physical activity, as activity measures are often based on subjective methods with known reporting problems. The high level of measurement error inherent in such methods undoubtedly leads to estimates of activity levels that are difficult to validate. However, with the new generation of electronic measurement instruments, there are clear possibilities for developing more accurate activity estimates. This in turn will strengthen our claims to understand the true level and nature of the health effects of physical activity.

In the final chapter of this section, van Sluijs and colleagues remind us that physical activity can be a double-edged sword. Taking three examples – sports injuries, risk of sudden cardiac death and the 'athletic triad' seen in some young female athletes – the risks of physical activity are identified and quantified. The chapter reminds us that much can be done to minimise risk, but also that realised risks can be devastating in some cases. Further, in a climate of evidence-based health policy, they establish a need to develop sensitive approaches in identifying *predictive* risk factors. Using a well-established process for linking realised risk to individual behaviour, they suggest ways for developing more effective risk management among free-living individuals.

CHAPTER 3

Epidemiology of Activity and Physical Health

RUPERT W. JAKES AND NICHOLAS J. WAREHAM

Chapter Contents

- Epidemiology and physical activity
- What is physical activity?
- How can physical activity be measured in population studies?
- Validation of physical activity questionnaires
- Descriptive epidemiology of activity
- Analytical epidemiology: associations of activity with health outcomes
- How do you decide whether an association is more or less likely to be causal?
- Studies of physical activity with mortality and specific disease endpoints
- Potential for prevention

This chapter is concerned with the nature of the relationship between physical activity and health, and the extent to which that relationship can be determined from epidemiological data. In order to understand and appropriately interpret such data, the reader needs to understand the strengths and weaknesses of the epidemiological methods that are employed. The chapter therefore starts with a description of the application of epidemiology to the study of physical activity, before proceeding to discuss the wealth of data that suggest that activity is an important determinant of health. The chapter concludes with some thoughts on the translation of epidemiological information into public-health intervention. This is not an easy step, and the responsible public-health practitioner needs to be able to critically appraise epidemiological

data very carefully before recommending action. This approach to the interpretation of data has been termed 'enlightened scepticism' by some and it is
this attitude that this chapter hopes to engender.

Epidemiology and physical activity

Epidemiology is the study of the distribution and determinants of health-
related states or events in specified populations, and the application of this
knowledge to the control of health problems (Last, 1995). Broadly speaking,
epidemiological studies can be divided into two major groups – descriptive
and analytical. In descriptive studies, data on the distribution of a health-
related behaviour or a health outcome is described in terms of the variation in
person, place or time. Such techniques can be applied to physical activity to
describe how patterns of activity vary between people in the same cultural setting, between people in different populations and in different time periods. If
this information is combined with other information about trends in health
outcomes, clues may be obtained about the link between activity and these
outcomes. However, this type of study can produce only clues; it can't generate
proof. For example, Prentice and Jebb used data from social surveys in the UK
to show that the prevalence or proportion of the population with obesity had
increased during a time-period in which physical activity, as measured by television viewing, had declined (Prentice & Jebb, 1995). From this data one might
infer that physical inactivity and obesity were causally linked. However, this
data is ecological and the inferences that can be drawn from them are not strong.
Many other factors have increased to a similar degree during this period, not
just television viewing. For example, if one were to plot membership of gyms
or fitness clubs during the same period, one would probably find that this had
increased steeply during the 1980s. Combined with the population prevalence
of obesity, one would then come to a completely different conclusion about
the link between physical activity and obesity. This limitation of the inferences
that can be drawn from population-level data is termed the ecological fallacy.
This problem arises because information about the possible cause of disease
(or exposure) is collected at the population-level. The data on the occurrence
of disease (or outcome) is taken from a sample of the same population, but
not the same individuals. As the link between exposure and outcome is very
indirect it can lead to false assumptions about the likelihood of causality, that
is, an ecological fallacy. It is this limitation that leads epidemiologists to
conduct analytical studies in order to investigate disease associations. In an
analytical study both the exposure and outcome are measured in the same
individuals. Even then the link between the exposure and the disease may not
be truly causal. Causality can never be proven, but associations may have certain
features that make this more or less likely. This chapter therefore describes the
Bradford Hill criteria which summarise the features of a disease association
that strengthen the inference of causality. Understanding whether physical

activity is causally linked to a health outcome is absolutely critical to the process of transferring epidemiological knowledge into preventive action. If there is no mechanistic link between physical activity and a health outcome, then however carefully an intervention is planned, it will not be effective in changing that outcome. This chapter provides a framework for examining the causal nature of the link between physical activity and health and summarises the key evidence linking activity with major health endpoints.

What is physical activity?

Physical activity is not an easy exposure to measure. An 'exposure' in an epidemiological study is the factor under examination that may be causally related to the outcome. Epidemiological methods have historically been designed for studies of much simpler exposures, for example cigarette smoking. It is worth briefly considering the difference in the complexity of assessing physical activity compared to smoking.

Differences between cigarette smoking and physical activity as epidemiological exposures

Cigarette smoking	Physical activity
• Unidimensional exposure – broadly speaking all cigarettes have the same effect	• Multidimensional exposure – physical activities differ greatly
• Can be reduced to a simple binary category that is, smokers/non-smokers	• Reduction to binary category is probably overly simplistic
• Reported cigarette consumption closely related to true consumption and can be tested by objective biomarker, for example serum cotinine	• Uncertain link between reported and true exposure – difficult to test with biomarker directly
• Among smokers a quantitative assessment of exposure can be made not allowing examination of dose–response relationships	• Quantification of activity is difficult and dose–response relationships are easy to study
• Stable behaviour. Habitual smoking behaviour easy to assess by asking about current behaviour	• Variable behaviour. Relationship between current or recent activity and habitual level is uncertain

The difficulties in measuring activity in populations have an impact on the strength of inference that can be drawn from epidemiological studies of activity. Unlike smoking, activity is a complex multi-dimensional exposure that cannot easily be reduced to a binary category. The subjective nature of most methods of defining exposure leads to uncertainties about whether true exposure is being measured or a biased estimate of it. In the case of smoking, biomarkers such as cotinine can be employed to demonstrate that reported and true exposures are closely related. For physical activity, such biomarkers are harder to employ. Smoking is also a stable behaviour. If one assesses smoking behaviour in a study today, then reported consumption will be closely related to the usual level. On the whole, this is not a behaviour that varies drastically from day to day. In addition, people have an idea about their usual consumption anyway and are able to average over time. Physical activity, by contrast, is much more variable and today's activity may not be related to usual activity, nor is it easy to ask individuals to average their activity over time.

How can physical activity be measured in population studies?

The most practical methods for measuring activity in large populations are questionnaires. They are relatively inexpensive and can be administered to populations without necessarily needing personal contact or the use of physiological measurement. One of the major drawbacks of using questionnaires to assess activity, however, is the accuracy with which they measure a particular sub-dimension of interest (for example, total energy expenditure, aerobic intensity, weight-bearing) and the degree to which the reporting of overall activity is biased. For example, an individual might complete a questionnaire and over-report all forms of activity undertaken and under-report the sedentary behaviours as a result of perceived beneficial levels of activity. If this under- and over-reporting is common to all individuals it is an *error*. However, if the degree of under- or over-reporting is different between individuals and is conditional on another factor (for example, access to recreational facilities), then the possibility of *bias* arises. In general, epidemiological, studies can allow for error, but bias is much harder to deal with.

 Chapter 5 (Measurement) considers the science supporting the many ways of measuring physical activity and exercise.

Questionnaires that have been used in large epidemiological studies include the Paffenbarger/Harvard Alumni questionnaire, the Tecumseh and Minnesota occupational and leisure-time activity questionnaires, the Nurses' Health Study questionnaire, the Framingham leisure-time physical activity questionnaire, the Zutphen physical activity questionnaire, the Baecke questionnaire and the EPIC (Norfolk) physical activity questionnaire (EPAQ2). The choice of a questionnaire for a particular study depends on several factors. There is no single questionnaire that is suitable for all purposes. Questionnaires differ in their length and complexity, their frame of reference, the targeted cultural context, the proposed target population and whether they are intended to summarise behaviour or produce an index of one of the underlying dimensions of activity. A questionnaire developed for the assessment of usual recreational activity in a study of middle-aged health professionals in the United States may not be a suitable choice for the measurement of activity in populations of a different age or social mix in a different cultural setting. Readers who wish to review the details of different physical activity questionnaires, their proposed target groups and published information on reliability and validity, may wish to consult the useful collection reported by Kriska and colleagues (Kriska & Caspersen, 1997).

Validation of physical activity questionnaires

The validity of a questionnaire is the extent to which the instrument assesses the true exposure of interest. This is not easy to assess and Table 3.1, provides a framework for asking questions that researchers ought to address before using a questionnaire (Rennie & Wareham, 1998).

What is the appropriate gold-standard technique for measuring physical activity?

Studies that report associations between activity and health often target energy expenditure as the principal exposure. It is therefore appropriate that the instrument with which one validates the questionnaire is the gold-standard method, or correlates highly with the gold-standard method for measuring energy expenditure. A number of instruments have been validated against other activity questionnaires, or activity diaries. In such cases caution should be exercised in interpreting the results since there is likely to be a degree of correlated error between the two. Similarly, activity instruments validated using estimated energy intake, using food frequency questionnaires or food diaries, might show similar levels of error as a result of biases in reporting of diet.

The two 'gold standard' methods of measuring energy expenditure are doubly labelled water or whole-body calorimetry. The doubly labelled water method

Table 3.1   Checklist for the validation of physical activity instruments

---

1. Has the dimension of physical activity that the instrument is purported to measure been clearly defined?

2. Does the validation method chosen measure the true exposure of interest and has it been applied in the same time frame of reference?

3. Has correlated error between the validation method and the physical activity instrument been avoided as far as possible?

4. Is there a close relationship between the validation method and the appropriate 'gold standard' instrument?

5. Is the sample chosen representative of the population to whom the physical activity instrument will be administered?

6. Have appropriate statistical techniques been employed to assess the validity of the physical activity instrument?

---

requires the ingestion of a quantity of water with known concentration of isotopes of hydrogen and oxygen. The labelled hydrogen and oxygen then leave the body as water (hydrogen and oxygen) or as carbon dioxide (oxygen). The production of carbon dioxide can then be calculated as the difference in elimination rates of the two isotopes. Using the respiratory quotient, oxygen uptake for the period can then be calculated (Prentice, 1990). This technique of estimating energy expenditure, although accurate, is expensive and so is not practical for use in large numbers of participants. Recent validation of three physical activity questionnaires using this method includes Philippaerts *et al.* (1999).

Whole body calorimetry is an alternative gold-standard method for estimating energy expenditure and uses a method of collecting all expired gases from an individual who is contained within a sealed room for a period of time. Again, this method makes a relatively accurate estimate of energy expenditure. However, the sealed chamber does not allow the individual to live in a 'free' state, and is not, therefore, relevant to epidemiological studies.

A number of physiological responses to activity are related to energy expenditure, including body temperature, blood pressure, ventilation, electromyography and heart rate (Montoye *et al.*, 1996). Monitoring heart rate in individuals in the free-living state has been used in epidemiological studies because of the relative ease with which it can be measured. It has been demonstrated that a linear relationship between heart rate and energy expenditure exists, above a particular heart rate. One of the difficulties in using this technique, however, is the imprecision of measuring energy expenditure at low levels of heart rate. It is possible to account for this, to some degree, by calculating the relationship between energy expenditure and heart rate for each individual. Estimation of energy expenditure using heart rate monitoring, with individual calibration (the flex heart rate method), correlates well with estimates of energy expenditure using doubly labelled water or whole body calorimetry (Ceesay *et al.*, 1989).

There are relatively few questionnaires that have been compared against these gold-standard objective methods. All too often questionnaires have been compared with other forms of self-report, such as diaries, introducing the potential for correlated error. Studies in the future will need to carefully select the appropriate validation instrument ensuring that errors are independent. In the evaluation of the EPAQ2 questionnaire, for example, a cohort of nearly 200 individuals completed heart rate monitoring for four days on four separate occasions at three-monthly intervals. At the end of this period the questionnaire was used. This repeated assessment of energy expenditure was available throughout the frame of reference of the questionnaire (Wareham *et al.*, in press).

How can the reliability of a physical activity questionnaire be assessed?

Reliability is also a necessary attribute of a questionnaire and one that is far easier to assess than validity. Reliability is the degree to which the results obtained by a measurement procedure can be replicated (Last, 1995). In using a questionnaire, for example, investigators ideally would recruit a sub-group of the study population to complete the questionnaire twice. The time interval should be long enough that the answers given on first completion cannot be recalled but short enough so that there is a high degree of overlap between the time frame of the questionnaire.

Why is it necessary to try to measure physical activity better?

Before discussing in detail the studies that attempt to demonstrate associations between physical activity and health, we need to consider why it is important to attempt to be more precise about how physical activity is assessed. Many epidemiological studies have relied on the assumption that the use of simple exposure measures leads to an underestimation of the true exposure–disease relationship provided the error in the measurement is non-differential[1] (Wareham & Rennie, 1998). There will usually be a degree of error in the measurement of exposure when using subjective measurement techniques and a lesser degree when using objective measures. *Differential* exposure measurement error occurs when exposure measurement error differs according to the disease or outcome being studied. One such example is recall bias. This occurs when those with a disease report exposures differently from the 'non-diseased' because of their knowledge or feelings about the disease and its symptoms. Recall bias may also be introduced if a data collector has knowledge about an individual's disease status (Armstrong *et al.*, 1994). When error is equal between the diseased and non-disease groups, there is *non-differential* exposure measurement error. Much of epidemiology has relied upon the assumption that error is non-differential. If this is the case, then the underlying relationships with disease endpoints are always stronger than those observed with simple exposure measures. This attenuation phenomenon is always seen when exposures are measured with non-differential error. It is this assumption that has led epidemiologists to be content with relatively inaccurate exposure methods because they can assume that the true relationship is at least as strong, but probably stronger, than that which has been observed. The approach using simple measures of exposure might be sufficient to demonstrate the overall importance of physical activity in its relation to health but it is inadequate as a basis for generating greater clarity about the exposure–disease relationship. It is also problematic if the assumption about the non-differential nature of the error is wrong.

Wareham and Rennie suggest five reasons that justify research aimed at improving the methods for assessing physical activity (Wareham & Rennie, 1998). First, since physical activity is a complex multi-dimensional exposure it is necessary to specify the dimension of physical activity that is of most importance for a particular health outcome. For example, seven prospective cohort studies concluded that physical activity, assessed using questionnaire-based methods, is protective for type-2 diabetes (Wareham & Rennie, 1998).

However, none of these studies measure occupational as well as recreational activity and this potentially hinders the process of translating their results into public health intervention. For example, the Nurses Health Study and the US Male Physicians Study base their assessment of physical activity on the responses to the question 'at least once a week do you engage in any regular activity similar to brisk walking, jogging, bicycling etc, long enough to work up a sweat?'. The validity of this assessment of physical activity is questionable since one of the cited validations compares the response to the score derived from the Harvard Alumni Activity Survey Questionnaire (Washburn *et al.*, 1990). In another validation this question about inducing sweat was 'validated' by comparing the results with a test of maximal oxygen uptake, a legitimate measure of fitness but not a direct measure of activity (Siconolfi *et al.*, 1985). So there is some debate as to which dimension of physical activity is being assessed.

Secondly, in order to make inferences and inform public health interventions, it is important to estimate the true effect size of the exposure–disease relationship.[2] The use of non-quantitative measures of physical activity does not allow assessment of dose–response relationships or tests of linearity and threshold effects. Again using an example in relation to diabetes, a physical activity index was used in the University of Pennsylvania Alumni Study and was based on the sum of energy costs of self-reported walking, stair climbing and recreational activity (Helmrich *et al.*, 1991). In this study, a 500 kcal/week increase in this index was associated with a 6 per cent reduction in the risk of developing diabetes in a model that also adjusted for body mass index, history of hypertension and parental history of diabetes.[3] The accuracy of the expected reduction of risk for each 500 kcal/week increase in the physical activity index is entirely dependent upon the quantitative validity of the index. As this instrument is not truly quantitative, the magnitude of the association is likely to be wrong, although the direction may well be correct. This would be a problem if you used this data to derive the expected benefit from an intervention that aimed to increase activity by 500 kcal/week.

Thirdly, many physical activity questionnaires are relevant only to the particular populations for which they were designed and so comparisons of activity patterns between countries or between different social or cultural groups within a country is difficult. This makes it difficult to compare international or geographical variation in physical activity patterns to variation in disease rates between the same regions.

Fourthly, objective measures of physical activity, as the introduction to this chapter suggests, would be of use in describing temporal trends in populations. Prentice and Jebb discuss the rise in prevalence of obesity in the UK using reasonable evidence on temporal trends in energy intake and the proportion of energy originating from dietary fat (Prentice & Jebb, 1995). However, their inferences about trends in energy expenditure are taken from changes in television viewing and car ownership. More direct evidence on trends in physical activity exists in the US and should become more available with successive publications of the Health Survey for England. A reported increase in leisure-time physical activity may be balanced by an opposite trend in work-related physical activity, which might have little effect on overall energy expenditure.

Finally, better measurement of physical activity would be useful in assessing the effect of interventions. Physical activity intervention studies may demonstrate an effect on a particular outcome; however, monitoring the means by which that effect was achieved is an important goal. Changes in energy expenditure are difficult to measure and this has meant that studies which have attempted to measure change objectively have concentrated on areas for which better techniques exist, such as cardio-respiratory fitness (Eriksson & Lindgarde, 1991). Recent health advice has been to increase participation from low-to-moderate intensity activity which will not result in measurable changes in fitness but will increase total energy expenditure.

Descriptive epidemiology of activity

Describing activity patterns and their relation to factors such as age, gender, social class, ethnicity, smoking and alcohol consumption in populations is a prerequisite to studying and understanding how activity is associated with health. The inter-relationships between physical activity and these other possible determinants of health become important when one moves from descriptive to analytical studies as these factors may introduce *confounding*. A confounding factor is one that has an association both with the exposure (activity) and the outcome (health) but is not part of the causal pathway linking exposure and outcome. Ignoring a major confounding factor can lead to the exaggeration or diminution of an exposure–disease relationship. The true picture can be revealed only when the effect of the confounding factor is diminished either at the design stage of an analytical study by restriction or matching or in the analysis by stratification, matching or adjustment[4] (Last, 1995). For example, some descriptive surveys show that smoking is associated with being physically inactive. Smoking has been proven elsewhere to be associated with adverse health events such as coronary heart disease (CHD). An analytical study of the association between physical inactivity and CHD might therefore find a positive association solely as a result of the common relationship between both the exposure and the outcome with the confounding factor (smoking). Only when the effect of smoking is adjusted for will the true association between physical inactivity and CHD be evident.

Cross-sectional surveys

A cross-sectional survey is designed to describe the distribution of an exposure and how it relates to other lifestyle factors at a particular point in time in a defined population. For example, it might be important to be able to describe

---

Box 3.1   Examples of population-based surveys

Temporal trends

- *Social Trends*
- *General Household Survey*
- *Health Survey for England*
- *Behavioural Risk Factor Surveillance System*

---

levels of activity by socio-economic group, smoking status or body-mass index, even though those variables might not be the principal variables of interest.

Series of cross-sectional studies, utilising individuals drawn at random from a population, provide data useful for looking at trends. The advantages of cross-sectional studies are that they are relatively uncomplicated to undertake and as a result large samples are often used. They are of great value to public-health doctors in assessing health status and for predicting health care needs.

Some examples of population-based surveys conducted on a regular basis are given in Box 3.1. Useful information regarding physical activities can be gleaned from such publications. In the UK, *Social Trends*, which was first published in 1970 by the Government Statistical Service, for example, provides information on time use in activities such as sleep, TV and radio, cooking, eating at home, personal care, gardening and do it yourself (DIY), care of others, and other home leisure (Office for National Statistics, 1998). It also describes participation in the most popular sports, games and other physical activities: walking, snooker/pool/billiards, cycling, swimming, soccer, and keeping fit. The *General Household Survey* and *Health Survey for England* provide similar types of information. The *Behavioural Risk Factor Surveillance System (BRFSS)* was established by the Center for Disease Control in the US in 1984. It is based on random digit dialling and is administered by telephone and now includes a physical activity module that takes about 10 minutes to complete. A number of standard physical activity indices have been developed using BRFSS data including duration (time spent a day or minutes a week), frequency (number of exercise sessions a week), intensity (estimated percentage of maximal cardio-respiratory capacity or METs (metabolic equivalents)) and estimated kcal burned (a function of the type of activity and its frequency).

Analytical epidemiology: associations of activity with health outcomes

Analytical epidemiological studies of physical activity and health attempt to compare activity levels of people with and without disease with a view to

---

Box 3.2   Types of epidemiological study

Descriptive studies

- Populations (ecological studies)
- Individuals (cross-sectional surveys)

Analytic studies

Observational studies

- Case-control studies
- Cohort studies
- Nested case-control studies

Randomised controlled trails

---

understanding how strongly they are linked. There are a number of study designs available that enable estimation of the risks associated with a disease outcome, each with strengths and weaknesses according to the degree to which one can attribute a causal role of activity in the development of disease (see Box 3.2).

Case-control studies

The case-control study utilises series of individuals who are identified as having a specific disease. These 'cases' are then compared with individuals, usually selected from a population comparable to that from which the patients were drawn, and who do not have the disease – the 'controls'. Matching cases and the controls according to variables such as age and gender may be used to diminish the effect of confounding. The exposure information, for example self-reported physical activity behaviour, is then assessed in cases and controls alike, along with information on other factors that might affect the outcome. The main advantage of such a study design is that cases can be identified quickly, making the study relatively inexpensive. Case-control studies are particularly useful for the evaluation of risks associated with rare disease. However, they are prone to selection and recall biases. By their very nature the assessment of the exposure takes place after the attribution of a disease label. An individual who has a disorder may well report an historical health-related exposure differently from someone who is, or considers themselves healthy. This is particularly true if the biological hypothesis under scrutiny is obvious.

Cohort studies

The cohort study is a more robust epidemiological design in which a defined group of individuals without disease are identified. In contrast to a case-control study, a cohort study is not affected by recall bias, since the assessment of the exposure pre-dates the development of the outcome. This also leads to a stronger inference about causality because the temporal sequence of cause and effect is clear. Measurements of physical activity and other covariates and confounding variables are made at recruitment to the study, and the cohort is then followed for the occurrence of disease. When a sufficient number of health events or outcomes[5] have occurred the incidence rate of disease according to different levels of physical activity can then be calculated and compared. Cohort studies have disadvantages as they require the measurement of exposure in a much larger number of individuals and the length of time needed to generate a sufficient number of health events is greater. Cohort studies are therefore expensive.

Nested case-control studies

This hybrid type of study is of a design similar to the case-control study but uses participants within a cohort study to identify the cases and controls. The difference to a normal cohort study is that the exposure measurements are analysed on only a small number of cases and controls who are included in the final analysis. This is efficient when the costs of analysing the exposure data are high. Thus this study design is cheap in this respect, but requires the time necessary for a cohort study. This design has the advantage that the cases and controls are drawn from a like population, with less selection bias. Nor is there a problem with recall bias.

Randomised controlled trials

The randomised controlled trial (RCT) is the gold-standard study design for evaluating interventions but it also plays a key role in establishing the causal link between physical activity and disease. The aim of such a study is to intervene by randomly allocating individuals either to a physical activity programme or to a control group.[6] The outcome variable is assessed both before the trial and following completion of the intervention, and a comparison made between the two groups. Randomisation helps reduce the effects of known confounding factors. However, the major advantage over other study designs is that randomisation also reduces the impact of unknown confounding factors. Physical activity trials not only tell us about the effectiveness of intervention but also contribute to the understanding of the causal nature of the physical activity–disease outcome relationship. Few studies of this nature are undertaken using physical activity as the intervention because of the difficulties in maintaining compliance in activity change. These studies are often of shorter duration and outcome measures are therefore usually intermediate for disease, such as blood pressure or weight change.

Systematic reviews

A single epidemiological study usually is unable to provide unequivocal evidence of an association between physical activity and disease; it merely contributes to the body of evidence. Systematic reviews of published literature are useful in summarising and consolidating the evidence. By combining the results of several studies from different populations that address the same fundamental question, the power of an association can be improved and a more accurate estimation of the true magnitude of effect can be made. Systematic reviews, although useful, are often subject to publication bias whereby journals tend to favour publishing results that show a positive effect of physical activity on disease.

Meta-analyses

Meta-analysis is a powerful technique, similar to that of a systematic review, that aims to identify all published and unpublished studies of a particular postulated association. It is preferable that the raw data for each individual, in each of the studies identified, is obtained and re-analysed to obtain a pooled estimate of the association. Meta-analyses are the gold-standard technique for pooling results from several studies and, providing all relevant studies are identified and included in the analysis, they provide the most accurate evidence of an association.

How do you decide whether an association is more or less likely to be causal?

Assuming that chance, bias and confounding are unlikely explanations for the finding of a study, we may be in a position to conclude that a valid statistical association exists between the exposure (that is, physical activity) and the disease. It is then necessary to assess whether this reported association is a result of cause and effect, since the presence of a statistical association alone does not imply causality. Based on the 1965 publication by Bradford Hill, Box 3.3 summarises the criteria that can be used to assess the degree to which the association is causal (Hill, 1965).

Box 3.3   Questions to be asked when interpreting an epidemiological study

Is the observed association statistically valid?

- Is this due to chance?
- Is this due to bias?
- Is this due to confounding?

To judge whether the association is causal:

- Is the association strong?
- Are the findings consistent with other studies?
- Does the exposure precede the disease?
- Is there biologic plausibility?
- Is there evidence of a biologic gradient?
- Is there evidence that the effect is reversible?

Studies of physical activity with mortality and specific disease endpoints

The opening sections of this chapter have considered the epidemiological method. The following section discusses the application of that method to studying the link between physical inactivity and health.

All-cause mortality

Relatively few studies have examined the association between physical activity and all-cause mortality. In order to have sufficient power, these studies are usually large and therefore, by necessity, have employed simple techniques for measuring physical activity. Associations have been demonstrated using measures of cardio-respiratory fitness, a marker of exercise training, and mortality. For example, compared with people who were most active, sedentary people experienced between a 1.2-fold to 2-fold increase in the relative risk of dying during the study follow-up period (Slattery & Jacobs, 1988; Sandvik *et al.*, 1993). The ratio of the incidence in the exposed, here the inactive, compared to the unexposed is the relative risk (RR). Incidence is the rate of occurrence of disease in a population. It is always characterised by being expressed in terms of events per unit time. It is therefore distinguished from prevalence, which is the proportion of a population affected by a disease at a given moment (point prevalence) or during a particular time interval (period prevalence). When the relative risk is high, the disease outcome is strongly associated with the exposure. When RR is less than 1 the exposure is protective. The RR is an estimate and therefore it has confidence limits. When this confidence interval (CI) includes 1.0 there is no statistically significant association. Using low cardio-respiratory fitness as the exposure measurement, one cohort study demonstrated a strong association with all-cause mortality in women (RR 5.35, 95 per cent CI, 2.44–11.73) and in men (RR 3.16, 95 per cent CI, 1.92–5.20). They found a weaker association between physical inactivity and mortality in men (RR 1.70, 95 per cent CI, 1.06–2.74), and no association for women (RR 0.95, 95 per cent CI, 0.54–1.70) (Blair *et al.*, 1993).

Associations are generally stronger for cardio-respiratory fitness than for reported physical activity (Blair *et al.*, 1989). However, studies of self-reported participation in physical activity have also demonstrated associations with risk of mortality. The Harvard Alumni Study is a large cohort study comprising men who matriculated as undergraduates between 1916 and 1950. Beginning in either 1962 or 1966, surviving alumni were sent health questionnaires periodically. In an analysis of 17 835 men who completed the 1977 questionnaire the authors calculated RR of all-cause mortality for a number of self-reported indices of physical activity, including distance walked, stairs climbed and participation in vigorous sports/recreation. Between 1977 and 1992 mortality rates were calculated and RR estimated by comparing the rates in different categories of activity. For example, comparing those who walked more than 20 km/week with those who walked less than 5 km/week the RR was 0.85 (95 per cent CI, 0.75–0.94). This means a reduced risk of dying, within the follow-up period, for those who reported walking further in 1977. Similarly, an RR of 0.82 (95 per cent CI, 0.74–0.91) was calculated for those who climbed more stairs (≥35 storeys/week) when compared with those who climbed fewer than ten storeys a week. When the participants were divided into five groups, according to the intensity of participation in vigorous activities, those in the most intensive group had a reduced risk of dying (RR 0.77, 95 per cent CI, 0.67–0.89) compared with those who participated in the least amount of vigorous activity (Lee & Paffenbarger, 2000). The results described here are statistically significant since the confidence limits do not include 1.0.

If physical activity is measured in each participant at more than one point in time within a cohort study it enables the effect of changing levels of physical activity on subsequent risk of mortality to be assessed. The Harvard Alumni Study and the Aerobics Center Longitudinal study are two examples. In the Harvard Alumni Study participants who took up moderately intense activity during the follow-up period (1962 or 1966, to 1977) had a lower death rate than those who reported no moderately intense activity at either the first or second assessment (RR 0.77, 95 per cent CI, 0.58–0.96) (Paffenbarger *et al.*, 1993). Although this observation contributes to the strength of the causal relationship this study is not a randomised design and so biases may be present in that those who took up activity may be different in other ways to those who remained sedentary. In addition, caution must be exercised in how results from a select group of well-educated men can be generalised to other populations. The Aerobics Center Longitudinal Study is a cohort study of 25 341 men and 7080 women, ranging from 20 to 88 years of age at the time of assessment, who attended the Cooper Clinic in Dallas, Texas. The cohort consisted mainly of white, well-educated participants. In one report on this cohort the study authors demonstrated that those men who improved their cardio-respiratory fitness, over an average of five years, had an RR of 0.56 (95 per cent CI, 0.41–0.75), compared to those who remained in the bottom quintile of cardio-respiratory fitness. As with the Harvard Alumni Study, the Aerobics Center Longitudinal Study used a selected group of participants, and therefore the generaliseability of the associations may be limited.

These studies of physical activity and all-cause mortality give an overall summary of the public-health importance of activity, but studies aimed at quantifying the effects of physical activity on the incidence and mortality from specific diseases provide greater insight into the biological mechanisms underlying these associations.

Summary of findings with physical activity and all-cause mortality: *The current data and studies available suggest that regular physical activity and higher cardio-respiratory fitness decrease overall mortality rates in a dose–response relationship.*

Cardiovascular disease

Cardiovascular disease, including coronary heart disease and stroke, although in decline, are still major causes of death in developed countries and are increasingly seen as a cause of death in developing countries. Most of the large epidemiological studies of physical activity and health have used cardiovascular disease or cardiovascular mortality as an endpoint, including the Framingham Study, the Canada Health Survey and the Harvard Alumni Study (Paffen-barger *et al.*, 1984; Kannel *et al.*, 1986; Arraiz *et al.*, 1992). Results vary between reporting an inverse association between level of physical activity and risk of cardiovascular disease and studies that found an inverse association for a moderately active group but a weaker effect in the vigorously active group. For studies focusing on the association between cardio-respiratory fitness and cardiovascular disease, results suggest an inverse dose–response relationship between fitness and risk of cardiovascular disease. These studies, apart from the Aerobic Center Longitudinal Study, used a single assessment of fitness and related this to cardiovascular disease. As with all-cause mortality, the Aerobic Center Longitudinal Study found that those who improved their cardio-respiratory fitness over a follow-up period had a lower risk of cardio-vascular mortality than those who showed no improvement in fitness (Blair *et al.*, 1995).

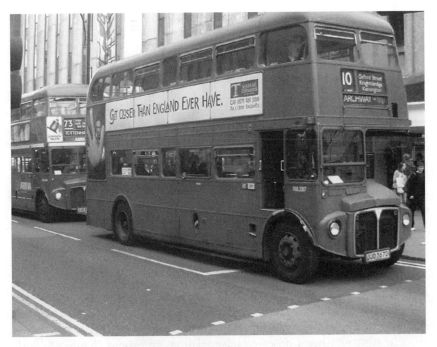

Illustration 3.1 Drivers and conductors of London double-decker buses gave us the first clues that physical activity is important for health.
(Photo: Chris Riddoch)

Coronary heart disease

One of the earliest studies to demonstrate an association between physical activity and coronary heart disease used a cohort of 31 000 male employees of the London Transport Executive aged between 35 and 64 years. Assessment of physical activity was, however, limited to an occupational classification. Bus conductors, who are on the whole more active, showed a reduced risk (RR 0.70) when compared to more sedentary bus drivers (Morris *et al.*, 1953).

More recently, Morris *et al.* incorporated a 48-hour recall of leisure-time physical activity as their criteria for physical activity, in a matched case-control study design among male civil servants. They found that those who participated in more vigorous activity had an RR of fatal or non-fatal coronary heart disease compared to the non-vigorous group (Morris *et al.*, 1973). In an analysis following the entire cohort, the same researchers found the age-adjusted risk of heart attack to be inversely associated with reported participation in vigorous activity defined using the 48-hour recall of leisure-time activity (Morris *et al.*, 1980). Paffenbarger and colleagues, using data from the Harvard Alumni Study, estimated energy expenditure from self-reported stair climbing, walking and participation in sports (Paffenbarger *et al.*, 1984). They reported a dose response with increasing index of physical activity and death due to coronary heart disease after adjustment for age, smoking and hypertension. Data from the British Regional Heart Study demonstrated an inverse association between self-reported activity on a six-point scale and heart attack although these findings were limited to those who reported moderate and moderately vigorous activity compared with sedentary individuals (Shaper & Wannamethee, 1991).

Data illustrating the association between cardio-respiratory fitness and risk of coronary heart disease is more consistent in demonstrating an inverse dose–response relationship (Sobolski *et al.*, 1987; Ekelund *et al.*, 1988; Hein *et al.*, 1992). The relative risk of coronary heart disease in these studies ranged from 1.2 to 3.2 when comparing those with low fitness to those with high fitness. A meta-analysis of studies of physical activity and coronary heart disease, conducted by Berlin and Colditz, calculated a pooled RR of 1.8 when comparing risk for the lowest level of physical activity with the highest, using studies considered to be of more sound methodological quality (Berlin & Colditz, 1990).

Stroke

Fewer studies have reported on the association between physical activity and stroke. Some of the earlier studies were not designed so that it was possible to determine whether a dose–response relationship existed (Kannel & Sorlie, 1979; Paffenbarger *et al.*, 1984; Wannamethee & Shaper, 1992). For the more recent studies that were designed in this way, half were able to detect dose–response relationships and half found either no association or a U-shaped association. In a study of women nurses in the US, Hu and colleagues report an inverse dose–response relationship between energy expenditure, estimated in METs using data from a questionnaire, and risk of stroke (Hu *et al.*, 2000). An RR of 0.66 (95 per cent CI, 0.47–0.91) for those in the highest quintile of energy expenditure when compared with the lowest quintile was reported and the effect was seen primarily for ischemic stroke.

Summary of findings with physical activity and cardiovascular disease: *The epidemiological evidence is strongly suggestive of an inverse association between physical activity or cardio-respiratory fitness and cardiovascular disease in general and coronary heart disease in particular. There is also evidence of a dose–response relationship. The association between physical activity and risk of stroke is less certain.*

Type-2 diabetes

Type-2 diabetes, formerly non-insulin-dependent diabetes mellitus, is a disease of increasing prevalence that is associated with premature death mainly from cardiovascular disease. Type-2 diabetes is the single biggest cause of preventable blindness in adults, and is a major risk factor for non-traumatic amputations and end-stage renal disease.

Ecological studies suggest a relationship between population levels of physical activity and prevalence of type-2 diabetes (King & Rewers, 1993). This is particularly true for populations such as the Pima Indians or Nauruans in whom lifestyles have changed rapidly. The high prevalence of diabetes in these groups has given rise to the thrifty genotype hypothesis in which a putative gene for diabetes is maintained in a population because it is advantageous to survival in times of food scarcity (Neel, 1962). However, when food is abundant and physical activity levels are low, this genetic predisposition becomes disadvantageous, leading to the high prevalence of diabetes among peoples who have adopted a westernised lifestyle. This theory may explain the emergence of type-2 diabetes and coronary heart disease among previously less-developed population who become westernised. The emergence of those disorders in populations that were previously affected mostly by infectious diseases and under-nutrition is sometimes termed the epidemiological transition. It is speculated that physical inactivity is a major cause for this change in disease patterning, but this remains to be proven. The evidence is supported by migration studies where those individuals who moved to developed areas had a higher prevalence of type-2 diabetes compared with those who remained (Kawate *et al.*, 1979; Hara *et al.*, 1983; Ravussin *et al.*, 1994).

Cross-sectional studies have reported an association between physical inactivity and type-2 diabetes (Dowse *et al.*, 1991; Ramaiya *et al.*, 1991; Kriska *et al.*, 1993). Other cross-sectional studies have reported the effects of physical activity on glucose intolerance in individuals without diabetes (Dowse *et al.*, 1991; Schranz *et al.*, 1991; Kriska *et al.*, 1993) and also with insulin values (McKeigue *et al.*, 1992; Feskens *et al.*, 1994; Regensteiner *et al.*, 1995; Wareham *et al.*, 2000) following a glucose load. These studies generally suggest that physical inactivity is associated with hyperinsulinaemia, a marker of insulin resistance, which is one of the key stages in the pathogenesis of type-2 diabetes.

Case-control studies that have looked at physical inactivity and type-2 diabetes have also demonstrated an inverse relationship, with Kaye and colleagues reporting that women who had high levels of physical activity had half the risk of disease than those who reported low levels of physical activity. Those who reported intermediate levels of activity had intermediate risk (Kaye *et al.*, 1991).

Stronger evidence comes from a variety of cohort studies that have reported on the risk of developing diabetes during a follow-up period. These include the Harvard Alumni Study, the Nurses Health Study and the Health Professionals Study. The Harvard Alumni Study reported an inverse dose–response relationship between levels of energy expenditure, estimated using a questionnaire, and the risk of developing type-2 diabetes (Helmrich *et al.*, 1991). The Nurses Health Study was not designed to detect the presence of a dose–response relationship, but showed a significantly reduced risk for those who reported one or more episodes of vigorous activity a week when compared to those who reported less than one episode of physical activity (Manson *et al.*, 1991). The Health Professionals' follow-up study is a cohort study that began in 1986 when 51 529 male US health professionals (dentists, optometrist, pharmacists, podiatrists, osteopaths, and veterinarians), aged 40–75 years, completed questionnaires regarding diet, physical activity and medical history. The study found a strong inverse linear relationship between increasing MET-hours a week, estimated using a detailed physical activity questionnaire, and development of type-2 diabetes. The RR of developing type-2 diabetes was 0.51 (95 per cent CI, 0.41–0.63) for those in the top quintile of physical activity compared with those in the bottom quintile (Hu *et al.*, 2001). In the same study a positive association between reported time spent viewing television and risk of developing type-2 diabetes was found (Hu *et al.*, 2001). After adjustment for age, smoking, physical activity, body-mass index and other confounding variables, individuals who watch, on average, more than 40 hours of television a week had an RR of 2.3 (95 per cent CI, 1.17–4.56) when compared with those who watched one hour a week.

Primary prevention trials can also add important evidence for the association between physical activity or inactivity and risk of developing diabetes. For example, a study in China that used an exercise intervention in people who were at high risk of developing diabetes demonstrated a lower incidence rate of diabetes, over a period of 8.5 years, in those who were prescribed exercise when compared with those who were not (Pan *et al.*, 1995). Similarly, a recent diet and exercise intervention study in 522 Finnish men and women (mean age 55 years) with impaired glucose tolerance demonstrated a 58 per cent reduction in the risk of developing diabetes over a mean follow-up period of 3.2 years (Tuomilehto *et al.*, 2001). However, as this was a combined intervention of diet and exercise, the precise impact of physical activity cannot be determined.

Summary of findings with physical activity and type-2 diabetes: *The epidemiological research strongly supports the existence of a protective effect of physical activity on the risk of type-2 diabetes. There is good supportive evidence of the biologic plausibility for the beneficial effects of activity on the observed effect.*

Cancer

Studies of physical activity and cancer have been limited mainly to colorectal cancer, breast cancer and prostate cancer. Generally, the evidence of an association has been less convincing than for other types of disease. However, a cohort study of Swedish men and women has shown increased risk of colon cancer for those who are least active in work and in leisure time with an RR of 3.6 (95 per cent CI, 1.3–9.8) compared to those who are most active (Gerhardsson *et al.*, 1988). In a nested case-control study using the same cohort, an RR of 1.8 (95 per cent CI, 1.0–3.4) was estimated when comparing least active with the most active (Gerhardsson *et al.*, 1990). In the Harvard College Alumni Study, Lee and co-workers found a significantly reduced risk (RR 0.5, 95 per cent CI, 0.27–0.93) of colon cancer when comparing high lifetime physical activity with inactivity (Lee *et al.*, 1991). The cohort study of male health professionals found a significant inverse relationship between increasing quintiles of activity and risk of colon cancer (Giovannucci *et al.*, 1995). The RR for the top quintile of activity compared to the bottom quintile was 0.53 (95 per cent CI, 0.32–0.88). There are, however, many studies that have found no association between activity and risk of colon cancer. Such negative associations could result from poor measurement of physical activity or from under-powered studies.[7]

One possible mechanism for the observed association between physical activity and colon cancer is an increase in prostaglandin synthesis. Strenuous physical activity increases prostaglandin F2 α, which in turn increases intestinal motility (Tutton & Barkla, 1980; Thor *et al.*, 1985). It is also postulated that physical activity decreases gastrointestinal transit time, which in effect reduces the length of contact between the potential carcinogens and the colon mucosa.

The results for breast cancer are similarly inconsistent in their findings. In one case-control study of Californian women with 545 cases and 545 controls, participation of more than 3.8 hours of leisure-time activity compared with none was associated with a reduced risk of in situ and invasive breast cancer (RR 0.42, 95 per cent CI, 0.27–0.64) (Bernstein *et al.*, 1994). However, in the Framingham Cohort Study, higher levels of activity were associated with increased incidence of breast cancer (RR 1.6, 95 per cent CI, 0.9–2.9) (Dorgan *et al.*, 1994). More recently, the Nurses Health Study, a cohort study of 121701 women aged 30–55 years at enrolment, published its findings on the incidence of breast cancer in relation to cumulative past physical activity and physical activity recorded at baseline (Rockhill *et al.*, 1999). The cohort was followed between 1977 and 1996, and the authors report participation in more than 7 hours a week of moderate and vigorous activity compared with less than one hour a week produced an RR of 0.82 (95 per cent CI, 0.70–0.97) for the occurrence of breast cancer.

Prostate cancer is the third cancer that has been widely studied. Results in relation to physical activity are again inconsistent. There are reports of significant inverse associations between activity and prostate cancer in the Harvard College Alumni Study and in a cohort of 13 000 Texan men (Lee *et al.*, 1992; Oliveria *et al.*, 1996). Other studies showed either a non-significant inverse association or no association. Again, it is likely that physical activity was measured poorly in these studies.

Summary of findings with physical activity and cancer: Epidemiological evidence of an association between physical activity and colon cancer is relatively consistent although there is minimal evidence for rectal cancer. Of the few studies of breast, prostate and other cancers, findings are generally inconsistent.

Osteoporosis and fracture

A positive association between physical activity and bone mineral density has been demonstrated in cross-sectional studies in which athletic young adults have a higher density of bone mineral than sedentary individuals (Grimston *et al.*, 1993; Kirchner *et al.*, 1996). Bone-mineral density has also been shown to vary according to the type of activity, for example in studies of weight-lifters, gymnasts, and according to daily energy expenditure in young individuals (Conroy *et al.*, 1993; Rubin *et al.*, 1993; Nichols *et al.*, 1994). Prolonged bed rest, immobility, or weightlessness causes a reduction in bone-mineral density (Donaldson *et al.*, 1970; Tilton *et al.*, 1980; Krølner *et al.*, 1983; Chestnut, 1993). A cross-sectional study of institutionalised subjects over the age of 70 years demonstrated a positive effect of physical activity on bone ultrasound parameters (Graafmans *et al.*, 1998). More recently, a population-based study reported beneficial effects of high-impact activity on bone ultrasound parameters in middle-aged men and women (Jakes *et al.*, 2001).

 Chapter 2 (Lifespan) explores how physical activity and exercise effects may differ across the lifecourse. Chapter 11 (Biology) describes the biological issues.

The biological basis for the study of the relationship between physical activity and bone mass is supported by animal studies. Lanyon and co-workers have examined the effects of functional loading, mechanical strain and applied dynamic loads on the structural competence of bone architecture and bone modelling and remodelling (O'Connor *et al.*, 1982; Lanyon, 1984; Rubin & Lanyon, 1984; Rubin & Lanyon, 1985; Lanyon, 1992). This work suggests that loading is the primary means by which this competence is established (Lanyon, 1996). It might also be the more diverse and unusual strain distributions that demonstrate more potent osteogenic potential (Lanyon, 1996). Studies in man have been hampered by the complexity of experimental design, by selection of specific population sub-groups and by the lack of precise physical activity measurement in observational epidemiological studies.

Summary of findings with physical activity and osteoporosis: *It appears that physical activity can build greater bone mass in early childhood and can help to maintain this in later life. There is also evidence that certain types of physical activity can reduce the rate of loss of bone mass in older age.*

Potential for prevention

Epidemiologists are primarily concerned with the prevention of disease. The ability to quantify the effects of lifestyle change or intervention on the risk of disease is important as it allows the potential for prevention to be quantified. Most of the examples of association in this chapter have been described in terms of RR. Attributable risk, by contrast, is a measure of association that tells us about the absolute effect of the exposure or the excess risk of disease in those exposed compared to those who are not exposed. It is defined as the difference between the incidence rates in those exposed and those who are not exposed. This difference can be expressed as a proportion of the total incidence of that disease to give an idea of the proportion of the risk that is

Table 3.2 Estimated population attributable risk of sedentary living for mortality from CHD for different population patterns of physical activity

Physical activity	RR	Baseline		Change in exposure	
		P_{exp} (%)	PAR (%)	P_{exp} (%)	PAR (%)
Sedentary	2.0	24	16	12	9
Irregular	1.5	54	18	39	14
Regular	1.2	10	1	32	2
Vigorous	1.0	12	–	17	–
			35		25

RR – relative risk; P_{exp} – prevalence of the exposure in the population; PAR – population attributable risk.

attributable to the exposure under scrutiny. This measure, the attributable-risk per cent, goes under a number of different names including the attributable fraction, the aetiologic or the preventable fraction.

Considering sedentary living as the exposure for the risk of coronary heart disease, colon cancer and diabetes, Powell and Blair use population-attributable risk per cent to estimate the percentage of deaths that theoretically would not occur if everyone were physically active. Population-attributable risk is related to both the RR and the proportion of the study population who are exposed. It increases when low levels of exposure prevalence are combined with a high relative risk of disease and also when the relative risk is low but the exposure is common (for example, sedentary lifestyle). Changes in population-attributable risk of sedentary behaviour and disease over time are more sensitive to changes in the prevalence of the exposure in the population than to the RR. The accuracy of the population-attributable risk is dependent upon the accuracy of the estimate of the prevalence of the exposure and the RR.

The potential for the reduction in the population-attributable risk by a population shift of increasing physical activity was estimated by Powell and Blair and is summarised in Table 3.2. This shows that if 50 per cent of people in each of the four categories on physical activity shifted to the next more active category, then a reduction in population-attributable risk of coronary heart disease of 10 per cent could be achieved.

These figures give a sense of the public health importance of physical inactivity. Efforts aimed at diminishing this burden are the topic of other chapters in this book.

In summary, this chapter has described the wealth of epidemiological information relating physical activity and inactivity to health. Although the focus has been on physical health (coronary heart disease, diabetes, cancer), physical activity also has effects on cognitive and psychological function, issues that are discussed elsewhere in this text. Viewing such data with the epidemiological perspective of 'enlightened scepticism' will allow researchers to critically appraise evidence and gauge the extent to which such data can form the basis for preventive action and to estimate the likely impact that this action will have.

Notes

1   Non-differential error occurs when the misclassification in the exposure variable is independent of the outcome. Differential error occurs when the misclassification is dependent upon the disease status.
2   The effect size of the exposure–disease relationship is an indication of its strength. It is measured by the odds ratio in a case-control and the RR in a cohort study.
3   Adjustment is undertaken by multivariate analysis where the effect of one factor is considered independently of other variables.
4   Restriction is a way of dealing with confounding simply by focusing only on one group of individuals. If gender were an important confounding factor, one could deal with it by focusing on only men or women (restriction). Alternatively, one could deal with it by analysing men and women separately (stratification). Finally if a case-control design were used, then cases and controls could be paired up so that they were of the same gender (matching).
5   One example of a health event or outcome in a cohort study would be a myocardial infarction.
6   Ideally individuals randomised to a control group in an RCT should not be aware which group they are in, nor should those researchers responsible for conducting outcome assessment (allocation concealment). This is obviously difficult, but not impossible, in physical activity interventions. Also control and intervention groups should receive the same amount of attention from the research team, otherwise any difference between them could be attributable to that attention rather than the effect of the intervention itself.
7   The power of a study is the probability of rejecting the null hypothesis even though it is true. It is principally related to size, as small studies may not be able to detect effects even though they are present.

References

Armstrong, B.K., White, E. & Saracci, R. (1994) *Principles of Exposure Measurement in Epidemiology*. New York: Oxford University Press.

Arraiz, G.A., Wigle, D.T. & Mao, Y. (1992) Risk assessment of physical activity and physical fitness in the Canada Health Survey Mortality Follow-up Study. *Journal of Clinical Epidemiology*, **45**: 419–428.

Berlin, J.A. & Colditz, G.A. (1990) A meta-analysis of physical activity in the prevention of coronary heart disease. *American Journal of Epidemiology*, **132**: 612–628.

Bernstein, L., Henderson, B.E., Hanisch, R., Sullivan-Halley, J. & Ross, R.K. (1994) Physical exercise and reduced risk of breast cancer in young women. *Journal of the National Cancer Institute*, **86**: 1403–1408.

Blair, S.N., Kohl, H.W., Paffenbarger, R.S., Clark, D.G., Cooper, K.H. & Gibbons, L.W. (1989) Physical fitness and all-cause mortality: a prospective study of healthy men and women. *Journal of the American Medical Association*, **262**: 2395–2401.

Blair, S.N., Kohl, H.W. & Barlow, C.E. (1993) Physical activity, physical fitness, and all-cause mortality in women: do women need to be active? *Journal of the American College of Nutrition*, **12**: 368–771.

Blair, S.N., Kohl, H.W., Barlow, C.E., Paffenbarger, R.S., Gibbons, L.W. & Macera, C.A. (1995) Changes in physical fitness and all-cause mortality: a prospective study of healthy and unhealthy men. *Journal of the American Medical Association*, **273**: 1093–1098.

Ceesay, S.M., Prentice, A.M., Day, K.C., Murgatroyd, P.R., Goldberg, G.R. & Scott, W. (1989) The use of heart rate monitoring in the estimation of energy expenditure: a validation study using indirect whole-body calorimetry. *British Journal of Nutrition*, **61**: 175–186.

Chestnut, C.H. (1993) Bone mass and exercise. *American Journal of Medicine*, **95**: (Suppl. 5A) S34–S36.

Conroy, B.P., Kraemer, W.J., Maresh, C.M., Fleck, S.J., Stone, M.H. & Fry, A.C. (1993) Bone mineral density in elite junior Olympic weightlifters. *Medicine and Science in Sports and Exercise*, **25**: 1103–1109.

Donaldson, C.L., Hulley, S.B., Vogel, J.M., Hattner, R.S., Bayers, J.H. & McMillan, D.E. (1970) Effect of prolonged bed rest on bone mineral. *Metabolism*, **19**: 1071–1084.

Dorgan, J.F., Brown, C., Barrett, M., Splansky, G.L., Kreger, B.E. & D'Agostino, R.B. (1994) Physical activity and risk of breast cancer in the Framingham Heart Study. *American Journal of Epidemiology*, **139**: 662–669.

Dowse, G.K., Zimmet, P.Z., Gareeboo, H., Alberti, K.G.M.M., Tuomilehto, J. & Finch, C.F. (1991) Abdominal obesity and physical inactivity as risk factors for NIDDM and impaired glucose tolerance, in Indian, Creole, and Chinese Mauritians. *Diabetes Care*, **14**: 271–282.

Ekelund, L.G., Haskell, W.L., Johnson, J.L., Whaley, F.S., Criqui, M.H. & Sheps, D.S. (1988) Physical fitness as predictor of cardio-vascular mortality in asymptomatic North American men: the Lipid Research Clinics Mortality Follow-up Study. *New England Journal of Medicine*, **319**: 1379–1384.

Eriksson, K.F. & Lindgarde, F. (1991) Prevention of type 2 (non-insulin-dependent) diabetes mellitus by diet and physical exercise. The 6-year Malmo feasibility study. *Diabetologia*, **34**: 891–989.

Feskens, E.J., Loeber, J.G. & Kromhout, D. (1994) Diet and physical activity as determinants of hyperinsulinemia: the Zutphen Elderly Study. *American Journal of Epidemiology*, **140**: 350–360.

Gerhardsson, M., Floderus, B. & Norell, S.E. (1988) Physical activity and colon cancer risk. *International Journal of Epidemiology*, **17**: 743–746.

Gerhardsson, M., Steineck, G., Hagman, U., Rieger, A. & Norell, S.E. (1990) Physical activity and colon cancer: a case-referent study in Stockholm. *International Journal of Cancer*, **46**: 985–989.

Giovannucci, E., Ascherio, A., Rimm, E.B., Colditz, G.A., Stampfer, M. & Willett, W.C. (1995) Physical activity, obesity, and risk for colon cancer and adenoma in men. *Annals of Internal Medicine*, **122**: 327–334.

Graafmans, W.C., Bouter, L.M. & Lips, P. (1998) The influence of physical activity and fractures on ultrasound parameters in elderly people. *Osteoporosis International*, **8**: 449–454.

Grimston, S.K., Willows, N.D. & Hanley, D.A. (1993) Mechanical loading regime and its relationship to bone mineral density in children. *Medicine and Science in Sports and Exercise*, **25**: 1203–1210.

Hara, H., Kawase, T., Yamakido, M. & Nishimoto, Y. (1983) Comparative observation of micro- and macroangiopathies in Japanese diabetics in Japan and USA. In: Abe, H. & Hoshi, M. (eds), *Diabetic Microangiopathy*. Basel: Karger.

Hein, H.O., Suadicani, P. & Gyntelberg, F. (1992) Physical fitness or physical activity as a predictor of ischaemic heart disease: a 17-year follow-up in the Gothenberg Male Study. *Journal of Internal Medicine*, **232**: 471–479.

Helmrich, S.P., Ragland, D.R., Leung, R.W. & Paffenbarger, R.S. (1991) Physical activity and reduced occurrence of non-insulin-dependent diabetes mellitus. *New England Journal of Medicine*, **325**: 147–152.

Hill, A.B. (1965) The environment and disease: association or causation? *Proceedings of the Royal Society of Medicine*, **58**: 295–300.

Hu, F.B., Leitzmann, M.F., Stampfer, M.J., Colditz, G.A., Willett, W.C. & Rimm, E.B. (2001) Physical activity and television watching in relation to risk for type 2 diabetes mellitus in men. *Archives of Internal Medicine*, **161**: 1542–1548.

Hu, F.B., Stampfer, M.J., Colditz, G.A., Ascherio, A., Rexrode, K.M., Willett, W.C. *et al.* (2000) Physical activity and risk of stroke in women. *Journal of the American Medical Association*, **283(22)**: 2961–2967.

Jakes, R.W., Khaw, K.-T., Day, N.E., Bingham, S., Welch, A., Oakes, S. *et al.* (2001) Patterns of physical activity and ultrasound attenuation by heel bone among Norfolk cohort of European Investigation of Cancer (EPIC Norfolk): population based study. *British Medical Journal*, **322**: 140–143.

Kannel, W.B. & Sorlie, P. (1979) Some health benefits of physical activity: The Framingham Heart Study. *Archives of Internal Medicine*, **139**: 857–861.

Kannel, W.B., Belanger, A., D'Agostino, R. & Israel, I. (1986) Physical activity and physical demand on the job and risk of cardiovascular disease and death: The Framingham Study. *American Heart Journal*, **112**: 820–825.

Kawate, R., Yamakido, M., Nishimoto, Y., Bennett, P.H., Hamman, R.F. & Knowler, W.C. (1979) Diabetes mellitus and its vascular complications in Japanese migrants on the island of Hawaii. *Diabetes Care*, **2**: 161–170.

Kaye, S.A., Folsom, A.R., Sprafka, J.M., Prineas, R.J. & Wallace, R.B. (1991) Increased incidence of diabetes mellitus in relation to abdominal adiposity in older women. *Journal of Clinical Epidemiology*, **44**: 329–334.

King, H. & Rewers, M. (1993) Global estimates for prevalence of diabetes mellitus and impaired glucose tolerance in adults. *Diabetes Care*, **16**: 157–177.

Kirchner, E.M., Lewis, R.D. & O'Connor, P.J. (1996) Effect of past gymnastics participation on adult bone mass. *Journal of Applied Physiology*, **80**: 225–232.

Kriska, A.M. & Caspersen, C.J. (1997) A collection of physical activity questionnaires for health-related research. *Medicine and Science in Sports and Exercise*, **29**: (Suppl. 6) S1–S205.

Kriska, A.M., Gregg, E.W., Utter, A.C., Knowler, W.C., Narayan, V. & Bennett, P.H. (1993) Association of physical activity and plasma insulin levels in a population at high risk for NIDDM. *Medicine and Science in Sports and Exercise*, **26**: (Suppl. 5) S121.

Kriska, A.M., LaPorte, R.E., Pettitt, D.J., Charles, M.A., Nelson, R.G. & Kuller, L.H. (1993) The association of physical activity with obesity, fat distribution, and glucose intolerance in Pima Indians. *Diabetologia*, **36**: 863–869.

Krølner, B., Toft, B., Nielsen, S.P. & Tøndevold, E. (1983) Physical exercise as prophylaxis against involutional vertebral bone loss: a controlled trial. *Clinical Science*, **64**: 541–546.

Lanyon, L.E. (1984) Functional strain as a determinant of bone remodeling. *Calcified Tissue International*, **36**: S56–S61.

Lanyon, L.E. (1992) Control of bone architecture by functional load bearing. *Journal of Bone and Mineral Research*, 7: (Suppl. 2) S369–S375.

Lanyon, L.E. (1996) Using functional loading to influence bone mass and architecture: objectives, mechanisms, and relationship with estrogen of the mechanically adaptive process in bone. *Bone*, **18**: (Suppl. 1) S37–S43.

Last, J.M. (ed.) (1995) *A Dictionary of Epidemiology*. 2nd ed. New York: Oxford University Press.

Lee, I.-M., Paffenbarger, R.S. & Hsieh, C.-C. (1991) Physical activity and risk of developing colorectal cancer among college alumni. *Journal of the National Cancer Institute*, **83**: 1324–1329.

Lee, I.-M., Paffenbarger, R.S. & Hsieh, C.-C. (1992) Physical activity and risk of developing prostatic cancer among college alumni. *American Journal of Epidemiology*, **135**: 169–179.

Lee, I.-M. & Paffenbarger, R.S. (2000) Associations of light, moderate, and vigorous intensity physical activity with longevity: The Harvard Alumni Health Study. *American Journal of Epidemiology*, **151**(3): 293–299.

McKeigue, P.M., Pierpoint, T., Ferrie, J.E. & Marmot, M.G. (1992) Relationship of glucose intolerance and hyperinsulinaemia to body fat pattern in south Asians and Europeans. *Diabetologia*, **35**: 785–791.

Manson, J.E., Rimm, E.B., Stampfer, M.J., Colditz, G.A., Willett, W.C. & Krolewski, A.S. (1991) Physical activity and incidence of non-insulin-dependent diabetes mellitus in women. *Lancet*, **338**: 774–778.

Montoye, H.J., Kemper, H.C.G., Saris, W.H.M. & Washburn, R.A. (1996) *Measuring Physical Activity and Energy Expenditure*. Champaign: Human Kinetics.

Morris, J.N., Chave, S.P.W., Adam, C., Sirey, C., Epstein, L. & Sheehan, D.J. (1973) Vigorous exercise in leisure-time and the incidence of coronary heart disease. *Lancet*, **1**(7799): 333–339.

Morris, J.N., Everitt, M.G., Pollard, R., Chave, S.P.W. & Semmence, A.M. (1980) Vigorous exercise in leisure time: protection against coronary heart disease. *Lancet*, **2**(8206): 1207–1210.

Morris, J.N., Heady, J.A., Raffle, P.A.B., Roberts, C.G. & Parks, J.W. (1953) Coronary heart disease and physical activity of work. *Lancet*, **2**: 1111–1120.

Nichols, D.L., Sanborn, C.F., Bonnick, S.L., Ben-Ezra, V., Gench, B. & DiMarco, N.M. (1994) The effects of gymnastics training on bone mineral density. *Medicine and Science in Sports and Exercise*, **26**: 1220–1225.

Neel, J.V. (1962) Diabetes mellitus: a thrifty genotype rendered detrimental by 'progress'? *American Journal of Human Genetics*, **14**: 353–362.

O'Connor, J.A., Lanyon, L.E. & MacFie, H. (1982) The influence of strain rate on adaptive bone remodelling. *Journal of Biomechanics*, **15**(10): 767–781.

Office for National Statistics (1998) *Social Trends*, London: The Stationery Office, **28**.

Oliveria, S.A., Kohl, H.W., Trichopoulos, D. & Blair, S.N. (1996) The association between cardiorespiratory fitness and prostate cancer. *Medicine and Science in Sports and Exercise*, **28**: 97–104.

Paffenbarger, R.S., Hyde, R.T., Wing, A.L. & Steinmetz, C.H. (1984) A natural history of athleticism and cardiovascular health. *Journal of the American Medical Association*, **252**: 491–495.

Paffenbarger, R.S., Hyde, R.T., Wing, A.L., Lee, I.-M., Jung, D.L. & Kampert, J.B. (1993) The association of changes in physical activity level and other lifestyle characteristics with mortality among men. *New England Journal of Medicine*, **328**: 538–545.

Pan, X., Li, G. & Hu, Y. (1995) Effect of dietary and/or exercise intervention on incidence of diabetes in 530 subjects with impaired glucose tolerance from 1986–1992. *Chinese Journal of Internal Medicine*, **34**: 108–112.

Philippaerts, R.M., Westerterp, K.R. & Lefevre, J. (1999) Doubly labelled water validation of three physical activity questionnaires. *International Journal of Sports Medicine*, **20**: 284–289.

Prentice, A.M. (ed.) (1990) *The doubly-labeled water method for measuring energy expenditure, technical recommendations for use in humans*. Vienna: Atomic Energy Agency.

Prentice, A.M. & Jebb, S.A. (1995) Obesity in Britain: gluttony or sloth? *British Medical Journal*, **311**: 437–439.

Ramaiya, K.L., Swai, A.B.M., McLarty, D.G. & Alberti, K.G.M.M. (1991) Impaired glucose tolerance and diabetes mellitus in Hindu Indian immigrants in Dar es Salaam. *Diabetic Medicine*, **8**: 738–744.

Ravussin, E., Bennett, P.H. & Valencia (1994) Effect of traditional lifestyle of obesity in Pima Indians. *Diabetic Medicine*, **17**: 1067–1074.

Regensteiner, J.G., Shetterly, S.M., Mayer, E.J., Eckel, R.H., Haskell, W.L. & Baxter, J. (1995) Relationship between habitual physical activity and insulin area among individuals with impaired glucose tolerance: the San Luis Valley Diabetes Study. *Diabetes Care*, **18**: 490–497.

Rennie, K.L. & Wareham, N.J. (1998) The validation of physical activity instruments for measuring energy expenditure: problems and pitfalls. *Public Health Nutrition*, **1(4)**: 265–271.

Rockhill, B., Willett, W.C., Hunter, D.J., Manson, J.E., Hankinson, S.E. & Colditz, G.A. (1999) A prospective study of recreational physical activity and breast cancer risk. *Archives of Internal Medicine*, **159**: 2290–2296.

Rubin, C.T. & Lanyon, L.E. (1984) Regulation of bone formation by applied dynamic loads. *Journal of Bone and Joint Surgery*, **66**: 397–402.

Rubin, C.T. & Lanyon, L.E. (1985) Regulation of bone mass by mechanical strain magnitude. *Calcified Tissue International*, **37**: 411–417.

Rubin, K., Schirduan, V., Gendreau, P., Sarfarazi, M., Mendola, R. & Dalsky, G. (1993) Predictors of axial and peripheral bone mineral density in healthy children and adolescents, with special attention to the role of puberty. *Journal of Pediatrics*, **123**: 863–870.

Sandvik, L., Erikssen, J., Thaulow, E., Erikssen, G., Mundal, R. & Rodahl, K. (1993) Physical fitness as a predictor of mortality among healthy, middle-aged Norwegian men. *New England Journal of Medicine*, **328**: 533–537.

Schranz, A., Tuomilehto, J., Marti, B., Jarrett, R.J., Grabauskas, V. & Vassallo, A. (1991) Low physical activity and worsening of glucose tolerance: results from a 2-year follow-up of a population sample in Malta. *Diabetes Research and Clinical Practice*, **11**: 127–136.

Shaper, A.G. & Wannamethee, G. (1991) Physical activity and ischaemic heart disease in middle-aged British men. *British Heart Journal*, **66**: 384–394.

Siconolfi, S.F., Lasater, T.M., Snow, R.C. & Carleton, R.A. (1985) Self-reported physical activity compared with maximal oxygen uptake. *American Journal of Epidemiology*, **122(1)**: 101–105.

Slattery, M.L. & Jacobs, D.R. (1988) Physical fitness and cardiovascular disease mortality: the US Railroad Study. *American Journal of Epidemiology*, **127**: 571–580.

Sobolski, J., Kornitzer, M., DeBacker, G., Dramaix, M., Abramowicz, M. & Degre, S. (1987) Protection against ischemic heart disease in the Belgian Physical Fitness Study: physical fitness rather than physical activity? *American Journal of Epidemiology*, **125**: 601–610.

Thor, P., Konturek, J.W., Konturek, S.J. & Anderson, J.H. (1985) Role of prostaglindins in control of intestinal motility. *American Journal of Physiology*, **248**: G353–G359.

Tilton, F., Degioanni, J.J.C. & Schneider, V.S. (1980) Long-term follow-up of skylab bone demineralization. *Aviat Space Environ Med*, 51(11): 1209–1213.

Tuomilehto, J., Lindström, J., Eriksson, J.G., Valle, T.T., Hämäläinen, H., Ilanne-Parikka, P. *et al.* (2001) Prevention of type 2 diabetes mellitus by changes in lifestyle among subjects with impaired glucose tolerance. *New England Journal of Medicine*, 344(18): 1343–1350.

Tutton, P.J.M. & Barkla, D.H. (1980) Influence of protaglandin analogues on epithelial cell proliferation and xenograft growth. *British Journal of Cancer*, 41: 47–51.

Wannamethee, G. & Shaper, A.G. (1992) Physical activity and stroke in British middle-aged men. *British Medical Journal*, 304: 597–601.

Wareham, N.J., Jakes, R.W., Rennie, K.L., Mitchell, J., Hennings, S. & Day, N.E. (in press) Validity and repeatability of the EPIC-Norfolk physical activity questionnaire. *International Journal of Epidemiology*.

Wareham, N.J. & Rennie, K.L. (1998) The assessment of physical activity in individuals and populations: Why try to be more precise about how physical activity is assessed? *International Journal of Obesity*, 22: (Suppl. 2) S30–S38.

Wareham, N.J., Wong, M.-Y. & Day, N.E. (2000) Glucose intolerance and physical inactivity: the relative importance of low habitual energy expenditure and cardiorespiratory fitness. *American Journal of Epidemiology*, 152: 132–139.

Washburn, R.A., Goldfield, S.R.W., Smith, K.W. & McKinlay, J.B. (1990) The validity of self-reported exercise-induced sweating as a measure of physical activity. *American Journal of Epidemiology*, 132: 107–113.

CHAPTER 4

Physical Activity and Mental Health

DAVID CARLESS AND GUY FAULKNER

Chapter Contents

- Introduction
- Evidence for the mental health benefits of physical activity
- Explanations for psychological changes
- Exploring physical activity and mental health
- Summary points

Introduction

Aims of the chapter

Mental health problems in many Western countries have increased to the point where traditional treatment provision is overstretched. This climate has generated interest in alternative mental health interventions and resulted in research being conducted to examine the potential of physical activity as a mental health intervention. Given that a comprehensive review of existing research is beyond the scope of a single chapter, we will instead provide a critical perspective on some important issues in physical activity and mental health research. Following a summary of current consensus in the field, we will focus specifically on what we consider to be the most pressing research questions concerning the use of physical activity as a therapeutic approach for people with mental health problems. We hope that this approach will provide the reader with a detailed and thorough understanding of current issues within this challenging field of research.

This chapter has three specific aims:

1. To summarise current consensus on physical activity and mental health research
2. To discuss potential mechanisms for mental health change through physical activity
3. To suggest alternative research perspectives for the future.

A mental health–illness perspective

The concepts of mental health and mental illness are often used interchange-ably. It is important to highlight that they should be differentiated. Mental health can be seen as the emotional and spiritual resilience which enables us to enjoy life and to survive pain, disappointment and sadness. It is a positive sense of well-being and an underlying belief in our own and others' dignity and worth (HEA, 1997). A mental health disorder is any health condition which is characterised by alterations in thinking, mood, or behaviour (or some combination thereof) associated with distress and/or impaired functioning (United States Department of Health and Human Services, 1999). Tudor (1996) argues that mental health and mental disorder should be seen as two separate continua (Figure 4.1) and that this should be reflected in research and practice. This has two main implications. First, it allows the possibility of having a diagnosis of mental illness but still attaining positive mental health. As such, it justifies the promotion of mental health to individuals with a mental illness rather than being overly fixated on treatment or prevention. Bryne *et al.* (1994) draw attention to the scarcity of literature that considers the possibility of an individual with a psychiatric illness achieving health or 'wellness' in con-trast to the more common focus on symptom control and medication issues. Second, mental health problems such as sub-clinical levels of depression or anxiety can affect us all without necessarily becoming a clinical, diagnosed condition. Consequently, mental health promotion has the capacity to improve the quality of life of clinical and non-clinical populations alike. As reflected in policy, the Department of Health has recognised the importance of mental health by identifying it as one of four key health outcomes in the national

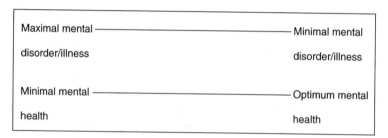

Figure 4.1 Mental Health and Mental Illness

health contract. They write that a national strategy 'must reflect more than just the absence of physical disease and be a basis for efforts which acknowledge a more rounded idea of good health' (DoH, 1999). Such identification is timely.

It has been estimated that one in four adults experiences some form of mental health problem in any one year (Goldberg, 1991), with some evidence that incidence is increasing (DoH, 1996). Depression is the most prevalent disorder with 5–10 per cent of the population estimated to be affected by clinical depression in most developed countries (Weismann & Klerman, 1992). Furthermore, depression is a greater worldwide disease burden than ischaemic heart disease, cerebrovascular disease and tuberculosis (Murray & Lopez, 1997). The cost of mental health problems is high. It is estimated that the direct and indirect costs of mental health problems for 1996–97 was over £32 billion in the UK, with estimates indicating that 80 million working days are lost each year due to anxiety and depression (Grant, 2000). In the United States, it is estimated that 15 per cent of the adult population uses some form of mental health service during the year. Eight per cent have a mental disorder; 7 per cent have a mental health problem (US DHHS, 1999). In 1996, the direct treatment of mental disorders, substance abuse, and Alzheimer's disease in the US cost $99 billion (Mark *et al.*, 1998). Poor mental health is not a trivial issue. Improving quality of life and reducing the financial burden imposed on health services by mental health problems has driven the consideration of alternative strategies for mental health promotion.

Physical activity is one alternative that has potential as an effective strategy for mental health promotion. Despite frequent reports of psychological benefits from regular exercisers and the intuitive holistic link between physical and mental well-being, researchers have only recently begun to systematically examine the impact of physical activity on mental health outcomes. The result of this research is that we now have a convincing evidence base that supports the existence of a strong link between physical activity and mental health (Morgan, 1997a; Biddle *et al.*, 2000). Fox *et al.* (2000) outline five potential benefits associated with the use of physical activity as an adjunctive strategy in improving the mental health of individuals. First, physical activity is cheap compared with the pharmacological treatment alternatives. Second, physical activity is associated with negligible adverse side-effects. Third, physical activity can be self-sustaining in that it can be potentially maintained across the lifecycle, unlike pharmacological and psychotherapeutic treatments which usually have a specified endpoint. Fourth, many non-drug treatments such as cognitive behavioural therapy can be expensive and often in short supply (Mutrie, 2000). Additionally, many patients report not wanting medication (Scott, 1996). Consequently, physical activity could be a cost-effective alternative for those preferring not to use medication or who cannot access therapy. Finally, physical activity should be promoted for physical health, regardless of whether it improves mental health. For example, depression and anxiety are significantly prevalent causes of physical illness and mortality throughout the world (APA, 1994). Additionally, many patients with chronic schizophrenia experience obesity, which is often associated with antipsychotic medication (Wetterling, 2001). The physical benefits alone, from regular physical activity in reducing morbidity and mortality in clinical populations, are sufficient justification for the inclusion of physical activity in programmes of rehabilitation. The consideration of physical activity as a strategy for mental health promotion has a sound rationale.

Evidence for the mental health benefits of physical activity

Existing evidence can be considered to fall within one of four avenues through which physical activity has the potential to impact upon mental health (Fox, 2000a):

- To prevent the onset of mental health problems
- To improve the mental well-being of the general public
- To improve the quality of life for people with mental health problems
- As treatment or therapy for existing mental illness.

Physical activity for prevention

The conclusions of a number of reviews concur that a lower incidence of mental health problems is observed among people who regularly participate in physical activity (Morgan, 1997a; Biddle *et al.*, 2000). However, this association does not in itself imply that physical activity prevented the development of mental health problems. Prospective epidemiological research is required in order to conclude with confidence that regular physical activity participation directly reduces the risk of mental health problems. Because studies of this kind are expensive and time-consuming to carry out, few have been conducted. However, Mutrie (2000) reports four longitudinal studies which examined the effect of regular physical activity on the incidence of depression at follow-up several years later. In all four studies, people who were more active at baseline reported a lower incidence of depression at follow-up. Mutrie concludes that current evidence indicates that physical activity has a protective effect against the development of depression. It may also be that physical activity offers some degree of anxiety protection on the basis of Taylor's (2000) conclusion that aerobically fit individuals generally have a reduced physiological response to psychosocial stressors. More research is required to investigate the extent that physical activity may be effective in preventing the onset of other types of mental health problems.

Physical activity to improve well-being in the general population

Participation in physical activity is consistently associated with positive affect and mood (Biddle, 2000). This relationship has been found in large population surveys and experimental studies. It would appear that physical activity does 'make you feel good' and, while this is an important outcome, it is also an important motivator for continued adherence. The 'feel good' phenomenon is also supported by the finding that single bouts of physical activity have a small-to-moderate effect on state anxiety (Taylor, 2000). Small but significant improvements in cognitive functioning have also been reported as a result of physical activity participation, although measurement difficulties for physical activity and cognitive functioning have hindered research in this area (Boutcher, 2000). Improvements in self-esteem and self-perceptions are further benefits that may be experienced through physical activity participation. Self-esteem is often regarded as the single most important indicator of psychological well-being, so any improvements in this area may be particularly significant. High self-esteem is associated with a number of important life-adjustment qualities whereas low self-esteem is associated with poor health behaviour decisions and is characteristic of many mental disorders such as depression (Fox, 1997). Fox (2000b) concluded that physical activity promotes physical self-worth and other important physical self-perceptions such as improved body image. For some people, in some situations, this generalises to improvements in global self-esteem. Given the vast array of factors that influence global self-esteem, it is probably optimistic to expect physical activity participation to reliably improve self-perceptions beyond the physical domain. However, direct links have been found between physical self-worth and mental health properties independent of global self-esteem (Sonstroem & Potts, 1996). Current consensus clearly supports an association between physical activity and numerous domains of mental health in the general population.

Physical activity for quality of life and coping with mental disorders

Among people with enduring mental health problems improved quality of life tends to enhance the individual's ability to cope with and manage their disorder. Physical activity has the potential to improve quality of life in people with mental health problems through two routes: physical and psychological. In terms of physical quality of life, we know that individuals with mental health problems have the same physical health needs as the general population. In certain clinical populations the physical health problems seen in the general population (such as obesity, hypertension, and low cardiovascular fitness) are exacerbated by the negative side-effects of commonly prescribed medications. This is a particularly serious problem for people with schizophrenia where the most effective medications result in considerable weight gain that tends to reduce treatment compliance (Green *et al.*, 2000). Because physical activity is an effective method of improving important aspects of physical health such as obesity, cardiovascular fitness, and hypertension (Bouchard *et al.*, 1994), it should be promoted to people with mental health problems for both general physical health and to counteract the side-effects of medication.

Preliminary evidence also suggests that regular physical activity improves positive aspects of mental health (such as psychological quality of life and emotional well-being) in people with mental disorders. Positive psychological effects from physical activity in clinical populations have been reported even among those individuals who experience no objective diagnostic improvement (Faulkner & Biddle, 1999). Improved quality of life is particularly important for individuals with severe and enduring mental health problems when complete remission may be unrealistic (Faulkner & Sparkes, 1999). The potential role of physical activity in reducing social exclusion is also a growing area of interest (HEA, 1999). While physical activity may have considerable direct health benefits, it may also influence health by reducing social isolation and increasing social interaction among isolated individuals or groups. This remains an under-researched area of study.

 Chapter 3 (Epidemiology) describes how epidemiologists address the health effects of physical activity and exercise.

Physical activity as treatment

Physical activity is emerging as an effective treatment or adjunct for directly tackling existing mental health problems in clinical populations. Currently, the strongest evidence concerns the use of physical activity as a treatment for depression, and a recent review found support for a causal link between physical activity participation and decreased depression (Mutrie, 2000). Meta-analyses generally report that physical activity has an effect size on depression comparable to that of other psychotherapeutic interventions (Mutrie, 2000). However, such optimism has been questioned on the basis of methodological weaknesses in existing research (Lawlor & Hopker, 2001). In terms of anxiety, evidence generally supports the existence of a positive effect through physical activity participation for both trait and state anxiety (Taylor, 2000). Although Taylor concluded that physical activity has a low-to-moderate anxiety reducing effect, he noted that the strongest effects were found in the best designed studies. At present, little evidence exists concerning the effects of physical activity on other mental health disorders, although it has been reported that physical activity is effective in treating the symptoms of certain psychoses such as schizophrenia (Faulkner & Biddle, 1999). Limited research also suggests that physical activity may be a useful adjunctive strategy for drug and alcohol rehabilitation (see Biddle & Mutrie, 2001).

Explanations for psychological changes

Despite the convincing evidence base there is still little consensus on the mechanisms or causes of the effects of physical activity participation on mental health. Although identification of significant relationships and subsequently the demonstration of causation through experimental trials provide evidence of a mental health effect, it is also important to identify the mechanisms through which these effects occur. The ability to explain how, why, and under what conditions psychological changes occur in response to physical activity allows the reliable prescription and management across varied mental health contexts. Understanding the mechanisms underpinning an individual's psychological responses to physical activity is therefore a prerequisite for further progress.

Plausible mechanisms for the effects of physical activity on mental health

Proposed mechanisms for mental health change through physical activity fall into one of three diverse perspectives: biochemical, physiological, or psychological. A summary of these mechanisms is provided in Table 4.1. At present no single mechanism adequately explains the diverse range of mental health effects that may be experienced through physical activity participation. The lack of precise understanding of psychological effects is not unique to physical activity interventions. Despite the acceptance and widespread use of certain anti-psychotic medications, for example, the biochemical basis for action for some drugs has not been clearly identified (Gerlach & Peacock, 1995). Similarly, attempts to identify the specific processes through which psychotherapies and behavioural therapies work has proved difficult, and in many studies the importance of patient and therapist characteristics is often overlooked (Garfield, 1998). A major reason for the lack of precise understanding of the effects of mental health interventions must lie in the complexity of mental health and disorder. According to the Surgeon General's Report (US DHHS, 1999):

> *Mental health and mental illness are dynamic, ever-changing phenomena. At any given moment, a person's mental status reflects the sum total of that individual's genetic inheritance and life experiences (p. 16).*

Because a diverse range of factors influence a person's mental health at any point in time it follows that a combination of triggers are likely to interact when

Table 4.1 Plausible mechanisms for mental health change through physical activity

Mechanism	Background and research evidence
Biochemical	
Opioids	β-endorphins have been the focus of media attention on the feelings of euphoria reported by some exercisers. Endogenous opioid peptides found in the blood during and following physical activity have been linked to this response. Research has not found this effect to be common among exercisers. It appears that high-intensity physical activity is necessary and research does not conclusively support any link between endorphins and mood. For further information see Hoffmann (1997).
Monoamines	Increased synthesis of central monoamines such as serotonin has been found in response to physical activity in humans and animals. However the effects of increased serotonin on psychological function is still unclear. For further discussion see Chaouloff (1997).
Norepinephrine	Norepinephrine neurons have been identified in the brain and linked to both depression and anxiety in some studies. However, this mechanism is yet to be fully explored in the physical activity context due to methodological problems (Dishman, 1997).
Physiological	
Improved cardiovascular and muscle function	Because physical fitness often improves with participation, epidemiological research has reported associations between physical fitness and psychological health. However, experimental research has not generally found improvements in fitness to be associated with mental health benefits. Fox *et al.* (2000) suggests that process factors linked with regular participation in physical activity seem to be more important to mental health change than improved fitness.
Thermogenesis and increased core body temperature	Increased core temperature decreases muscle tension with reductions in anxiety has been hypothesised, but there has been little support for this from the literature (Biddle & Mutrie, 2001).
Psychological	
Improved social interaction and support	Physical activity offers a diverse range of social interaction possibilities. Often, the opportunity for positive social interaction and support are missing for those with mental disorders such as depression. Physical activity conducted in a supportive group environment may be particularly important for mental health improvements in these individuals (Biddle & Mutrie, 2001).
Sense of autonomy and personal control	Psychologists generally recognise the importance of autonomy and self-determination to psychological health. Physical activity offers a potential area where meaningful control can be taken over health behaviours. It may be that autonomy gained through physical activity generalises to other areas of life through feelings of empowerment (Fox, 1997).
Improved perceptions of competence	Specific physical self-perceptions have been shown to be related to physical self-worth in general (Fox, 1990). In turn, physical self-worth has direct mental health links (Sonstroem & Potts, 1996) and is related to global self-esteem. Existing research suggests that competence and self-perceptions can be improved through physical activity and that this can have a positive mental health effect (Fox, 1997).
Enhanced body image and self-acceptance	Body image has been found to be strongly related to self-esteem, particularly in women (Davis, 1997). Additionally, body image concerns may be relevant to individuals receiving medication. The improvement in body composition possible through physical activity, coupled with improved self-acceptance, is a potentially effective route to improving psychological well-being.

Distraction or 'time-out'	Bahrke and Morgan's (1978) distraction hypothesis suggests that physical activity works as a distraction from the worries and stresses of daily life, inducing positive emotions and reducing anxiety. For example, when comparing running therapy with verbal therapy for the relief of depression, Greist *et al.* (1979) suggested that 'depressive cognitions and affect seldom emerge during running, and when they do, they are virtually impossible to maintain' (p. 45).

an individual experiences a mental health problem. It appears that 'the causes of most mental disorders lie in some combination of genetic and environmental factors, which may be biological or psychosocial' (US DHHS, 1999, pp. 16–17). In accepting that both biological and psychosocial factors cause mental disorders it is also necessary to acknowledge that both biological and psychosocial changes might lead to the remittance of a disorder. For example, if a person's depression is caused by a combination of social, environmental, and biochemical factors then it is likely that improvements in any combination of these factors could explain remission. The difficulty in pinning down a single mechanism to explain the mental health benefits of physical activity is likely to be connected to the complex, individual causes of mental illness.

Alternative mechanisms for mental health change: a process approach

The range of factors that influence occurrence and recovery from mental disorder, in combination with the problems of specific mechanisms already discussed, suggests that attempts to identify a single mechanism for the mental health benefits of physical activity may be futile. Although an understanding of mental function at the biochemical level might ultimately be useful, two arguments suggest that an alternative focus is currently more appropriate. First, all mental functions and psychological processes are, at the most fundamental level, carried out by chemical processes. In other words, thought processes and emotional responses are dependent on chemical or physical changes in the brain for their expression (US DHHS, 1999). This situation applies equally in mental health and illness. That chemical or physical changes underlie the expression of mental illness does not imply that chemical or physical factors *caused* the disorder (Bedi, 1999). Because biological and psychosocial factors interact to determine mental health, a sole focus on biochemical change is insufficient to adequately explain changes in mental functioning. Second, as previously discussed, the biochemical changes triggered by medications are only partly understood, yet pharmacological interventions are widely used to good effect. The same is true for physical activity; the appropriate employment of physical activity as a means of improving mental health is not dependent on specifying chemical change within the brain.

An alternative approach to understanding the causes or mechanisms of psychological change through physical activity is to adopt a *process* orientation. The process of mental health change as a result of physical activity participation must allow for the diverse biological and psychosocial factors that determine an individual's mental health. The isolation of a specific mechanism cannot realistically address the large number of potential psychological influences that may be experienced through physical activity. It is more realistic for a process-oriented approach to allow for the broad range of potential influences and therefore provide a more complete explanation of the causes of psychological change. This is particularly pertinent when we consider that psychological benefits have been found independent of changes in physical fitness. Process factors related to physical activity participation, in contrast to changes in physiological parameters, appear more salient in promoting mental health (Fox, 1999).

Given that mental health and mental disorder can be seen as existing on two separate continua (see Figure 4.1), similar factors have the potential to result in improved mental health for both individuals with mental disorders and the general population. Several recent theories, including the psychobiological theory of personality (Cloninger *et al.*, 1994) have been proposed to explain mental health and psychological function from this perspective. These theories all take a process-oriented approach in that they include a diverse range of factors that have been suggested to affect mental health. Although these new developments have not yet been examined in physical activity situations, they have the potential to explain the effects of physical activity interventions on mental health. It may be that the diverse range of possible biological and psychosocial benefits that can be experienced through physical activity makes these broader process-oriented explanations relevant to physical activity contexts.

Psychobiological theory of personality

Cloninger and colleagues' (1994) psychobiological theory of personality integrates the psychosocial and biological aspects of mental health identified in the Surgeon General's Report (US DHHS, 1999) and offers an explanation for changes in mental health. In this theory, mental health is conceptualised as being dependent on the interaction of two developmentally separate components of personality: *temperament* and *character* (Cloninger *et al.*, 1994). Temperament 'refers to biases in automatic responses to emotional stimuli and is moderately heritable and stable throughout life regardless of culture or social learning' (Cloninger *et al.*, 1999, p. 34). Temperament is conceived as being largely genetically determined and therefore more related to traditional personality theories where personality is viewed as being relatively unchangeable. The second component, character, 'refers to individual differences in our voluntary goals and values, which are based on insight learning of intuitions and concepts about ourselves, other people, and other objects' (Cloninger & Svrakic, 1997, p. 121). Character is developmentally changeable, that is, it is determined by psychosocial factors such as experiential learning and environmental influences. This component is therefore of more direct interest in the physical activity context.

Recent research has investigated temperament and character in mental health contexts such as depression, alcohol dependence, and psychoses. Although temperament has been found to link with certain types of disorder (Reichter *et al.*, 2000) and response to certain medications (Joyce *et al.*, 1994), it has been character that has predicted the presence and risk of a mental disorder (Cloninger *et al.*, 1999; Hansenne *et al.*, 1999; Peirson & Heuchert, 2001). Two specific aspects of character have been found to be particularly important: self-directedness (autonomy and perceptions of control) and co-operativeness (perceived interpersonal relations). Individuals reporting low levels of self-directedness and co-operativeness have been found to be more likely to experience a mental disorder (Cloninger *et al.*, 1999). Because character profile is responsive to experiential learning and social or environmental factors, improvements in self-directedness and co-operativeness represent a potential mechanism to explain mental health improvements through any behavioural or psychological intervention. The broad range of psychosocial phenomena included in psychobiological theory (such as individual predisposition, influence of environmental factors, learning experiences, and life events) suggests that this theory might offer a more comprehensive account of the psychological benefits experienced through participation in physical activity.

True self-esteem

Recent theoretical advances suggest that in addition to improved self-esteem being a potential outcome of physical activity, self-esteem may act as a psychosocial mechanism that explains the effects of physical activity on mental health. One recent self-esteem theory offers a potentially enlightening perspective on explaining the psychological benefits of physical activity. Deci & Ryan (1995) identify two alternative forms of self-esteem that have differing effects on mental health. *True* self-esteem is most closely related to positive mental health and well-being and is dependent on meeting and balancing three fundamental needs: autonomy, relatedness, and competence. The authors propose that failure to meet and balance these needs will result in either low self-esteem or *contingent* self-esteem, resulting in a fragile, insecure sense of self (Deci & Ryan, 1995).

Of particular interest in Deci and Ryan's theory is that all three of the basic needs are commonly reported outcomes of physical activity interventions (Fox, 1997) and are often unmet among individuals with mental disorders. Autonomy, or perceptions of personal control, is reported to be frequently lacking particularly among people with depression where feelings of power-lessness and helplessness are common (Seligman, 1975). Physical activity offers a potential avenue where meaningful control can be gradually taken as the individual assumes responsibility for the organisation of his or her physical activity schedule. Relatedness to other people is often missing for individuals with mental disorders who might report feelings of isolation or difficulty in maintaining close or social contact with friends and family (US DHHS, 1999). The provision of physical activity in a supportive group environment represents one approach to providing opportunities for positive social interaction that may be valuable. Finally, perceptions of competence may be low among people with mental illness and physical activity has well-documented positive effects on perceived competence, particularly in areas related to physical abilities (Fox, 1997). Although no research has as yet applied Deci and Ryan's theory to phys-ical activity and mental health settings, it has clear similarities to Cloninger's psychobiological theory in that both acknowledge the central importance of autonomy and inter-relations with others in achieving mental health.

Stress sensitivity

Salmon (2001) has recently proposed an alternative explanation for the anti-depressive and anxiolytic effects of physical activity. In this theory Salmon proposes that participation in physical activity is initially experienced as an aversive stimulus but sensitivity to the stress of physical activity is reduced as a result of repeated participation. Through a process of Pavlovian association, reduced sensitivity to physical activity-specific stress is thought to result in a general resistance to other stressors or disruptions. This general reduction in sensitivity to stress is theorised to result in a protective effect against anxiety and depression that may explain the finding from longitudinal research that habitual physical activity reduces the risk of future mental illness. Salmon (2001) proposes:

> *The particular value of exercise might therefore be that it is a controllable stressor. On this basis, to maximise clinical benefit, participants' perception of being in control of the exercise regime should be maximised (p. 51).*

The identification of personal control is in agreement with the theories discussed above and when combined with recent commentaries (Fox, 1997; Biddle & Mutrie, 2001) suggests that this dimension of exercising may be particularly important for achieving psychological benefits.

A major drawback of stress sensitivity theory is the view that initial physical-activity experience should be perceived as aversive in order to have a positive mental health effect (Salmon, 2001). Existing research indicates clearly that physical activity perceived as aversive, uncomfortable or unpleasant, has a negative impact on physical activity adoption and adherence, particularly among people beginning to exercise (Rejeski, 1994). It is evident that if mental health benefits are to be realised from physical activity (in any population) the individual must maintain participation. Given the difficulties of adoption and adherence in clinical populations, it seems clear that stress-sensitivity theory offers important challenges for understanding the initiation of regular, frequent physical activity.

Individual specificity

The diversity of explanations for the mental health benefits of physical activity parallels the broad range of factors that influence mental health and disorder. It is possible that psychological, biochemical and physiological factors are all partly responsible for mental health change in different contexts or that an interaction of psychosocial and genetic factors results in change. Given the diverse genetic and psychosocial determinants of mental health and the broad range of psychological stimuli that can be experienced through physical activity, any comprehensive explanation must be flexible and broad enough to cover many possible scenarios. In reality, it currently appears that Salmon (2001) is correct in his view that no single theory is likely to adequately explain the mental health benefits of physical activity.

To date, the most satisfying conclusion in the mechanisms debate has been offered by Fox (1999). In acknowledging the huge diversity of potential triggers (such as physical activity type, environment, social context) and individual circumstances (such as state of mental health, needs, preferences, and personal background), Fox suggests that several mechanisms most likely operate in concert with the precise combination are highly individual-specific. That is, different processes operate for different people at different times. It is from this perspective that we propose future research should be conducted in order to *include* as many aspects of the 'physical activity experience' as possible. Rather than focusing on specific mechanisms for mental health change, we suggest that it is currently more important to allow for *individual* variation through the adoption of an appropriately broad theoretical stance and adopting suitably inclusive and sensitive research methods.

Exploring physical activity and mental health

The randomised controlled trial

From the 1990s into the new millennium UK government documents, including *Our Healthier Nation* (DoH, 1999), all emphasise the role of evidence-based practice as being at the centre of effective planning and delivery of health services. Evidence-based practice is defined by its adherents as the 'conscientious, explicit and judicious use of current best evidence in making decisions about the care of individual patients' (Sackett *et al.*, 1996, p. 71). Such evidence is principally gathered through randomised controlled trials (RCT):

> *It is when asking questions about therapy that we should try to avoid the non-experimental approaches, since these routinely lead to false-positive conclusions about efficacy. Because the randomised trial, and especially the systematic review of several randomised trials, is so much more likely to inform us and so much less likely to mislead us, it has become the 'gold standard' for judging whether a treatment does more good than harm (Sackett et al., p. 72).*

Random selection of participants and random assignment to treatments is the most effective means of controlling threats to internal and external validity, while the inclusion of a control group rules out the possibility that something other than the experimental treatment (for instance, exercise) has influenced the outcome.

As an example, Blumenthal *et al.* (1999) compared the effects of physical activity treatment and drug treatment in a sample of older individuals. After recruitment, initial screening and assessment by clinical psychologists blind to treatment allocation, 156 men and women (M=57 years) meeting DSM (Diagnostic Symptoms Manual)-IV criteria for major depressive disorder were randomly assigned to one of three treatment groups: (a) a physical activity group consisting of three supervised physical activity sessions (30 minutes of continuous cycle ergometry or brisk walking/jogging at 70–85 per cent heart rate reserve) a week for 16 consecutive weeks; (b) antidepressant therapy (sertraline, a selective serotonin reuptake inhibitor); or (c) a combination of physical activity and antidepressants. Randomisation was stratified according to the severity of depression. After 16 weeks, all groups exhibited significant reductions in symptoms of depression and there were no significant differences across groups. Additionally, the percentage of patients no longer classified as clinically depressed did not differ across the three treatment groups. A ten-month follow-up (Babyak *et al.*, 2000) found that improvements persisted for at least six months after treatment termination. Self-reported participation in physical activity during the follow-up period was inversely related to the incidence of depression at ten months. Each 50-minute increment in physical activity a week was associated with a 50 per cent decrease in the odds of being classified as depressed. Overall, this important and well-designed study suggests that physical activity is an effective and robust treatment for patients with major depression, at least for those inclined to take part! The finding that physical activity was equally efficacious to a standard drug treatment has important financial implications.

This study also contributes to a growing body of evidence supporting the efficacy of physical activity as an adjunctive treatment for depression (see Mutrie, 2000). However, less is known regarding the effectiveness of such interventions in community settings. What is the likely effect of physical activity on clinical patients in everyday practice? RCT's answer 'a circumscribed set of questions and issues related to outcome rather than to process, and to efficacy rather than effectiveness' (Roth & Parry, 1997, p. 370). Efficacy describes what works in the clinical-trial setting while effectiveness refers to what works in typical clinical-practice settings. That is, the external validity or general-isability of such trials has been questioned. In the case of physical activity, a recurring weakness is the reliance on volunteers (Lawlor & Hopker, 2001). As Babyak *et al.* (2000) wrote, 'we presume that these participants believed physical activity to be a credible treatment modality for depression and were favourably inclined toward participation' (p. 637). Burbach (1997) has pointed to the need to distinguish between those who are referred to specialised mental health services as they are likely to be more severely impaired. How acceptable would physical activity be to a clinically depressed client presenting for treatment? How should physical activity be effectively delivered to depressed clients given the low rates of physical activity compliance in the general population?

Additionally, if the mechanisms underpinning an antidepressant effect are specific to the individual, as previously discussed, then participants who are allocated to their non-preferred treatment or mode of physical activity are less likely to experience psychological benefit and may drop out. This differential attrition itself introduces a non-random element into the design, and those who complete physical activity programmes may be atypically receptive, which further reduces the generalisability of findings (Roth & Parry, 1997). An unexpected finding in the aforementioned study was that combining physical activity with medication conferred no additional advantage over either treatment alone. The authors suggest that one of the positive psychological benefits of physical activity is the development of personal mastery and self-esteem (Babyak *et al.*, 2000, p. 636):

> *It is conceivable that the concurrent use of medication may undermine this benefit by prioritising an alternative, less self-confirming attribution for one's improved condition. Instead of incorporating the belief 'I was dedicated and worked hard with the exercise program; it wasn't easy, but I beat this depression', patients might incorporate the belief that 'I took an antidepressant and got better'.*

In other words, we have a positive outcome but what actually happened? Such questions remain largely speculative through the RCT design. Issues related to mechanisms and dynamics of change are untouched. Furthermore, what else was happening in the lives of participants? How does the social context and the relative impact of other life circumstances, such as marital status or occupational opportunities, mediate the relationship between physical activity participation and depression? It may be that a case-study approach to evaluation might be at least as rewarding as a randomised controlled trial (Riddoch *et al.*, 1998) in that wider, often unintended, outcomes of an intervention can be ascertained. The consideration of alternative methodological approaches can complement the findings of research trials by exploring individuals' experiences of process and effectiveness.

A qualitative approach

Mutrie (1997) wrote that qualitative[1] methods may 'hold the key to a better understanding of the mechanisms underlying the effect of physical activity on life quality' providing a 'richer, more informed view' (p. 307). Qualitative research comprises a wide range of research approaches but it is usually characterised by a rich description and a narrative style to more closely represent the experience of participants. It is ideally suited to understanding the process by which events and actions take place and how views and attitudes change over time (Maxwell, 1996). For example, longitudinal involvement in the 'field' of study offers an opportunity to explore perceptions of physical activity, the motives and barriers to involvement and its role in promoting psychological well-being alongside the narrative of participants' lives. An important objective may be to discover and 'understand naturally occurring phenomena in their naturally occurring states' (Patton, 1980, p. 41).

Faulkner & Sparkes (1999) report a qualitative study investigating the effects of an physical activity programme on the lives of three individuals with schizophrenia within a residential setting. An experimental approach was considered impractical for two main reasons. Firstly, there were only a small number of residents living in the hostel and self-report inventories for psychotic patients may not be reliable. Secondly, given the heterogeneity of schizophrenia, issues of comorbidity and the often vastly differing individual pharmacological interventions, ascertaining base levels or generalising results can also be difficult. Consequently, an ethnographic approach incorporating intensive, long-term observation and participation in the natural setting, and interviews with participants and their main key workers, was deemed most suitable. After a period of familiarisation, three patients participated in a ten-week physical activity programme based within their hostel accommodation. Triangulating the different data sources captured a contextual picture of physical activity in the lives of these individuals. For example, improved behaviour was observed on days of physical activity in comparison to days of inactivity while participants self-reported physical activity as a beneficial distraction from auditory hallucinations. Given the 'immersion' in the setting, it was possible to ascertain that there were no other changes in participants' lives other than involvement in the physical-activity programme. Arguably, in a form of internal validity,[2] such benefits were clearly associated with the physical activity programme. In particular, the *process* of exercising (rather than the exercise *per se*), through the provision of distraction and social interaction, created a new, external social world for participants. Staff were also enthusiastic about the benefits of the programme for their clients. Despite planing, the clinical condition of participants gradually deteriorated when staff could not maintain the programme.

Overall, this study found evidence to support the use of physical activity as an adjunct treatment for schizophrenia but that consideration must also be given to the systemic and attitudinal barriers that hinder the development of such opportunities (see Faulkner & Biddle, 2001).

Such studies carry their own challenges, but they are sensitive to the individual, capture the context in which physical activity – irrespective of how this is contextualised – are experienced and can illuminate mechanisms of change. Readers will note the sample size of three as opposed to 156 in the Blumenthal *et al.* (1999) study. By its very nature, qualitative research usually utilises a small sample which limits notions of generalisation. Faulkner & Sparkes (1999) drew on the words of Sears (1992) to discuss such an imbalance:

> *The power of qualitative data, however, lies not in the number of people interviewed but in the researcher's ability to know well a few people in their cultural contexts. The test of qualitative inquiry is not the unearthing of a seemingly endless multitude of unique individuals but illuminating the lives of a few well chosen individuals. The ideographic often provides greater insight than the nomothetic (p. 148).*

A point emphasised by Chadwick (1997), a psychiatrist still 'recovering from psychosis':

> *It could indeed be that the scientific scenario of 'demonstrably effective procedures' and 'empirically confirmed fact' so characteristic of evidence-based medicine is not all there is to helping recovering psychotic people and indeed may not even be the most important thing at all. At the individual level, the unexpected and the coincidental can be the most powerful catalysts of health (p. 583).*

Given that the experience of physical activity is likely to be unique then a methodology that accounts for the individual deserves recognition.[3]

 Chapter 7 (Inactivity) details how physical activity and exercise can be promoted to individuals.

Best of both worlds?

Quantitative and qualitative approaches have different concerns and highly contrasting strengths and weaknesses. We would argue that it is the integration and awareness of a diversity of approaches that will further understanding in exercise science in general, and physical activity and mental health in particular. The area of physical activity and mental health remains under-researched and the existing research does have weaknesses (see Morgan, 1997b; Fox, 2000; Lawlor & Hopker, 2001). Most of these methodological weaknesses, however, are not

Table 4.2 Potential research issues

Qualitative	Quantitative
Motives and barriers to physical activity of different clinical populations	Adherence to physical activity and psychological outcomes
Client acceptance of physical activity as a therapeutic modality	Interventions (for example, exercise counselling) and programme delivery
Mechanisms of change	Differential impact of different styles of physical activity behaviour (for example, fitness training versus accumulate 30 minutes of moderate intensity physical activity a day) on measures of mental health
Perceptions of exercise held by mental health professionals	Barriers to promotion by health care staff
Benefits of exercise in under-researched client groups (for example, acquired immune deficiency syndrome, schizophrenia, cancer or social inclusion)	Motivational consequences of mental health benefit on future participation

foreign to the fields of psychopharmacology (Jacobs, 1999) and psychotherapy (Roth & Parry, 1997). Yet, it is within an emerging area of research that a rich diversity of methodological approaches has much to offer. When conditions make clinical trials difficult, qualitative research can evaluate programmes in naturalistic settings via observation, and patient and staff perception of benefits.

Action research may be particularly insightful in such circumstances (see Gilbourne, 1999). Additionally, longitudinal research of a qualitative nature can best incorporate a process approach to understanding the mechanisms of action. Using these methodologies may allow exploration of which mechanisms operate for whom and under what conditions. At the same time, randomised controlled trials remain a necessity. In particular, ascertaining the cost-effectiveness of physical activity interventions is a priority. Further trials comparing physical activity in conjunction with and in contrast to Cognitive Behavioural Therapy (CBT) and medication are also needed. Table 4.2 lists additional examples of important research issues that should be investigated in the future. Depending on the research objectives, they could be addressed using any number of methodological approaches in combination or isolation. An inclusive and complementary approach to research will not only develop our evidence base but also our evidence-based *practice*.

Summary points

- A strong evidence base exists to support the psychological and mental health benefits of physical activity among the general population and for those with mental disorders.

- Mental health and illness should be conceptualised as separate continua. Improved mental health is a valid goal for both people with mental illness and for the general population.
- As yet we do not understand the mechanisms for the mental health benefits of physical activity. Proposed mechanisms have so far been unsuccessful in integrating the broad range of psychosocial and genetic factors that impact upon mental health.
- A broader process-oriented approach to explaining psychological change is advocated on the basis of allowing for the diverse stimuli possible through physical activity, the varied factors that determine mental health, and the individual-specific nature of psychological change.
- To move the field forward the inclusion of alternative research perspectives is recommended. Qualitative studies with a focus on change at the individual level permit greater insight and understanding of person-level changes than are possible through a randomised controlled trial.

Notes

1 Locke (1989) wrote that 'at best, qualitative research is a field characterized by zesty disarray' (p. 2). The term qualitative is an umbrella for a wide (dis)array of methodological tools that generally produce non-quantitative data through participant observation, focus groups or interviews. However, assumptions about the nature of reality and knowledge may vary widely among researchers of different orientations. Readers are referred to Sparkes (1992) for an introduction to these issues.
2 Criteria for judging qualitative research are not necessarily parallel to those often represented in quantitative research (for example, internal and external validity). See Sparkes (1998) for further discussion.
3 Readers are referred to Biddle *et al.* (2001) for a further discussion of qualitative research within exercise and sport psychology.

References

American Psychiatric Association (1994) *Diagnostic and Statistic Manual of Mental Disorders (4th ed.)*. Washington, DC: Author.

Babyak, M., Blumenthal, J.A., Herman, S., Khatri, P., Doraiswamy, M., Moore, K., Craighead, E., Baldewicz, T.T. & Krishnan, K.R. (2000) Exercise treatment for major depression: Maintenance of therapeutic benefit at 10 months. *Psychosomatic Medicine*, **62**: 633–638.

Bahrke, M.S. & Morgan, W.P. (1978) Anxiety reduction following exercise and meditation. *Cognitive Therapy and Research*, **2**: 323–334.

Bedi, R.P. (1999) Depression: an inability to adapt to one's perceived life distress? *Journal of Affective Disorders*, **54(1–2)**: 225–234.

Biddle, S.J.H. & Mutrie, N. (2001) *Psychology of Physical Activity: Determinants, Well-being and Interventions*. London: Routledge.

Biddle, S.J.H., Markland, D., Gilbourne, D., Chatzisarantis, N.L.D. & Sparkes, A.C. (2001). Research methods in sport and exercise psychology: Quantitative and qualitative issues. *Journal of Sports Sciences*, **19**: 777–809.

Biddle, S.J.H. (2000) Emotion, mood and physical activity. In: Biddle, S.J.H., Fox, K.R. & Boutcher, S.H. (eds) *Physical Activity and Psychological Well-being*. London: Routledge.

Biddle, S.J.H., Fox, K.R. & Boutcher, S.H. (eds) (2000) *Physical Activity and Psychological Well-being*. London: Routledge.

Blumenthal, J.A., Babyak, M.A., Moore, K.A., Craighead, E., Herman, S. *et al.* (1999) Effects of exercise training on older patients with major depression. *Archives of Internal Medicine* **159(19)**: 2349–2356.

Bouchard, C., Shepherd, R.J. & Stephens, T. (eds) (1994) *Physical Activity, Fitness and Health: International Consensus Proceedings*. Champaign, IL: Human Kinetics.

Boutcher, S.H. (2000) Cognitive performance, fitness, and aging. In: Biddle, S.J.H., Fox, K.R. & Boutcher, S.H. (eds) *Physical Activity and Psychological Well-being*. London: Routledge.

Burbach, F.R. (1997) The efficacy of physical activity interventions within mental health services: Anxiety and depressive disorders. *Journal of Mental Health*, 6: 543–566.

Byrne, C., Brown, B., Voorberg, N. & Schofield, R. (1994) Wellness education for individuals with chronic mental illness living in the community. *Issues in Mental Health Nursing*, **15**: 239–252.

Chadwick, P.K. (1997) Recovery from psychosis: Learning more from patients. *Journal of Mental Health*, 6: 577–588.

Chaouloff, F. (1997) The serotonin hypothesis. In: Morgan, W.P. (ed.) *Physical Activity and Mental Health*. Washington, DC: Taylor and Francis, pp. 179–198.

Cloninger, C.R., Svrakic, D.M., Bayon, C. & Przybeck, T.R. (1999) Measurement of psychopathology as variants of personality. In: Cloninger, C.R. (ed.) *Personality and Psychopathology*. Washington, DC: American Psychiatric Press.

Cloninger, C.R. & Svrakic, D.M. (1997) Integrative psychobiological approach to psychiatric assessment and treatment. *Psychiatry*, **60(2)**: 120–141.

Cloninger, C.R., Przybeck, T.R., Svrakic, D.M. & Wetzel, R.D. (1994) *The Temperament and Character Inventory (TCI): A Guide to its Development and Use*. St Louis, MO: Washington University Press.

Davis, C. (1997) Disability, identity, and involvement in sport and exercise. In: Fox, K.R. (ed.) *The Physical Self: From Motivation to Well-being*. Champaign, IL: Human Kinetics, pp. 257–286.

Deci, E.L. and Ryan, R.M. (1995) Human autonomy: The basis for true self-esteem. In: Kernis, M. (ed.) *Efficacy, Agency, and Self-esteem*. New York: Plenum Press.

Department of Health (1996) *Attitudes to Mental Illness: Summary Report*. Unpublished.

Department of Health (1999) White paper. *Saving Lives: Our Healthier Nation*. London: HMSO.

Dishman, R.K. (1997) The norepinephrine hypothesis. In: Morgan, W.P. (ed.) *Physical Activity and Mental Health*. Washington, DC: Taylor and Francis, pp. 199–212.

Faulkner, G. & Biddle, S. (1999) Exercise as an adjunct treatment for schizophrenia: A review of the literature. *Journal of Mental Health*, **8(5)**: 441–457.

Faulkner, G. & Biddle, S. (2001) Exercise as therapy: It's just not psychology! *Journal of Sports Sciences*, **19(6)**: 433–444.

Faulkner, G. & Sparkes, A. (1999) Exercise as therapy for schizophrenia: An ethnographic study. *Journal of Sport and Exercise Psychology*, **21(1)**: 52–69.

Fox, K.R. (2000a) Physical activity and mental health promotion: The natural partnership. *International Journal of Mental Health Promotion*, **2(1)**: 4–12.

Fox, K.R. (2000b) The effects of exercise on self-perceptions and self-esteem. In: Biddle, S.J.H., Fox, K.R. & Boutcher, S.H. (eds) *Physical Activity and Psychological Well-being*. London: Routledge.

Fox, K.R. (1999) The influence of physical activity on mental well-being. *Public Health Nutrition*, **2(3A)**: 411–418.

Fox, K.R. (ed.) (1997) *The Physical Self: From Motivation to Well-being*. Champaign, IL: Human Kinetics.

Fox, K.R. (1990) *The Physical Self-Perception Profile Manual*. DeKalb, IL., Office for Health Promotion, Northern Illinois University.

Fox, K.R., Boutcher, S.H., Faulkner, G. & Biddle, S.J.H. (2000) The case for exercise in the promotion of mental health and psychological well-being. In: Biddle, S.J.H., Fox, K.R. & Boutcher, S.H. (eds) *Physical Activity and Psychological Well-being*. London: Routledge.

Garfield, S.L. (1998) Some comments on empirically supported treatments. *Journal of Consulting and Clinical Psychology*, **66(1)**: 121–125.

Gerlach, J. & Peacock, L. (1995) New antipsychotics: the present status. *International Clinical Psychopharmacol.*, **10**: 39–48.

Gilbourne, D. (1999) Collaboration and reflection: Adopting action research themes and processes to promote adherence to changing practice. In: Bull, S.J. (ed.) *Adherence Issues in Sport and Exercise*. Chichester: Wiley, pp. 239–263.

Goldberg, D. (1991) Filters to care – model. In: Jenkins, R. & Griffiths, S. (eds) *Indicators for Mental Health in the Population*. London: HMSO.

Grant, T. (2000) *Physical Activity and Mental Health: National Consensus Statements and Guidelines For Practice*. London: Health Education Authority.

Green, A.I., Patel, J.K., Goisman, R.M., Allison, D.B. & Blackburn, G. (2000) Weight gain from novel antipsychotic drugs: Need for action. *General Hospital Psychiatry*, **22**: 224–235.

Greist, J.H., Klein, M.H., Eischens, R.R., Faris, J., Gurman, A.S. & Morgan, W.P. (1979) Running as treatment for depression. *Comprehensive Psychiatry*, **20**: 41–54.

Hansenne, M., Reggers, J., Pinto, E., Kjiri, K., Ajamier, A. & Ansseau, M. (1999) Temperament and character inventory (TCI) and depression. *Journal of Psychiatric Research*, **33**: 31–36.

Health Education Authority (1997) *Mental Health Promotion: A Quality Framework*. Health Education Authority.

Hoffmann, P. (1997) The endorphin hypothesis. In: Morgan, W.P. (ed.) *Physical Activity and Mental Health*. Washington, DC: Taylor and Francis, pp. 163–177.

Jacobs, D.H. (1999) A close and critical examination of how psychopharmacotherapy research is conducted. *The Journal of Mind and Behavior*, **20**: 311–350.

Joyce, P.R., Mulder, R.T. *et al.* (1994) Temperament predicts clomipramine and desipramine response in major depression. *Journal of Affective Disorders*, **30**(1): 35–46.

Lawlor, D.A. & Hopker, S.W. (2001) The effectiveness of exercise as an intervention in the management of depression: Systematic review and meta-regression analysis of randomised controlled trials. *British Medical Journal*, **322**: 763.

Locke, L. (1989) Qualitative research as a form of scientific inquiry in sport and physical education. *Research Quarterly for Exercise and Sport*, **60**: 1–20.

Mark, T., McKusick, D., King, E., Harwood, H. & Genuardi, J. (1998) *National Expenditures for Mental Health, Alcohol, and Other Drug Abuse Treatment, 1996*, Rockville, MD: Substance Abuse and Mental Health Services Administration.

Maxwell, J.A. (1996) *Qualitative Research Design*. Sage: California.

Morgan, W.P. (ed.) (1997a) *Physical Activity and Mental Health*, Washington, DC: Taylor and Francis.

Morgan, W.P. (1997b) Methodological considerations. In: Morgan, W.P. (ed.) *Physical Activity and Mental Health*. Washington, DC: Taylor and Francis, pp. 3–32.

Murray, C.J.L. & Lopez, A.D. (1997) Global mortality, disability, and the contribution of risk factors: Global Burden of Disease Survey. *Lancet*, **349**: 1436–1442.

Mutrie, N. (1997) The therapeutic effects of exercise on the self. In K. Fox (ed.) *The Physical Self: From Motivation to Well-being*. Champaign, IL: Human Kinetics, pp. 287–314.

Mutrie, N. (2000) The relationship between physical activity and clinically defined depression. In: Biddle, S.J.H., Fox, K.R. & Boutcher, S.H. (eds) *Physical Activity and Psychological Well-being*. London: Routledge.

Patton, M.Q. (1980) *Qualitative Evaluation Methods*. California: Sage.

Peirson, A.R. & Heuchert, J.W. (2001) The relationship between personality and mood: comparison of the BDI and the TCI. *Personality and Individual Differences*, **30**(3): 391–399.

Reichter, J., Eisemann, M. *et al.* (2000) Temperament and character during the course of unipolar depression among inpatients. *European Archives of Psychiatry and Clinical Neuroscience*, **250**(1): 40–47.

Rejeski, W.J. (1994) Dose-response issues from a psychosocial perspective. In: Bouchard, C., Shepherd, R.J. & Stephens, T. (eds) *Physical Activity, Fitness and Health: International Consensus Proceedings*, Champaign, IL: Human Kinetics.

Riddoch, C., Puig-Ribera, A. & Cooper, A. (1998) *Effectiveness of Physical Activity Promotion Schemes in Primary Care: A Review*. London: Health Education Authority.

Roth, A.D. & Parry, G. (1997) The implications of psychotherapy research for clinical practice and service development: Lessons and limitations. *Journal of Mental Health*, **6**: 367–380.

Sackett, D.L., Rosenberg, W.M.C., Gray, J.A.M., Haynes, R.B. & Richardson, W.C. (1996) Evidence based medicine: What it is and what it isn't. *British Medical Journal,* **312**: 71–72.

Salmon, P. (2001) Effects of physical exercise on anxiety, depression, and sensitivity to stress: A unifying theory. *Clinical Psychology Review,* **21(1)**: 33–61.

Scott, J. (1996) Cognitive therapy of affective disorders: A review. *Journal of Affective Disorders,* **37**: 1–11.

Sears, J. (1992) Researching the other/searching for self: Qualitative research on (homo)sexuality in education. *Theory into Practice,* **31**: 147–156.

Seligman, M.E.P. (1975) *Helplessness: On Depression, Development, and Death.* New York: W.H. Freeman.

Sonstroem, R.J. & Potts, S.A. (1996) Life adjustment correlates of physical self-concepts. *Medicine and Science in Sports and Exercise,* **28(5)**: 619–625.

Sparkes, A. (1992) The paradigms debate: an extended review and a celebration of difference. In A. Sparkes (ed.) *Research in Physical Education and Sport: Exploring Alternative Visions,* London: The Falmer Press.

Sparkes, A. (1998) Validity in qualitative inquiry and the problem of criteria: Implications for sport psychology. *The Sport Psychologist,* **12**: 363–386.

Taylor, A.H. (2000) Physical activity, anxiety, and stress. In: Biddle, S.J.H., Fox, K.R. & Boutcher, S.H. (eds) *Physical Activity and Psychological Well-being.* London: Routledge.

Tudor, K. (1996) *Mental Health Promotion: Paradigms and Practice.* London: Routledge.

United States Department of Health and Human Services (1999) *Mental Health: A report of the Surgeon General.*

Weismann, M.M. & Klerman, G.L. (1992) Depression: Current understanding and changing trends. *Annual Review of Public Health,* **13**: 319–339.

Wetterling, T. (2001) Bodyweight gain with atypical antipsychotics: A comparative review. *Drug Safety,* **24**: 59–73.

CHAPTER 5

Objective Measurement of Physical Activity

ASHLEY COOPER

Chapter Contents

░ Physical activity and health

░ Objective measurement of physical activity and energy expenditure

░ Applications of objective activity measurement

░ Summary

Accurate measurement is crucial to our understanding of the relationship between physical activity and health. Imagine that you are unwell and your doctor prescribes a drug to make you better. The doctor tells you that overall the drug is known to be beneficial, but too little may have no effect and too much may do you harm. The doctor also tells you that he/she does not know how large a dose you should take, or how often, or for how long to treat your symptoms. You would not find this an acceptable situation, yet it reflects our understanding of the relationship between activity and health. We know that people who are more physically active are healthier – they live longer, have less chance of developing major diseases and have better mental health – yet until recently we have not been able to say with confidence how much activity is necessary to achieve this healthy state, or how vigorous that activity needs to be. The reason for this is that, unlike a drug, the dose of which can be measured very accurately, we have not been able to measure physical activity with precision.

However, that situation is changing. Developments in technology, particularly miniaturisation and increased capacity for data storage, have resulted in the development of a new generation of instruments that hold the promise of dramatically improving our ability to measure activity. Some of these instruments allow us to measure not only the volume and intensity of activity, but also to investigate patterns of activity that may be associated with health outcomes. This chapter will describe these new instruments and illustrate the types of information they can give us using examples from current research. We will examine the basic principles of the instruments, describe the range of uses to which they can be put, and discuss their strengths and weaknesses.

Physical activity and health

Physical activity and prevention of disease

Over the past two decades it has become clear that lack of physical activity is a major risk factor for premature mortality and the development of chronic diseases such as coronary heart disease and type-2 diabetes mellitus (US Department of Health and Human Services, 1996). The strongest evidence for these associations comes from studies where large populations of initially healthy people have been regularly assessed over many years, completing questionnaires to describe their physical activity and health status (normally assessed as development of chronic illness). These longitudinal studies have consistently shown that the least physically active individuals have the highest risk of chronic illness and premature mortality. Relatively small amounts of regular physical activity, equivalent to walking briskly for 30 minutes each day, appear to provide significant protection from the development of such diseases. Furthermore, since much of the activity that people report is intermittent, such as stair climbing, it appears that this beneficial physical activity can be accumulated throughout the day (Lee *et al.*, 2000).

What more then do we need to know about this relationship? There are many questions that remain unanswered – what is the dose–response relationship between physical activity and risk of disease or alteration in risk factors for disease, is either volume or intensity of activity more important in achieving health benefits, can activity be accumulated throughout the day or must it be done in sustained bouts? These issues have recently been the topic of a major symposium published in a supplement to *Medicine and Science in Sports and Exercise* (Volume 33: 6 (Supplement) 2001) and will not be discussed in depth. However accuracy of physical activity measurement underpins many of the issues central to this topic. To appreciate the limitations in our knowledge of the physical activity–health relationship and to understand the need for better measurement we must understand what we mean by 'physical activity'.

 Chapter 3 (Epidemiology) describes the importance of distinguishing the specific doses of physical activity and/or exercise that influence specific health indices.

Definition of physical activity

Physical activity is a complex behaviour that incorporates all the activities of daily living. Defined as 'any bodily movement that results in an increase in energy expenditure above resting levels' (Caspersen *et al.*, 1985), physical activity has dimensions of volume (how much activity is done in total), duration (how long a bout of activity might be), frequency (number of bouts of activity), intensity (how hard the activity is) and mode (the type of activities carried out). To understand which of these components is important for a particular health outcome requires the consistent and accurate measurement of each dimension. In addition, the many diverse areas of everyday physical activity – exercise, sport and recreation, occupational activity, non-sport, non-occupational activity – all need to be accounted for in understanding the activity–health relationship. Thus the ideal instrument for measuring physical activity should be able to accurately measure each dimension of activity throughout a long enough period to encompass all the domains of everyday activity.

Indirect measurement of physical activity using questionnaires

The majority of large-scale studies of the relationship between physical activity and health outcomes rely upon the individual participants to recall their daily activities by answering a questionnaire. Questionnaires are widely used in such studies as they are easy to use, cheap to administer and do not influence behaviour. In its simplest form, the physical activity questionnaire may be a short one-to-four item instrument for use in surveys where only simple activity classifications are required (for example, active as opposed to inactive). However, to understand the activity–health relationship, more complex instruments are used to investigate the different dimensions and domains of physical activity. Questionnaires may be tailored to a population, for example to an ethnic group, clinical population or particular age range, by utilising questions particular to those individuals, or may be designed to answer a particular research question by, for example, investigating occupational activity in detail. A comprehensive discussion of the use of questionnaires in a range of populations may be found in a special issue of *Research Quarterly for Exercise and Sport* (Volume 71, Supplement to No. 2, June 2000).

Limitations of questionnaires

It is attractive to tailor a questionnaire to address a particular issue, but this approach is not helpful in understanding the physical activity–health relationship overall, since many different questionnaires have been used in the literature, making it difficult to draw comparisons between studies. There are a number of reviews of the more common questionnaires (Montoye *et al.*, 1996;

Sallis & Saelens, 2000), and a useful resource is a collection of thirty-two commonly used questionnaires where each questionnaire is provided with instructions for administration and analysis, and a summary of reliability and validity studies is provided (Kriska & Caspersen, 1997). This list is by no means comprehensive, and it can be seen that the questionnaires differ in several ways:

- Mode of administration (self-completed or interviewer administered)
- Time frame over which activity is assessed (for example, 24 hours, past week, 'usual' week)
- Dimensions of activity that are assessed (for example, assessment of sedentary behaviour is rare (Sallis & Saelens, 2000))
- Domains of activity that are assessed (for example, occupational, recreational, sport, commuting)
- Outcome variables (for example, energy expenditure, activity score, and so on).

In addition to these differences in design, questionnaires have a number of further limitations (Montoye *et al.*, 1996). People find it relatively easy to recall attending programmed activities, such as sports and exercise classes (Montoye *et al.*, 1996), but their recall of the precise amount of time spent in exercise during those periods is less good. For example, a respondent may report 90 minutes of football, but could not describe how much of that time was spent running. Similarly, recall of the amount of time spent in sporadic, non-programmed, low-intensity activities, such as walking or occupational activity is poor, particularly in children or the elderly (Sallis & Saelens, 2000). In addition to difficulties of recall, social desirability bias (the perceived desirability of being physically active) can lead to over-reporting of physical activity (Warnecke *et al.*, 1997). As a consequence of these limitations, questionnaires are generally found to correlate well with other measures of vigorous or moderately intense physical activity, but are generally less accurate when measuring light-to-moderate intensity activity.

Physical activity and energy expenditure

It is important to recognise that physical activity is a behaviour that results in energy expenditure, and the most important source of variation in energy expenditure between individuals (when adjusted for body size) is physical activity. Consequently, in addition to understanding the relationship between physical activity and health outcomes, the role of energy expenditure also needs to be understood. Indeed, recent evidence has suggested that energy expenditure *per se* may be more predictive of health-related outcomes than the specific type of physical activity that produces increased energy expenditure (Lee *et al.*, 2000).

A conceptual model of the relationship between movement, physical activity and energy expenditure has recently been proposed (Lamonte & Ainsworth,

2001). In this model, a global construct of movement has two dimensions, physical activity and energy expenditure, each of which may be measured in a number of different ways. The extrapolation of these measurements to units of energy expenditure before analysing the potential effects on health parameters will facilitate interpretation of physical activity data and comparisons between studies.

To enable comparison of studies using different questionnaires or populations, specific physical activities may be converted to estimates of energy expenditure using the *Compendium of Physical Activities* (Ainsworth *et al.*, 2000b). The compendium is an instrument developed to facilitate the coding of questionnaires and provides the energy cost of an extensive range of activities performed in various settings. It is a valuable and widely used instrument, but has drawbacks to its use. Since the energy cost of an activity will vary depending on how it is carried out, respondents must accurately assess activity intensity. This is difficult as perception of intensity may vary with fitness, fatigue or the interpretation of instructions given by the researcher. Similarly, programmed, vigorous activities are likely to be accurately recalled, but low-intensity activities form the bulk of physical activity energy expenditure, and will be poorly reported. Additionally, the compendium is based mostly upon data from healthy male adults, and its use in other populations may not be appropriate. Given these limitations, it is not surprising that questionnaires generally show poor validity against criterion measures of energy expenditure (Sallis & Saelens, 2000).

Public health implications

Despite their limitations, questionnaires have been an important tool in demonstrating the associations between physical activity, energy expenditure and health. The concept that regular, moderate intensity activity could provide significant protection from the development of disease, and that activity could be accumulated throughout the day, revolutionised both the field of exercise and health science and the promotion of physical activity in the early 1990s. Until that time it had been believed that activity of an intensity sufficient to improve cardio-respiratory fitness was required to achieve health benefits, and there was concern that the majority of the population was unwilling to participate in activities of that intensity on a regular basis, if at all. The realisation that moderate activity confers significant health benefits has been adopted by health promoters and public-health organisations in many countries. Guidelines now recommend the accumulation of at least 30 minutes of moderate-intensity activity on most days of the week for health (Pate *et al.*, 1995; Department of Health, 1996; US Department of Health and Human Services, 1996).

However, many questions remain unanswered about the precise relationship between physical activity and health at the population level. Current data suggests that the dose–response relationship may differ for different disorders.

For example, a linear dose–response relationship is seen between physical activity and risk of coronary heart disease, with greater amounts of activity conferring increased protection (Barinaga, 1997). However, such a relationship is not seen for stroke. Many studies designed to detect a dose–response gradient have failed to do so, and there is some suggestion of a non-linear 'U-shaped' relationship, with a higher risk of stroke associated with higher/more vigorous activity levels than with more moderate activity (Kohl, 2001).

What then is the optimal prescription for public health – is being physically active sufficient to provide health benefits regardless of intensity, or does activity need to be above a particular intensity to elicit an effect? In other words, is it more effective to carry out a few brief bouts of daily vigorous activity, such as stair climbing, or longer periods of moderate activity such as walking, or are both equally effective? These issues are topics of current debate, and there are no clear answers. Given the reluctance or inability of people to be regularly active, there is a need to identify the least invasive and disruptive physical activity prescription that achieves significant health benefits. To accurately understand a specific dose–response relationship both the outcome (disease state or mortality) and the exposure (physical activity) of interest must be accurately measured (Lamonte & Ainsworth, 2001). With regard to the physical activity–health relationship, population studies have utilised binary measures (well/unwell, dead/alive) of disease state which can be accurately measured, but the complexity of physical activity as a behaviour and the limitations of questionnaires used in such studies means that the exposure is poorly measured. The development of instruments designed to accurately record activity volume, intensity and duration over many days offers greater accuracy in measuring the different dimensions of physical activity, and will allow us to investigate the relationship between physical activity patterns and health in greater detail (Wareham & Rennie, 1998).

Physical activity and risk factors

The development of chronic diseases such as coronary heart disease, hypertension and type-2 diabetes and acute events such as myocardial infarction or stroke are normally preceded by many years of abnormalities in a number of biochemical and physiological parameters, for example blood-lipid profile and glucose metabolism. An extensive body of literature has demonstrated that physically inactive individuals have a less healthy risk factor profile than active individuals, and that increasing physical activity is effective in favourably modifying many of these risk factors (US Department of Health and Human Services, 1996). However, despite a considerable volume of research, as evidenced by the epidemiological studies the precise dose–response relationships between physical activity dimensions and changes in risk factor status are poorly understood. The prescription of moderate intensity activity has been adopted for the treatment of disorders such as hypertension and type-2 diabetes (Joint National Committee on Prevention, Detection, Evaluation and Treatment of High Blood Pressure, 1997; American Diabetes Association, 1998; Ramsay *et al.*, 1999) but in many instances the efficacy of this prescription remains to be determined (Cooper *et al.*, 2000; Kelley & Goodpaster, 2001).

There is thus an urgent need to better understand the dose–response relationships between the varying dimensions of physical activity and a range of important health outcomes, both at the population level to inform public-health recommendations, and at the individual level for the prevention and treatment of specific disorders. To achieve this requires more accurate measurement of physical activity, probably in a number of discrete dimensions. Examples of physical activity dimensions that are likely to be associated with health include:

- Overall activity volume (total physical activity energy expenditure)
- Time spent in activities of differing intensity (sedentary, light, moderate, hard, very hard)
- Duration of continuous bouts of activity of moderate or greater intensity
- Spontaneous physical activity.

A more complete understanding of these aspects of activity will underpin not only the effective promotion of physical activity for public health, but will also inform the design of research studies into the efficacy and effectiveness of physical activity for the treatment of disease (Wareham & Rennie, 1998). New, objective measures of physical activity offer us the opportunity to investigate the physical activity–health relationship in greater detail than ever before.

Objective measurement of physical activity and energy expenditure

Questionnaires are thus indirect measures of physical activity and energy expenditure, and are prone to a number of methodological shortcomings. Fortunately, a number of alternative methods are now available that allow the direct measurement of physical activity and/or energy expenditure. Direct measurement of physical activity and energy expenditure can be achieved by the doubly labelled water and direct calorimetry methods. Both of these provide accurate assessments against which other methods can be compared, but have practical limitations that mean that they are not appropriate for most studies. The technique of indirect calorimetry is a widely used method for establishing the energy cost of individual activities. Most commonly used in laboratory studies of walking, running and cycling, the development of portable instruments has allowed the energy cost of 'lifestyle' activities such as gardening and housework to be assessed (Hendelman *et al.*, 2000).

More useful for the majority of studies are heart-rate monitoring and, more recently, the use of motion sensors to measure actual bodily movement. Both techniques allow the measurement of physical activity over periods long enough to be representative of normal daily life with minimal discomfort to the participants. This potential for the time-resolved measurement of activity volume, intensity and duration opens the door to investigations for which questionnaires are inappropriate or insufficiently accurate, and also provides a means to increase the accuracy with which the relationship between activity and health outcomes can be measured.

Doubly Labelled Water (DLW)

The doubly labelled water method is considered to be the most accurate method for measurement of total energy expenditure in free-living individuals. The technique uses the stable (non-radioactive) isotopes deuterium ($^2H_2$) and ^{18}O and has been used to assess human energy expenditure under laboratory and field conditions (Montoye et al., 1996). The technique has been reviewed in detail (Speakman, 1998), and will be described only briefly. An individually weighed oral dose of water enriched with deuterium and ^{18}O is given and sequential urine samples are taken over a period of days to monitor the disappearance of the isotopes from the body, while the subject goes about their normal daily activities. The technique relies on the observation that the oxygen in body water is in complete isotopic equilibrium with the oxygen expired in CO_2. Thus while ^{18}O is lost as water and CO_2, deuterium is lost from the body as water alone, and, consequently, the differential rate of disappearance of the two isotopes gives a measure of CO_2 production. The rate of isotope disappearance depends upon the individual's level of physical activity. Measurement of isotope disappearance is made over as few as three days in extremely active subjects or as many as 30 days in the sedentary elderly. For 'normal' active adults, a period of 14 days is usually used.

The DLW method measures total energy expenditure over a period of 1–3 weeks, and thus can provide a good estimate of average daily energy expenditure. Together with an estimate of basal metabolic rate, the energy expenditure for physical activity can be calculated (activity energy expenditure=total energy expenditure – BMR). However, there are a number of limitations to this technique. The main limitation is the restricted supply, and hence high cost, of the ^{18}O isotope. At the time of writing (2002), a dose of DLW costs £2.60 per kg body weight, a price that is restrictive for large-scale studies. In addition, the analysis of samples using gas-isotope mass spectrometry is also a complex and expensive task. Consequently the DLW technique is usually restricted for use in small studies to provide an estimate of the accuracy of other measures of physical activity, and has also been used for the validation of questionnaire, heart rate and accelerometer methods. However, while providing a good estimate of average energy expenditure, it does not give any information about day-to-day variability in energy expenditure, nor does it differentiate the duration, frequency or intensity of specific physical activities.

Calorimetry

The rate of heat production by an individual is directly proportional to their metabolic rate. Direct calorimetry is the most accurate method for measuring energy expenditure via heat production. Measurements take place in a specially constructed chamber called a whole-body calorimeter and will always be carried out in a specialised research institute, since the equipment and methodology required is highly complex and expensive. While well suited to experimental studies of energy metabolism, this technique cannot study energy expenditure in free living conditions, and experiments using this procedure are now relatively uncommon.

A second, more straightforward technique called indirect calorimetry is much more widely used. This technique does not measure heat production directly, but relies on the direct relationship between oxygen consumption and heat produced (Powers & Howley, 2001). Measuring oxygen consumption therefore provides an accurate estimate of metabolic rate. This method can be carried out both within the confines of the laboratory and in the field, although the constraints of the equipment (particularly the need to wear a face mask) mean that measurement periods are rather short and the measurement procedure has an impact upon natural behaviour. Nonetheless indirect calorimetry provides accurate minute-by-minute measurements of energy expenditure and is commonly used to derive equations that allow the output of measures such as accelerometers to be expressed in terms of energy expenditure.

The above techniques both provide accurate estimates of energy expenditure, but in each case have significant limitations to their use for assessing physical activity and energy expenditure in free-living individuals. While DLW allows people to carry out their normal, everyday activities, it does not allow a time-resolved picture of activity levels to be developed. In contrast, indirect calorimetry can provide temporal information about activity volume, duration and intensity, but does not allow normal daily activities to be continued without interference from the instrumentation required. Neither is therefore widely applicable as field measures of physical activity.

Heart rate monitoring

Heart rate (HR) has commonly been employed as an objective method of assessing physical activity as there is a strong positive association between HR and energy expenditure during large-muscle dynamic exercise. Under controlled laboratory conditions, there is a linear relationship between HR and oxygen uptake ($\dot{V}O_2$) over a wide range of exercise intensities, particularly between heart rates of 110 bpm and 150 bpm.

HR monitoring would appear to be an ideal method for measuring physical activity in the field. Heart-rate monitors consist of an elasticated chest strap containing a transmitter and a receiver that is usually worn as a wrist watch. The monitors are small and relatively cheap but also robust and designed to function under many conditions, including use during water-based activities. The method is non-invasive and is generally well accepted by participants and can be used in both children and adults. The monitors are also able to give information on the pattern of physical activity. The latest monitors allow sampling over five-second to one-minute intervals, for a period of between 22 and 260 hours, depending upon the sampling interval chosen. The data can then be downloaded to a personal computer for analysis, providing information on the various components of physical activity, including frequency, intensity and duration.

However, there are a number of disadvantages to the technique. HR monitoring does not measure activity directly, but rather an individual's physiological response to activity. Consequently, factors that influence HR, such as emotional stress, high ambient temperature, body position and food intake are potential sources of error (Melanson & Freedson, 1996). This is a particular problem at lower HR levels, and it is unfortunate that most people spend most of their day in this zone. In addition, the HR–$\dot{V}O_2$ relationship is affected by a number of factors, including the type of muscular contraction employed, fatigue, hydration state and relative size of the exercising muscle mass, with arm exercise eliciting a higher HR than leg exercise at the same $\dot{V}O_2$, due to the relatively smaller size of the arm musculature (McArdle *et al.*, 1991; Montoye *et al.*, 1996). While reproducibility of HR within subjects has been shown to be quite high, comparison of HR between individuals may be problematic because of individual differences in fitness, fatness, age and gender. Finally, estimation of energy expenditure from HR data may provide another source of error, depending upon the technique used. This is discussed below.

Estimation of energy expenditure from HR data

Various techniques have been used for using HR data to estimate energy expenditure. The simplest method determines the number of minutes spent within defined HR 'zones' to provide an estimate of the amount of time spent in activities of varying intensities. This may then be used to estimate energy expenditure from metabolic tables, though the accuracy of this method is poor. An improvement on this approach is to determine the number of minutes spent above a certain percentage of HR reserve (HRR = maximal HR − resting HR). The heart-rate-reserve method allows comparison of individuals with different fitness levels since %HRR can be directly validated against %$\dot{V}O_2$ reserve (the difference between maximal $\dot{V}O_2$ and resting $\dot{V}O_2$) (Powers & Howley, 2001). In the laboratory a strong 1:1 relationship between %HRR and %$\dot{V}O_2$ reserve has been demonstrated for treadmill exercise (Swain *et al.*, 1998), and there is a strong linear relationship between the two measures over a wide range of activities, including domestic, occupational and recreational activity (Strath *et al.*, 2000). This indicates that this method of analysing HR data agrees closely with measured energy expenditure in field-based settings.

A third approach to estimating energy expenditure from HR data is to derive individual HR–$\dot{V}O_2$ calibration curves in the laboratory for each participant (the FLEX HR method). Although the relationship between HR and $\dot{V}O_2$ is linear over a wide range of exercise intensities, at the lower end of the range the linearity between energy expenditure and HR is lost (Freedson & Miller, 2000). In addition, there is a wide inter-individual variation in the slope of the relationship due to individual differences in fitness – a fit subject can perform the same work load at a lower HR than an unfit subject, although the oxygen consumption is the same. It is difficult, therefore, to establish a single regression equation that applies to all individuals. The FLEX HR technique produces an individual calibration curve for each participant by simultaneously monitoring HR and oxygen consumption during exercise at different intensities and while lying down, sitting and standing. The slope of the regression line derived from sedentary activities is significantly different from that derived from exercise, and the FLEX HR is defined as the point where the two slopes diverge. The FLEX HR can then be used to discriminate between rest and physical activity during monitoring, and the calibration curve used to translate HR above the FLEX HR into energy expenditure. Below the FLEX HR, resting metabolic rate is used to determine energy expenditure.

The FLEX HR method is the most accurate way to estimate energy expenditure from HR data, but there are limitations. The regression line derived for individual calibration in the laboratory is specific to the activity performed, and thus may not accurately represent the cardiovascular response associated with activity under free living conditions. In addition, the calibration technique is time-consuming, taking at least 45 minutes to complete for each subject, sometimes leading to the practice of using group calibration curves that will introduce further error.

A number of studies have compared the FLEX HR method of assessing energy expenditure against criterion measures. Energy expenditure estimated using the FLEX HR method has been shown not to differ significantly from metabolic rate measured by indirect calorimetry (Spurr *et al.*, 1988). Comparisons with DLW have demonstrated high individual variation, but when examined on a group basis by amalgamating individual results (not by use of group calibration curves) estimates are within 10 per cent of DLW values (Livingstone *et al.*, 1992; Bassett, 2000).

HR monitoring is thus a valuable technique for the minute-by-minute analysis of physical activity. The utility of the technique for measuring energy expenditure in large-scale studies is limited by the need for individual calibration, although it has recently been suggested that energy expenditure can be estimated in epidemiological studies without the need for full individual calibration using a combination of simple measurements and HR monitoring (Rennie *et al.*, 2001).

Motion sensors

Motion sensors are mechanical and electronic devices that detect motion or acceleration of a limb or trunk, depending on where the monitor is attached to the body. In contrast to HR monitoring, motion sensors provide a direct measurement of physical activity. There are two main types of motion sensors – pedometers and accelerometers.

Pedometers

Pedometers (often called step counters) rely upon vertical movements of the body to trigger a switch (either mechanical or electrical) each time a step is taken, thus allowing the total number of steps taken to be counted. Pedometers are also able to provide an estimate of the distance walked by incorporating a measure of stride length, and some instruments can provide a crude estimate of energy expenditure if body weight is incorporated. Energy expenditure measurements from a pedometer are most accurate when walking comprises most of an individual's activity.

Pedometers are generally worn at the waist, clipped onto the user's waistband, although they may also be worn on the wrist or ankle. The main advantages of pedometers are that they are small and inexpensive, but until recently they have been seen as relatively inaccurate instruments, particularly at low and high walking speeds. In early instruments, differences in spring tension led to high variability between instruments (models and units) making comparisons between studies difficult, although recent improvements in technology and quality control has led to improvements in both reliability and validity (Bassett *et al.*, 1996, 2000). The most accurate of the currently available instruments, the Yamax Digi-Walker (model DW-500), has been reported to be accurate for counting steps on concrete pavements to within 1 per cent of the actual steps recorded and was also very accurate over a range of walking speeds, providing distance estimates within 3 per cent of the actual at 67 and 80 m·min^{-1} and within 10 per cent of the actual at 54 and 94 m·min^{-1} (Bassett *et al.*, 1996). The Digi-Walker has also been evaluated as a tool for assessing moderate intensity overground walking (on an indoor track) (Hendelman *et al.*, 2000). Steps recorded were highly correlated with walking speed (r=0.86) and $\dot{V}O_2$ (r=0.75) for speeds ranging from 63 to 111 m·min^{-1}.

This data confirms that pedometry may be useful for the assessment of total activity if walking is the predominant form of activity.

However, the pedometer has limited application for measuring habitual physical activity for several reasons. Pedometers do not provide any temporal information about activity patterns, as they do not store data over a specified time interval. Additionally, they are not very sensitive to physical activity that does not involve locomotion or to activity that involves the upper body. Finally, since pedometers are not sensitive to changes in speed, and stride length is longer when, for example, running than when walking, more steps will be accumulated when walking rather than running a fixed distance. In a study comparing the steps required to cover a mile at walking (15 min a mile), jogging (10 min a mile) and running (8 min a mile) speeds, male participants recorded 1875, 1606 and 1307 steps respectively (Welk *et al.*, 2000b). The corresponding values for females were 1996, 1662 and 1330 steps. This study found that the mean number of steps differed significantly by pace for both males and females, and significant gender differences were observed for the walk and jog paces, though not for running.

Although limited for the detailed assessment of habitual physical activity, the pedometer is potentially useful in establishing overall levels of activity. The previous study (Welk *et al.*, 2000b) estimates that approximately 4000 steps are required to fulfil the current health-related physical activity guidelines of 30 minutes a day of moderate intensity activity (roughly equivalent to walking at 4 mph). However, since most people will accumulate many steps in just going about their normal activities, this figure cannot be used to categorise a person as active. Studies conducted in Japan have concluded that a figure of 10 000 steps a day is a more appropriate target for health (Yamanouchi *et al.*, 1995). This value has been confirmed in a study designed to determine the number of steps an active individual might accumulate, where participants wore the Digi-Walker for seven days under two conditions. In the first condition, they recorded their daily number of steps; in the second they removed the pedometer for any structured moderately vigorous to vigorous activity, for example running. The average daily scores were 11 603 when all activity was included, and 8265 when only light and moderate activity were included, giving support to the idea that an individual achieving 10 000 counts a day will be meeting health guidelines. However it should be noted that individual variability was high in this study. These studies thus provide target values that can be used, for example, in intervention studies where participants can be given specific pedometer goals that can be monitored very easily.

The pedometer has not been widely used for the assessment of physical activity in free living populations. The pedometer has been shown to be able to differentiate between various levels of occupational activity in adults, with those in inactive occupations recording approximately 7000 steps a day compared with 9800 to 10 800 steps a day for those in heavy work (Sequeira *et al.*, 1995). Those individuals who reported 'fitness training' were found to have mean step counts of 10 200 to 10 500 regardless of occupational activity.

The small and unobtrusive nature of pedometers suggests that they may be a valuable means of measuring physical activity in children. A study using the Digi-Walker to evaluate physical activity in children found a correlation of $r=0.78$ between pedometer steps and oxygen uptake during treadmill walking, and an equally encouraging correlation between steps and both oxygen uptake ($r=0.92$) and heart rate ($r=0.88$) was observed for unstructured, low-intensity play activities (Eston *et al.*, 1998). This suggests that the Digi-Walker is an effective measure of children's physical activity in the field.

Accelerometers

Pedometers are relatively simple and cheap, but accelerometers range in complexity and cost, from a basic instrument able to measure overall energy expenditure to more sophisticated instruments able to give minute-by-minute activity readings in three planes, over a period of several days or weeks. In contrast to the pedometer, accelerometers measure the acceleration and deceleration of the body when moving. Since vigorous activity produces greater accelerations than gentle activity, these instruments provide a measure of overall activity volume, including activity of different intensities.

A number of accelerometers are available that measure acceleration either in the vertical plane only (uni-axial accelerometers) or in vertical, horizontal and lateral planes (tri-axial accelerometers).

Uni-axial as opposed to tri-axial accelerometers

Both uni-axial and tri-axial accelerometers provide comparable assessments of free-living physical activity. This view is supported by the fact that the instruments correlate highly with each other – usually in excess of $r=0.90$ – suggesting that they measure similar elements of physical activity. This is not surprising, as for the great majority of bodily movements, movements involving non-vertical planes are almost always accompanied by movement in the vertical plane.

It is beyond the scope of this chapter to discuss all the available accelerometers, and a list of instruments and key references is provided in Table 5.1 for the interested reader. The most commonly used accelerometers in recent years have been the Tracmor, Tritrac R3D, Caltrac™ and CSA 7164. Of these, the Tracmor is not commercially available, and the Tritrac has been superseded by the smaller RT3 for which no validation data is currently available. The following discussion will focus on the Caltrac™ and CSA 7164 as examples of widely used instruments that have different functionality. The Caltrac™ is a relatively old instrument that has been used in many studies and provides an overall measurement (that is, not time-resolved) of energy expenditure in physical activity. In contrast, the CSA 7164 is probably the most widely used of the current generation of instruments, and provides minute-by-minute

Table 5.1 Commonly used accelerometers in physical activity research

Name	Type	References
Caltrac[TM]	Uni-axial	Haymes & Byrnes (1993) and Montoye *et al.* (1996)
CSA 7164	Uni-axial	Tryon & Williams (1996) and Freedson *et al.* (1998)
Kenz	Uni-axial	Yamada & Baba (1990) and Bassett *et al.* (2000)
Biotrainer	Uni-axial	Welk *et al.* (2000a)
Actilume	Uni-axial	Freedson & Miller (2000)
Tritrac R3 D	Tri-axial	Nichols *et al.* (1999) and Jakicic *et al.* (1999)
RT3	Tri-axial	
Tracmor	Tri-axial	Bouten *et al.* (1994, 1996) and Levine *et al.* (2000)

measurement of physical activity that requires regression equations to be derived for conversion of data to energy expenditure estimates.

The Caltrac[TM] accelerometer

The Caltrac[TM] accelerometer is a relatively small device ($70 \times 70 \times 20$ mm) that was one of the first commercially available accelerometers. On its front panel a liquid crystal display provides feedback to the user and a number of buttons are provided for programming. The instrument is worn clipped to a belt at the user's waist. The instrument is uni-axial and detects vertical motion via movement of a piezo electric bender element that is mounted in a cantilever beam position. When the body accelerates vertically the beam moves and a charge is produced proportional to the force exerted. The area under this acceleration-deceleration wave form is integrated and summed to provide a raw score. Before use, the user's height, weight, age and gender are entered via buttons on the front of the instrument, and this data is used to calculate resting metabolic rate using standard formulae (Montoye *et al.*, 1996; Bassett *et al.*, 2000). When movement occurs the metabolic cost of the activity is calculated from this data and the magnitude of the accelerations using an unpublished algorithm. The instrument can display different energy expenditure parameters in kilocalories, including total energy expenditure and energy expenditure from physical activity alone, updated at two-minute intervals.

The reliability of the Caltrac[TM] has been investigated in many studies in a range of populations. Inter-instrument reliability of two Caltrac[TM] instruments worn on the left and right hips during treadmill exercise was $r = 0.89$ indicating that different instruments provide similar data. Overall the test–retest reliability of the Caltrac[TM] is generally good in laboratory studies in both adults and children ($r = 0.7$ to $r = 0.93$), but is highly variable in field studies ($r = 0.3$ to $r = 0.91$)

(Montoye *et al.*, 1996). This is likely to be due both to limitations in the instrument and to changes in the physical activity of the subjects between the two measures. The Caltrac™ has also been validated against a range of other measures, where it tends to overestimate the energy cost of brisk walking and slow jogging by 25–50 per cent, but underestimates the cost of most lifestyle activities (Bassett, 2000). Despite this, reasonable correlation ($r = 0.3$–0.7) with HR and physical activity questionnaires (Montoye *et al.*, 1996), and good correlation with DLW ($r = 0.83$) (Gardner & Poehlman, 1998) and indirect calorimetry for treadmill running ($r = 0.71$) (Haymes & Byrnes, 1993) have been reported.

Although the results of validity studies of the Caltrac™ are variable, it is generally seen as an acceptable instrument for measuring physical activity. There are, however, a number of limitations to its use. Firstly, the exposed buttons on the front of the instrument can be deliberately or inadvertently pushed by the participants. We have found that it is easy for participants to switch the instrument to 'cycle mode', where the energy expenditure values appear to be increased approximately 2.5-fold. If this occurs, it causes a significant difference in the results produced by the instrument, and failure to identify this problem may be a major source of error in some studies. To avoid this the buttons must be protected from accidental knocks and inquisitive children's fingers!

A second limitation of the Caltrac™ is that it has no capacity to store minute-by-minute data, providing only a total measure of physical activity at the time when it is read. Consequently participants need to record the values shown in the Caltrac™ display in an activity log to provide a crude form of time-resolved information. Values recorded at the beginning and end of each day, and before and after each exercise bout or activity, can be used to provide an estimate of daily energy expenditure in physical activity, and the energy expenditure in individual activities respectively. This does however increase the reporting burden on the participant, but can provide a useful means of promoting increased physical activity and measuring compliance to a physical activity programme.

The CSA 7164 accelerometer

The CSA accelerometer is a small ($51 \times 8 \times 15$ mm) uni-axial accelerometer that detects motion in the same way as the Caltrac™, through movement of a piezo electric bender element. A technical description of the instrument can be found in Tryon & Williams, 1996. The instrument is usually worn around the user's waist, positioned over the hip, but may also be worn on the wrist (Swartz *et al.*, 2000). The instrument has no external controls and does not provide feedback to the wearer. It is programmed through an infrared interface attached to a personal computer, and data is downloaded in the same way. The instrument samples movement ten times a second, and sums this data over a user-defined period of time, usually one minute, providing an output of movement counts a minute. When set to record at one-minute epochs, the instrument can collect and store data for a period of 22 days. A useful facility is that the instrument can also operate as a pedometer, simultaneously collecting data on the number of steps walked as well as activity counts. In this dual channel mode the data collection period is halved.

Only one study has validated the CSA 7164 against DLW. Ekelund *et al.* (2001) monitored 26 children (9.1 ± 0.3 years) for 14 consecutive days using the CSA 7164, and simultaneously measured total energy expenditure using DLW. Activity counts were found to be significantly correlated both with total energy expenditure ($r = 0.39$) and activity energy expenditure ($r = 0.54$). In studies utilising indirect calorimetry as the criterion method, the CSA 7164 has demonstrated a high correlation between oxygen consumption and activity counts in children ($r = 0.87$) (Trost *et al.*, 1998) and adults ($r = 0.88$) (Freedson *et al.*, 1998) walking on a treadmill. Similarly good test–retest reliability ($r = 0.85$) during treadmill walking has been demonstrated in adults (Welk *et al.*, 2000a).

Use of the CSA to estimate energy expenditure

In each of the above studies, a linear relationship was demonstrated between the counts recorded when walking at different speeds and energy expenditure. This enables equations to be developed that predict energy expenditure (MET level) from CSA counts. In addition, these equations can be re-ordered to derive CSA count ranges that correspond to different intensity categories: moderate (≥ 3 to < 6 METs), hard (≥ 6 to < 9 METs) and very hard (≥ 9 METs). The mean CSA counts that differentiate between each intensity category are termed 'cut points', and can be used to determine the amount of time spent in the various categories in assessing multiple days of continuous activity recording. It should be noted that these 'cut points' differ between adults and children and between children of different ages. A number of different regression equations have been derived (Freedson *et al.*, 1998; Trost *et al.*, 1998; Hendelman *et al.*, 2000; Swartz *et al.*, 2000; Ekelund *et al.*, 2001) in addition to that provided by the manufacturers of the CSA (Computer Science and Applications, 1998).

The accuracy of the regression equation used to derive energy expenditure from CSA data obviously has a major impact on the accuracy of the CSA for describing physical activity intensity. Since accelerometers cannot detect increased energy expenditure due to a gradient (Melanson & Freedson, 1995; Fehling *et al.*, 1999), it raises the possibility that laboratory-derived values are not applicable to those that would be obtained in the field. The ability to collect minute-by-minute physical activity data in parallel with measurement of energy expenditure using portable metabolic systems allows us to address this issue.

Three studies have recently investigated the validity of the CSA for assessment of energy expenditure in the field by comparing energy expenditure predicted from accelerometer data with actual values. Using CSA calibration curves derived for each participant (rather than a generic regression equation), the relationship between the CSA estimates and metabolic cost of walking, golf, house cleaning and gardening has been investigated (Hendelman *et al.*, 2000). For walking, correlation between the accelerometer and energy expenditure was good ($r=0.77$) but for all activities combined (as a model of normal daily activity) the correlation was reduced ($r=0.59$). The intensity of the individual lifestyle activities was significantly underestimated by the CSA by between 30.5–56.8 per cent, with the degree of under prediction lowest in two activities that involve walking (golf and lawn-mowing). Although predominantly walking-based activities, it is suggested that they may have been underestimated due to the difference in terrain used in derivation of the calibration curves (track walking), during the activity (grass) and by extra weight bearing (pulling golf cart, pushing mower).

A second study investigating the accuracy of the CSA for estimating the intensity of lifestyle activities (various housework and gardening activities) using published prediction curves, found higher correlations between the CSA and calorimetry for treadmill walking ($r=0.85$) than for lifestyle activities (housework and gardening; $r=0.48$), and an underestimation of intensity by the CSA of 42–67 per cent (Welk *et al.*, 2000a).

To determine the influence of using different prediction equations, Bassett *et al.* (2000) compared the energy cost of 28 lifestyle activities measured by indirect calorimetry with predicted values from CSA counts derived using three different regression equations. Similar moderate correlation ($r=0.62$) between the predicted and measured values was achieved using equations derived from theoretical considerations (Computer Science and Applications, 1998) and from calibration curves established in the field (Hendelman *et al.*, 2000); that derived from treadmill studies (Freedson *et al.*, 1998) was less good.

Accuracy of CSA 'cut points'

The above studies suggest that the protocol and type of activities used to determine the 'cut points' corresponding to specific intensity levels may greatly affect the values, owing to the differences in the count–$\dot{V}O_2$ relationship for different activities. In comparing the cut points developed from treadmill studies with those from walking on a track, discrepancies of several thousand counts were observed for moderate activity, raising the potential for misclassification (Hendelman *et al.*, 2000). To examine this further Ainsworth *et al.* (2000a) compared the time spent in daily physical activity over 21 days in 83 adults completing an activity log and wearing a CSA. Three different CSA cut-point methods were used and showed modest to good agreement for time spent in different intensity categories ($r=0.43–0.94$).

It thus appears that the accuracy of the energy expenditure estimate derived from the CSA (and consequently of 'cut points') is dependent both upon the accuracy of the prediction equation used to derive it and upon the type of activity performed. This may be due to the inability of accelerometers to detect increased energy cost of activities involving upper-body movement, added weight bearing (carrying, lifting and so on) or graded or soft surfaces.

How many days of measurement are required to be representative of 'normal' physical activity?

Under free-living conditions, individuals may participate in many different types and amounts of activity each day, and measurement of activity over a single day is unlikely to represent the overall activity level of an individual. This is particularly true of weekdays and weekend days. A number of studies have investigated how many days of monitoring are required to provide a representative measure of 'usual' physical activity. Using the Caltrac™ accelerometer, it has been shown that for adults scores differ between weekdays and weekend days, and that a sampling period of at least 5–6 days is required to minimise variability (Gretebeck & Montoye, 1992). Using the CSA accelerometer between four and five days of monitoring have been shown to be necessary to achieve a reliability of 0.80 for children aged 7–10 years (Trost *et al.*, 2000). Older children (aged 12–16 years) exhibit greater day-to-day variability in their physical activity and between eight and nine days of monitoring is required to achieve the same reliability.

Applications of objective activity measurement

Instruments for the objective measurement of activity have great potential for increasing our understanding of the relationship between activity and health in a number of ways not previously achievable.

Patterns of activity

The ability to collect data each minute for periods of up to 3 weeks allows us, for the first time, to investigate the patterns of physical activity of individuals as they go about their normal life, for example to compare activity at work or school with activity during leisure time in the evening or at weekends. Figure 5.1, for example, shows the physical activity pattern of a class of 10-year-old children during a schoolday. A CSA accelerometer was used to collect minute-by-minute data, and that was then averaged into 15-minute periods. The graph clearly shows the peaks of activity during the day – before school (8:30 to 9:00), at morning break (10:45), at lunch break (12:00 to 13:00) and immediately after school (15:00 to 15:30). The graph also shows that girls are consistently less active than boys in this sample.

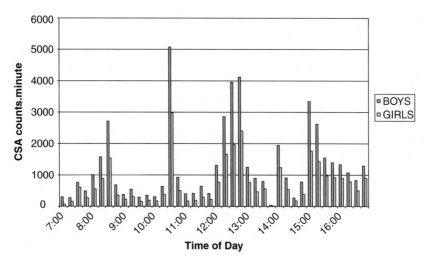

Figure 5.1 Physical activity pattern of 10-year-old children on a schoolday

Group differences

Many physical activity questionnaires are relevant only to the population for which they were designed, and this makes comparison between different countries or different social or cultural groups difficult. Similarly, even within a relatively homogeneous group there may be selective under- or over-reporting. For example, sedentary people may report being more active than they really are due to a perceived social pressure to be active (social-desirability bias). The ability to measure the physical activity of different groups of people with equal precision overcomes this major disadvantage.

Prescription of physical activity

The facility of some objective measures of activity such as the Digi-Walker and Caltrac™ to provide instant feedback to the wearer (through a visual display) makes it possible to individualise prescriptions of physical activity. The development of the self-confidence to be an exerciser is a critical factor in people becoming more physically active. To develop such self-confidence (often called self-efficacy) individuals need to have successful experiences of increasing their activity, and this relies upon monitoring their activity and then setting realistic, achievable physical activity goals. Accelerometers and pedometers are increasingly being used in this role, to promote physical activity. Individualised prescription of lifestyle activity and implementation of behaviour change strategies to increase self-efficacy for exercise using an accelerometer for feedback have been shown to be effective in achieving the adoption and maintenance of regular physical activity (Andersen *et al.*, 1999).

 Chapter 7 (Inactivity) discusses how behaviour change can be facilitated.

Special populations

The majority of questionnaires are designed for use with healthy adults, and are most accurate when used with better-educated groups of people. Much of the data relating physical activity to health outcomes is derived from such groups, for example University alumni or those in professional groups. However, relatively little is known about the physical activity levels of people who do not fit this profile and who may encounter difficulties in completing sometimes complex questionnaires. To address this issue, a number of questionnaires have been designed specifically for use with, for example, children or older people. Cognitive ability varies with age, and both children and older people can suffer from problems of inaccurate recall. Additionally, there are other groups, for example, blind people, mentally impaired people and those with learning difficulties about whose activity very little is known due to problems with questionnaire completion. The use of objective methods overcomes these problems, and offers the opportunity for greater understanding of physical activity and health relationships in these important groups.

Use in longitudinal studies

At the time of writing, the expense of the more sophisticated accelerometers has limited their use in large studies, and especially longitudinal studies. The time-scale required to relate physical activity to development of disease means that the outcomes of such studies are some years away. However, the influence of physical activity on risk factors for disease can be used as predictors of disease development, and a number of studies are under way using accelerometers to investigate these relationships over time.

One of the first studies to utilise this approach is the European Youth Heart Study. This study is designed to investigate the relationships between physical activity and risk factors for cardiovascular disease in children (aged 9 and 15 years at baseline) recruited from five European countries. One thousand children from each country have completed a battery of baseline measurements including physical activity (assessed by accelerometry) and the major CVD risk factors. These measurements will be repeated at five-year intervals in order to track the changes in risk factors and how they relate to physical activity. Figure 5.2 shows an example of the relationships that precise measurement can reveal. Comparison of physical activity quintile and fasting plasma insulin

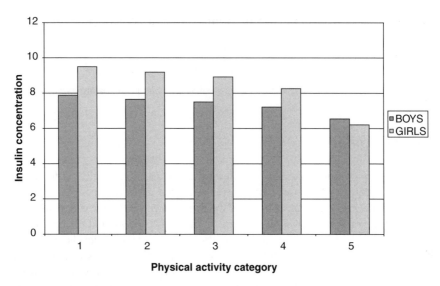

Figure 5.2   Relationship between physical activity category measured with the CSA accelerometer and serum insulin concentration in nine-year-old Danish children

level in 293 nine-year-old Danish children (139 boys and 154 girls) shows a graded reduction in plasma-insulin levels with increasing levels of physical activity. The effect is seen in both genders, but is much greater in the girls at the lowest activity levels, which may help develop a closer understanding of the dose-response relationship at different stages of the lifecourse.

Limitations of accelerometers

Accelerometers offer us the opportunity to investigate physical activity patterns in greater detail and accuracy than has previously been achievable, but they are not able to measure all activities. Activity involving predominantly upper-body movement such as resistance exercises and many household and occupational activities are poorly registered, even by tri-axial instruments. Similarly, accelerometers are unable to measure water-based activity, and do not reflect true activity levels when used for cycling. Of particular importance is the recent understanding of the potential role of spontaneous physical activity in the maintenance of normal body weight. In a study of 16 normal-weight individuals who were overfed by 1000 kcal a day for eight weeks, it was found that a significant amount of the excess energy intake was dissipated by increased spontaneous physical activity, for example fidgeting, and that those participants who had the greatest increase in spontaneous physical activity accumulated least extra fat mass (Levine *et al.*, 1999). Such activity would not be registered by instruments such as an accelerometer.

Summary

The development of new objective instruments for the measurement of physical activity in free-living individuals offers us the opportunity to understand the relationship between activity and health outcomes better than in the past. The ability to measure the volume, duration and intensity of activity in detail over a prolonged period should allow us to better recommend activity programmes that would be effective in the prevention and management of ill health. In addition, the use of feedback from these instruments will allow us to monitor individual achievement of physical activity targets, to encourage not only the adoption but also the maintenance of a more active and hopefully healthier lifestyle.

References

Ainsworth, B.E., Bassett Jr, D.R., Strath, S.J., Swartz, A.M., O'Brien, W.L., Thompson, R.W., Jones, D.A., Macera, C.A. & Kimsey, C.D. (2000a) Comparison of three methods for measuring the time spent in physical activity. *Medicine and Science in Sports and Exercise*, **32**: (Suppl.) S457–S464.

Ainsworth, B.E., Haskell, W.L., Whitt, M.C., Irwin, M.L., Swartz, A.M., Strath, S.J., O'Brien, W.L., Bassett Jr, D.R., Schmitz, K.H., Emplaincourt, P.O., Jacobs Jr, D.R. & Leon, A.S. (2000b) Compendium of Physical Activities: an update of activity codes and MET intensities. *Medicine and Science in Sports and Exercise*, **32(9)**: (Suppl.) S498–S516.

American Diabetes Association (1998) Clinical practice recommendations. Diabetes Mellitus and exercise. *Diabetes Care*, **21**: (Suppl. 1) S41–S44.

Andersen, R.E., Wadden, T.A., Bartlett, S.J., Zemel, B., Verde, T.J. & Franckowiak, S.C. (1999) Effects of lifestyle activity versus structured aerobic exercise in obese women; a randomised trial. *Journal of the American Medical Association*, **281(4)**: 335–340.

Barinaga, M. (1997) How much pain for cardiac gain? *Science*, **276**: 1324–1327.

Bassett, D.R., Ainsworth, B.E. & Leggett, S.R. (1996) Accuracy of five electronic pedometers for measuring distance walked. *Medicine and Science in Sports and Exercise*, **28**: 1071–1077.

Bassett, D.R. (2000) Validity and reliability issues in objective monitoring of physical activity. *Research Quarterly for Exercise and Sport*, **71(2)**: 30–36.

Bassett, D.R., Ainsworth, B.E., Swartz, A.M., Strath, S.J., O'Brien, W.L. & King, G.A. (2000) Validity of four motion sensors in measuring moderate intensity physical activity. *Medicine and Science in Sports and Exercise*, **32**: (Suppl.) S471–S480.

Bouten, C.V., Verboeket-Van De Venne, W.P.H.G., Westerterp, K.R., Verduin, M. & Janssen, J.D. (1996) Daily physical activity assessment: comparison between movement registration and doubly labeled water. *Journal of Applied Physiology*, **81(2)**: 1019–1026.

Bouten, C.V., Westerterp, K.R., Verduin, M. & Janssen, J.D. (1994) Assessment of energy expenditure for physical activity using a triaxial accelerometer. *Medicine and Science in Sports and Exercise*, **26(12)**: 1516–1523.

Caspersen, C.J., Powell, K.E. & Christenson, G.M. (1985) Physical activity, exercise and physical fitness: Definitions and distinctions for health-related research. *Public Health Reports*, **100**: 126–130.

Computer Science and Applications (1998) *Activity Monitor Operator's Manual Model 7164 Multimode Release 1.24E*. Shalimar, FL, Computer Science and Applications Inc.

Cooper, A.R., Moore, L.A.R., McKenna, J. & Riddoch, C.J. (2000) What is the magnitude of the blood pressure response to a programme of moderate intensity exercise? Randomised controlled trial among sedentary adults with unmedicated hypertension. *British Journal of General Practice*, **50**: 958–962.

Department of Health (1996) Strategy statement on physical activity. London, Department of Health.

Ekelund, U., Sjostrom, M., Yngve, A., Poortvliet, E., Nilsson, A., Froberg, K., Wedderkopp, N. & Westerterp, K. (2001) Physical activity assessed by activity monitor and doubly labelled water in children. *Medicine and Science in Sports and Exercise*, **33**(2): 275–281.

Eston, R.G., Rowlands, A.V. & Ingledew, D.K. (1998) Validity of heart rate, pedometry and accelerometry for predicting the energy cost of children's activities. *Journal of Applied Physiology*, 362–371.

Fehling, P.C., Smith, D.L., Warner, S.E. & Dalsky, G.P. (1999) Comparison of accelerometers with oxygen consumption in older adults during exercise. *Medicine and Science in Sports and Exercise*, **31**: 171–175.

Freedson, P.S., Melanson, E. & Sirard, J. (1998) Calibration of the Computer Science and Applications Inc. accelerometer. *Medicine and Science in Sports and Exercise*, **30**(5): 777–781.

Freedson, P.S. & Miller, K. (2000) Objective monitoring of physical activity using motion sensors and heart rate. *Research Quarterly for Exercise and Sport*, **71**(2): 21–29.

Gardner, A.W. & Poehlman, E.T. (1998) Assessment of free-living daily physical activity in older claudicants: Validation against the doubly labeled water technique. *Journal of Gerontology: Medical Sciences*, **53A**(4): M275–M280.

Gretebeck, R. & Montoye, H.J. (1992) Variability of some objective measures of physical activity. *Medicine and Science in Sports and Exercise*, **24**: 1167–1172.

Haymes, E.M. & Byrnes, W.C. (1993). Walking and running energy expenditure estimated by Caltrac and indirect calorimetry. *Medicine and Science in Sports and Exercise*, **25**(12): 1365–1369.

Hendelman, D., Miller, K., Baggett, C., Debold, E. & Freedson, P.S. (2000) Validity of accelerometry for the assessment of moderate intensity physical activity in the field. *Medicine and Science in Sports and Exercise*, **32**(9): (Suppl.) S442–S449.

Jakicic, J.M., Winters, C., Lagally, K., Ho, J., Robertson, R.J. & Wing, R.R. (1999) The accuracy of the TriTrac-R3D accelerometer to estimate energy expenditure. *Medicine and Science in Sports and Exercise*, **31**(5): 147–754.

Joint National Committee on Prevention, Evaluation and Treatment of High Blood Pressure. (1997) The Sixth Report of the Joint National Committee on Prevention, Detection, Evaluation and Treatment of High Blood Pressure. *Archives of Internal Medicine*, **157**: 2413–2446.

Kelley, D.E. & Goodpaster, B.H. (2001) Effects of exercise on glucose homeostasis in Type 2 diabetes mellitus. *Medicine and Science in Sports and Exercise*, **33**(6): (Suppl.) S495–S501.

Kohl III, H.W. (2001) Physical activity and cardiovascular disease: evidence for a dose-response. *Medicine and Science in Sports and Exercise*, **33**(6): (Suppl.) S472–S483.

Kriska, A.M. & Caspersen, C.J. (1997) A collection of physical activity questionnaires for health-related research. *Medicine and Science in Sports and Exercise*, **29**(6): (Suppl.).

Lamonte, M.J. & Ainsworth, B.E. (2001) Quantifying energy expenditure and physical activity in the context of dose-response. *Medicine and Science in Sports and Exercise*, **33**(6): (Suppl.) S370–S378.

Lee, I.M., Sesso, H.D. & Paffenbarger, R.S. (2000) Physical activity and coronary heart disease risk in men. Does duration of exercise episodes predict risk? *Circulation*, **102**: 981–986.

Levine, J.A., Eberhardt, N.L. & Jensen, M.D. (1999) Role of non-exercise activity thermogenesis in resistance to fat gain in humans. *Science*, **283**: 212–214.

Levine, J.A., Baukol, P.A. & Westerterp, K.R. (2000) Validation of the Tracmor triaxial accelerometer system for walking. *Medicine and Science in Sports and Exercise*, **33**(9): 1593–1597.

Livingstone, M.B., Coward, W.A., Prentice, A.M., Davies, P.S., Strain, J.J., McKenna, P.G., Mahoney, C.A., White, J.A., Stewart, C.M. & Kerr, M. (1992) Daily energy expenditure in free-living children: comparison of heart-rate monitoring with the doubly labeled water method. *American Journal of Clinical Nutrition*, **56**: 343–352.

McArdle, W., Katch, F. & Katch, V. (1991) *Exercise Physiology*. London, Lea and Febiger.

Melanson, E. & Freedson, P.S. (1995) Validity of the Computer Science and Applications, Inc. (CSA) activity monitor. *Medicine and Science in Sports and Exercise*, **27**(6): 934–940.

Melanson, E.L. & Freedson, P.S. (1996) Physical activity assessment: a review of methods. *Critical Reviews in Food Science and Nutrition*, **36**: 385–396.

Montoye, H.J., Kemper, H.C.G., Saris, W.H.M. & Washburn, R.A. (1996) *Measuring Physical Activity and Energy Expenditure.* Champaign, Il., Human Kinetics.

Nichols, J.F., Morgan, C.G., Sarkin, J.A., Sallis, J.F. & Calfas, K.J. (1999) Validity, reliability and calibration of the Tritrac accelerometer as a measure of physical activity. *Medicine and Science in Sports and Exercise*, **31(6)**: 908–912.

Pate, R.R., Pratt, M., Blair, S.N., Haskell, W.L., Macera, C.A., Bouchard, C. *et al.* (1995) Physical activity and public health: a recommendation from the Centers for Disease Control and Prevention and the American College of Sports Medicine. *Journal of the American Medical Association*, **273**: 402–407.

Powers, S.K. & Howley, E.T. (2001) *Exercise Physiology. Theory and Application to Fitness and Performance.* London, McGraw-Hill.

Ramsay, L.E., Williams, B., Johnston, G.D., MacGregor, G.A., Poston, L., Potter, J.F., Poulter, N.R. & Russell, G. (1999) Guidelines for management of hypertension: report of the third working party of the British Hypertension Society. *Journal of Human Hypertension*, **13**: 569–592.

Rennie, K.L., Hennings, S.J., Mitchell, J. & Wareham, N.J. (2001) Estimating energy expenditure by heart-rate monitoring without individual calibration. *Medicine and Science in Sports and Exercise*, **33(6)**: 939–945.

Sallis, J.F. & Saelens, B.E. (2000) Assessment of physical activity by self-report: status, limitations, and future directions. *Research Quarterly for Exercise and Sport*, **71(2)**: 1–14.

Sequeira, M., Rickenbach, M., Wietlisbach, V., Tullen, B. & Schutz, Y. (1995) Physical assessment using a pedometer and its comparison with a questionnaire in a large population survey. *American Journal of Epidemiology*, **142**: 989–999.

Speakman, J.R. (1998) The history and theory of the doubly labeled water technique. *American Journal of Clinical Nutrition*, **68**: 932S–938S.

Spurr, G.B., Prentice, A.M., Murgatroyd, P.R., Goldberg, G.R., Reina, J.C. & Christman, N.T. (1988) Energy expenditure from minute-by-minute heart-rate recording: comparison with indirect calorimetry. *American Journal of Clinical Nutrition*, **48**: 552–559.

Strath, S.J., Swartz, A.M., Bassett Jr, D.R., O'Brien, W.L., King, G.A. & Ainsworth, B.E. (2000) Evaluation of heart rate as a method for assessing moderate intensity physical activity. *Medicine and Science in Sports and Exercise*, **32**: (Suppl.) S465–S470.

Swain, D.P., Leutholtz, B.C., King, M.E., Haas, L.A. & Branch, J.D. (1998) Relationship between heart rate reserve and %VO2 reserve in treadmill exercise. *Medicine and Science in Sports and Exercise*, **30**: 318–321.

Swartz, A.M., Strath, S.J., Bassett Jr, D.R., O'Brien, W.L., King, G.A. & Ainsworth, B.E. (2000) Estimation of energy expenditure using CSA accelerometers at hip and wrist sites. *Medicine and Science in Sports and Exercise*, **32(9)**: (Suppl.) S450–S456.

Trost, S.G., Pate, R.R., Freedson, P.S., Sallis, J.F. & Taylor, W.C. (2000) Using objective physical activity measures with youth: How many days of monitoring are needed? *Medicine and Science in Sports and Exercise*, **32(2)**: 426–431.

Trost, S.G., Ward, D.S., Moorehead, S.M., Watson, P.D., Riner, W. & Burke, J.R. (1998) Validity of the Computer Science and Applications (CSA) activity monitor in children. *Medicine and Science in Sports and Exercise*, **30**: 629–633.

Tryon, W.W. & Williams, R. (1996) Fully proportional actigraphy: a new instrument. *Behavior Research Methods, Instruments, and Computers*, **28(3)**: 392–403.

US Department of Health and Human Services (1996) *Physical Activity and Health: A Report of the Surgeon General.* Atlanta, GA, US Department of Health and Human Services, Centers for Disease Control and Prevention, National Center for Chronic Disease Prevention and Health Promotion.

Wareham, N.J. & Rennie, K.L. (1998) The assessment of physical activity in individuals and populations: Why try to be more precise about how physical activity is assessed? *International Journal of Obesity*, **22**: (Suppl. 2) S30–S38.

Warnecke, R.B., Johnson, T.P., Chavez, N., Sudman, S., O'Rourke, D.P., Lacey, L. & Horm, J. (1997) Improving question wording in surveys of culturally diverse populations. *Annals of Epidemiology*, **7**: 334–342.

Welk, G.J., Blair, S.N., Wood, K., Jones, S. & Thompson, R. (2000a) A comparative evaluation of three accelerometry-based physical activity monitors. *Medicine and Science in Sports and Exercise*, **32(9)**: (Suppl.) S489–S497.

Welk, G.J., Differding, J.A., Thompson, R.W., Blair, S.N., Dziura, J. & Hart, P. (2000b) The utility of the Digi-Walker step counter to assess daily physical activity patterns. *Medicine and Science in Sports and Exercise*, **32(9)**: (Suppl.) S481–S488.

Yamada, S. & Baba, Y. (1990) Assessment of physical activity by means of a calorie counter combined with an accelerometer. *Japanese Journal of Industrial Health*, **32**: 253–257.

Yamanouchi, K., Shinozaki, T., Chikada, K., Toshihiko, N., Katsunori, I., Shimizu, S., Ozawa, N., Suzuki, Y., Maeno, H., Kato, K., Oshida, Y. & Sato, Y. (1995) Daily walking combined with diet therapy is a useful means for obese NIDDM patients not only to reduce body weight but also to improve insulin sensitivity. *Diabetes Care*, **18**: 775–778.

CHAPTER 6

Risks of Physical Activity

ESTHER M.F. VAN SLUIJS, EVERT A.L.M. VERHAGEN,
ALLARD J. VAN DER BEEK, MIREILLE N.M. VAN POPPEL
AND WILLEM VAN MECHELEN

Chapter Contents

- Introduction
- Benefits of physical activity
- Risks of physical activity
- Minimising risk and maximising benefits
- Recommendations for future research

Introduction

Studies performed in the 1980s and 1990s confirm the health benefits of regular physical activity, which is a concept with foundations in antiquity. The effects of physical activity on certain individual health conditions, the precise dose of activity required for specific benefits, the role (if any) of intensity of effort, and the elucidation of biological pathways through which physical activity contributes to health, are topics still under research. Although these topics remain to be clarified, it is now clear that regular physical activity reduces the risk of morbidity and mortality from several chronic diseases. It also increases physical fitness, which leads to improved function and health.

However, in addition to having health-enhancing properties, participating in physical activity and, more precisely, in sports activities also carries risks. These risks can be biomechanic (for example, injury and adverse effects on bone), cardiovascular (ranging from discomfort to transient risk of sudden cardiac death) or combined (for example, the female athlete triad: the inter-relationship of eating disorders, amenorrhea and osteoporosis in the female athlete). The occurrence of these three types of health problems in the physically active population is low. In an athletic population, however, the chances of the occurrences grow with an increasing level of physical activity. Sudden cardiac death, for instance, has a low incidence of one cardiac arrest per 20 000 exercisers a year. However, the risk of sudden cardiac death during vigorous exercise is 5 to 56 times greater than during normal activities (Siscovick *et al.*, 1984). The actual prevalence of the female triad is unknown in both the general and the athlete population. However, data on eating disorders in the female athlete population suggest the existence of a large problem. The prevalence of anorexia nervosa and bulimia nervosa is as high as 4–39 per cent in a female athlete population, where it is between 0.5–5 per cent in the general population (Sanborn, 2000). Taking the risks of physical activity into account, individuals might adopt a 'decision-balance' approach in deciding whether it is 'worth' continuing with activity or becoming less or more active. Risk is therefore a perception that may guide an individual's physical activity behaviour.

In this chapter the benefits of physical activity will be discussed briefly. Most attention will be given to the risks of physical activity, including sports. The focus will be on injuries, the female triad, and sudden cardiac arrest. However, these are not the only risks associated with involvement in physical activity and sports. We acknowledge the risks of, for example, performance-enhancing drugs, but we view this as beyond the scope of this chapter. After discussing the risks, strategies for preventing these risks will be proposed.

Benefits of physical activity

Smoking, excessive alcohol intake and nutrition (for example, a too high intake of dietary fat or an excessive intake of polyunsaturated fatty acids, or both) are considered 'classic' independent risk factors for multi-causal chronic disease. The role of physical inactivity as an independent lifestyle risk factor has been the subject of debate and controversy. This debate seems, however, to have come to an end with the publication of consensus statements (for example, Pate *et al.*, 1995) and policy documents (for example, Anonymous, 1996) on the health benefits of a physically active lifestyle.

Not only will the individual person's health benefit from a reduced risk of the chronic diseases, like coronary heart disease (CHD), hypercholesterolaemia, hypertension, stroke, non-insulin dependent diabetes mellitus (NIDDM) and certain forms of cancer, but the public-health status of a nation will also benefit from a physically active lifestyle. The public-health burden of a sedentary lifestyle can be quantified by calculating the population attributable risk (PAR) of such a lifestyle. PAR is an estimate of the proportion of the public-health burden caused by a particular risk factor, for example, a sedentary lifestyle. By calculating PAR we may estimate the proportion of deaths from chronic diseases (CHD, NIDDM, cancer, and so on) that would not occur if everyone in a population was sufficiently physically active (Powell & Blair, 1994). To calculate PAR, we need to know the relative risk (as a measure of the strength of the relation between a risk factor and the (public) health burden) and the prevalence of the risk factor. The 'true' relative risk is constant, because it is biologically determined and will therefore not change, even though estimates of relative risk may change because of improvement of scientific measurement (Powell & Blair, 1994). Consequently, changes in PAR are highly dependent on changes in prevalence.

Based on available information on both relative mortality risks and prevalence of a sedentary lifestyle, Powell and Blair (1994) estimated the PAR of sedentary living for mortality from CHD, colon cancer and diabetes mellitus to be 35 per cent, 32 per cent and 35 per cent, respectively, meaning that 35 per cent of the CHD deaths, 32 per cent of the colon cancer deaths and 35 per cent of the diabetes mellitus deaths could, theoretically, be prevented if everyone was vigorously active. Recently in the Netherlands (Ruwaard & Kramers, 1997), similar PAR calculations were made for chronic disease mortality, not only for a sedentary lifestyle, but also for other lifestyle-related risk factors. The following calculations are based on the most recent Dutch population data. For CHD the following PARs were calculated for men and women respectively: smoking 42 per cent and 44 per cent, saturated fatty acid intake (exceeding 10 per cent of total energy intake) 13 per cent and 12 per cent, obesity (body mass index $> 30 \text{kg/m}^2$) 13 per cent and 15 per cent, and sedentary lifestyle 40 per cent and 40 per cent. From these PARs it seems that for CHD mortality the public-health burden caused by a sedentary life-style is at least of the same magnitude as the public-health burden caused by smoking and about three times as great as the burden caused by obesity and the excess intake of saturated fatty acids. From a public-health perspective it may be more appropriate to encourage a physically active lifestyle, second only to the restriction of smoking habits, than to emphasise further improvement of the dietary habits or reductions in body weight. Stimulating a physically active lifestyle has other related benefits: a physically active lifestyle (that is, regular exercise) helps to maintain body weight, leads to favourable dietary habits, and leads to a decline in the number of smokers (Vuori & Fentem, 1995). Knowing this, it seems that stimulating a physically active lifestyle is the individual's and the public health's best buy.

Risks of physical activity

In the new public health move toward greater physical activity, low-to-moderate intensity physical activities are promoted in order to reduce the health risks of a sedentary lifestyle (Pate *et al.*, 1995). Just as the health benefits from physical activity seem to grow with an increase in physical activity, so do the risks attached to physical activity, as depicted in Figure 6.1. When talking about physical activity and health benefits one usually means light-to-moderate daily activities (for example, walking and cycling). It might be obvious that the risks of such low-to-moderate physical activities are relatively low.

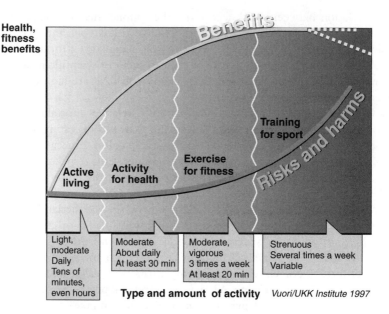

Figure 6.1   Health fitness benefits

However, more vigorous physical activity and, in particular, sports participation, is not without risk, whether the individual is an elite athlete or is involved only recreationally. In this chapter, therefore, when talking about risks of physical activity, it is chosen to target the more intense physical activities (that is, exercise for fitness and training for sport).

 Chapter 11 (Biology) explores the detail of biological responses to different physical activity and exercise loads.

Where people are encouraged to engage in physical activity for the many health benefits, attempts to reduce the inherent risks of the more vigorous of these activities are obviously warranted. Sports injuries, for instance, cause significant discomfort and disability, reduce short-term productivity, and are responsible for substantial medical expense. Furthermore, where physical activity becomes more vigorous and professionalised, athletes demand more of their bodies, and being physically active may even cause chronic health problems. Finally, the transient risk of sudden cardiac arrest is one of the most hazardous, direct complications of vigorous exercise. Before giving suggestions for risk prevention and risk reduction, the magnitude of the mentioned 'physical activity' problems should be addressed.

Sports injuries

One way of looking at the sports-injury problem is by considering the absolute number of sports injuries from data in a specific location. According to the most recent count in the Netherlands, on a population of about 16 million, a total of 2.9 million injuries were registered in 1992–1993. Of all these injuries, 1.1 million required medical attention (Schmikli *et al.*, 1995). Sport-specific numbers are given in Table 6.1. Absolute numbers, however, do not give a precise representation of the injury risk of each particular sport. Given the popularity of soccer in the Netherlands and the total number of participants in this sport, it is not a surprising to find that in absolute numbers soccer is the most 'dangerous' sport. However, a better way of looking at injuries is by calculating the number of injuries per 1000 hours of sports participation, that is, the injury incidence. Injury-incidence numbers give a more precise estimate of the actual risk of injury when participating in a particular sport. The injury-incidence numbers in Table 6.1 show that indoor soccer has the highest injury risk in the Netherlands. Furthermore, karate and tae kwon do, with an absolute number of only 63 500 injuries, together have an equal injury risk to that of soccer.

Each sport has its own injury types and causes. In this light, prevention should be focused on the specific risk factors and injuries inherent to the sport. For instance, soccer players make hard cuts, sharp turns off a planted foot, and intense contact with the ball and other players. This makes players more vulnerable to acute lower-extremity injuries, especially in the knee and ankle. As in soccer, acute lower-extremity injuries are the most common injuries in volleyball. There is general agreement that these acute volleyball injuries result from frequent jumping and landing, as well as striking the leg on the floor during defensive manoeuvres. The upper extremity is particularly

Table 6.1 Sport specific injury numbers; estimated total number of injuries, absolute number of injuries medically treated, and injury incidence (number of injuries per 1000 hours of sports participation)

Type of sport	Number of injuries	Numbers of medically treated injuries	Number of injuries/1000 hours
Soccer	797 000	328 000	5.5
Volleyball	190 000	78 500	3.6
Outdoor tennis	156 500	59 500	1.5
Indoor soccer	134 000	41 000	6.2
Hockey	130 500	63 500	5.5
Fitness	115 500	59 500	1.8
Gymnastics	104 500	48 500	2.7
Indoor tennis	89 500	48 500	3.5
Horse-riding	74 500	33 500	1.6
Karate/tae kwon do	63 500	18 500	5.5

Table 6.2   Various sports and their main injury risk factors

Soccer	Previous injury (Ekstrand & Tropp, 1990)
	Players' position (Jörgenson, 1984)
	Playing surface (Ekstrand & Nigg, 1989)
Volleyball	Jumping technique
	Position
	Playing surface
Tennis	Shoulder strength
	Equipment
	Playing surface
	Muscle imbalance
Hockey	Physical characteristics
	Aggressive play
	Equipment
Gymnastics	Previous injury
	High lumbar curvature
	Protection
Karate/tae kwon do	Physical characteristics
	Technique (Wirtz *et al.*, 1988)
	Equipment
	Opponent
	Skill level (Zandbergen, undated)

susceptible to injury (acute and chronic) in tennis, because of the use of the racquet and its effect on the dominant arm. It is beyond the scope of this chapter to discuss risk factors and injury types for each sport in full detail (for full detail information the reader is referred to Renström, 1993 and 1994). Therefore, in Table 6.2 the most common risk factors are presented for various sports.

Female triad

Professional athletes are under intense pressure to perform. Many, especially female, athletes experience pressure from the coach, peers and family to have a low percentage of body fat. Female athletes may believe that a low percentage of body fat increases their performance and improves their appearance. Athletes are known as driven people who are willing to make extreme sacrifices to accomplish their goals, but for female athletes this willingness can drive them to unhealthy behaviour, which can lead to what is referred to as 'the female triad'. The female triad is a combination of three interrelated conditions that are associated with athletic training: disordered eating, amenorrhea and osteoporosis.

The term 'disordered eating' refers to a wide spectrum of abnormal patterns of eating, which range in severity from restricting food intake; to using diet pills, diuretics, or laxatives; to having periods of binge eating and purging; to having anorexia nervosa or bulimia nervosa at the extreme end of the spectrum

Table 6.3   Diagnostic criteria for anorexia nervosa and bulimia nervosa

---

Diagnostic criteria for anorexia nervosa

A. Refusal to maintain body weight at or above 85 per cent of normal weight for age and height.
B. Intense fear of gaining weight or becoming fat, although underweight.
C. Disturbance in the way in which one's body weight or shape is experienced, undue influence of body weight or shape on self-evaluation, or denial of the seriousness of the current low-body weight.
D. In post-menarchal females, amenorrhea.

Diagnostic criteria for bulimia nervosa

A. Recurrent episodes of binge eating. An episode of binge eating is characterised by the following:

  1. Eating, in a discrete period (for example, within any 2-hour period), an amount of food that is definitely larger than most people would eat during a similar period of time under similar circumstances.
  2. A sense of lack of control over eating during the episode (for example, a feeling that one cannot stop eating or control what or how much one is eating).

B. Recurrent inappropriate compensatory behaviour to prevent weight gain, such as self-induced vomiting; misuse of laxatives, diuretics, enemas, or other medications; fasting; or excessive exercise.
C. The binge eating and inappropriate compensatory behaviours occur, on average, at least twice a week for 3 months.
D. Self-evaluation is unduly influenced by body shape and weight.
E. The disturbance does not occur exclusively during episodes of anorexia nervosa.

Source: American Psychiatric Association (2000) Diagnostic and Statistical Manual of Mental Disorders, Fourth Edition, Text Revision, Washington DC.

(Sanborn *et al.*, 2000). Athletes may start simply by monitoring food intake, progressing to restricting food such as fats or red meats, evolving to limiting the food (and calorie) intake, and finally to voluntary starvation. The prevalence of eating disorders in the general population is 0.5–1.0 per cent for anorexia nervosa and 1–5 per cent for bulimia nervosa (for example, Sanborn *et al.*, 2000; Putukian, 1998), though these are most likely underestimations. In athletes, the prevalence of disordered eating has been reported to be between 4 per cent and 39 per cent for meeting the DSM-IV criteria of anorexia nervosa and bulimia nervosa (Petrie *et al.*, 1993) and has been reported as high as 62 per cent for pathogenic weight control behaviour (Rosen & Hough, 1988) (see Table 6.3 for DSM-IV criteria). However, these prevalences are based on self-report, which may underestimate their real prevalence in the female athlete population.

The second aspect of the female athlete triad, amenorrhea, refers to the delayed onset or the absence of menstrual bleeding. The inability to initiate a menstrual cycle (menarche) before the age of 16 years is called 'primary amenorrhea', whereas the cessation of the menstrual cycle function after menarche has occurred is termed 'secondary amenorrhea'. Both primary and secondary amenorrhea have a higher prevalence in female athletes, as compared to the general population. The prevalence in the general population ranges from 2 to 5 per cent, whereas in an athlete population prevalences have been reported of 3.4–66 per cent. The highest frequencies of amenorrhea have been found among dancers and long-distance runners (Vereeke West, 1998),

Table 6.4 Female athletes at high risk for developing (parts of) the female triad according to the American College of Sports Medicine (Otis *et al.*, 1997)

Female athletes at high risk for developing (parts of) the female triad according to the American College of Sports Medicine (ref in Vereeke West):

- Sports in which performance is subjectively scored (for example, dance, figure skating and gymnastics)
- Endurance sports favouring participants with a low body weight (for example, distance running, cycling and cross-country skiing)
- Sports in which body contour-revealing clothing is worn for competition (for example, volleyball, swimming, diving and running)
- Sports using weight categories for participation (for example, horse racing, martial arts and rowing)
- Sports in which prepubertal body habitus favours success (for example, figure skating, gymnastics and diving).

but all female athletes training at high intensities are at risk (A list of the athletes at risk, identified by the ACSM, is given in Table 6.4). The pathophysiology of exercise-induced amenorrhea is complex, with varied contributions of a lowered percentage of body fat, body-weight loss, and emotional and physical stress. Although amenorrhea is more prevalent in a population with a co-existing eating disorder, Loucks and Horvath (1985) showed that there is no specific body-fat percentage below which regular periods cease. Some athletes with amenorrhea regain their periods after resting, even without regaining body weight or body fat. These findings suggest that amenorrhea is not caused solely by low body weight or body fat, and other important factors must be considered.

Osteoporosis is the final component of the female athlete triad. Osteoporosis is defined as the loss of bone-mineral density (BMD) and the inadequate formation of bone, which can lead to increased bone fragility and an increased risk of fracture. Premature osteoporosis puts the female athlete at risk of stress fractures as well as more devastating fractures of the hip or vertebral column (Hobart & Smucker, 2000). Amenorrheic athletes have been shown to have low bone mass, though the prevalence of osteoporosis among athletes is unknown (Sanborn *et al.*, 2000). In women, accelerated bone loss usually starts at menopause, when they experience a 3 per cent per year bone loss for an average of ten years, after which the rate of bone loss slows to normal levels (0.3–0.5 per cent a year). Among young athletes osteoporosis can result in bone mass loss of 2–6 per cent a year, with the total loss of bone during adolescence reaching up to 25 per cent of initial levels. A young athlete may acquire the bone mass of a 60-year-old, with a subsequent three-fold risk of stress fractures. This accelerated bone loss is the result of oestrogen deficiency and subsequent bone resorption (Vereeke West, 1998). The concern is that the bone loss during early age is partly irreversible, although research shows that regaining periods can result in increases in BMD. A significant increase in BMD is found in women decreasing their training intensity and regain their periods. However, these athletes will reach a level that is far below normal bone mass for their age and presumably will never reach this normal level again (Keen, 1997).

Sudden cardiac arrest

One of the most hazardous complications of vigorous exercise is the transient risk of sudden death during or directly after vigorous exercise, which raises concerns regarding the cardiac safety of exercise. The numbers of sudden deaths during exercise are small; data from autopsies shows that 0.35–0.5 per cent of all sudden deaths were attributable to exercise, while there was less than one death per one million exercise hours in middle-aged men (Vuori, 1995). The incidence rates of sudden death during vigorous exercise are estimated at one cardiac arrest per 20 000–45 000 exercisers a year (Siscovick *et al.*, 1984; Mosterd, 1999). These figures indicate that the absolute risk is low among apparently healthy middle-aged and older adults. But every death occurring during vigorous exercise is one too many and therefore this risk of physical activity should be discussed as well.

It should be stressed that total mortality is less among physically active people than among inactive people. At the same time, there is an increased risk for sudden death or myocardial infarction during physical activity, as compared with inactivity (Jensen-Urstad *et al.*, 1995). The mechanisms behind this counter-intuitive phenomenon are complex and not fully known, making the cause (and thus the prevention) of sudden cardiac arrest multifactoral. Pathophysiological evidence suggests that exercising increases the oxygen consumption of the heart muscle while also shortening diastole and coronary perfusion time. In this process a transient oxygen deficiency may be evoked at the subendocardial level, which is worsened by abrupt cessation of activity (Franklin, 1999). A shortage of blood in the heart muscle (myocardial ischaemia) can alter depolarisation, repolarisation and conduction velocity, triggering serious ventricular arrhythmia, which in extreme cases may be the forerunner of ventricular tachycardia or fibrillation. Another cause of sudden death may be plaque rupture or acute coronary thrombosis, although the reasons why strenuous activity may cause this are unknown (Franklin, 1999). Further, the mechanisms responsible for exercise-related sudden death differ with the age of the athlete. Most deaths in young athletes (<35 years) are congenital and cardiovascular in nature, the most common being hypertrophic cardiomyopathy (46 per cent), followed by coronary artery abnormalities (19 per cent). In contrast, most sudden deaths during exercise in older athletes (>35 years) are attributed to coronary artery disease (Futterman & Myerburg, 1998).

 Chapter 11 (Biology) further explores biological responses to different physical activity and exercise loads.

When discussing this risk of vigorous physical activity, one must be aware of the intensity of the physical activities and the health status of the people engaged in these activities. To answer to the question 'Is strenuous exercise worth the risk?' Siscovick *et al.* (1984) studied the incidence of sudden death during vigorous exercise, paying special attention to the initial level of habitual physical activity. They showed that the relative risk of sudden cardiac arrest among men with low levels of habitual activity was 56 times greater during exercise compared to other times in their lives. Among men with the highest levels of habitual physical activity this risk was also elevated, but only by a factor 5. In addition, Siscovick *et al.* (1984) also studied the overall risk of sudden death (during and not during vigorous physical activity) and showed that men with high levels of habitual physical activity had a risk of sudden cardiac arrest that was only 40 per cent of that in the risk habitual sedentary men. These results support the hypothesis that physical activity both protects against and provokes cardiovascular events (Franklin, 1999).

Minimising risk and maximising benefits

Knowing these three risks associated with vigorous physical activity, and, in particular, sports participation raises the question of whether being physically active or participating in sports is as healthy as might be believed or hoped. It is, but to lead a healthy, physically active life one must minimise the risks in order to maximise the benefits. In this last section we will discuss strategies to minimise these risks.

Injury prevention

Measures to prevent injuries should not stand by themselves. They should form part of what might be called a sequence of prevention (van Mechelen, 1992) (Figure 6.2). First, the problem must be identified and described in terms of incidence and severity of sports injuries. Second, the factors and mechanisms that play a part in the occurrence of sports injuries have to be identified. The third step is to introduce measures that are likely to reduce the future risk and/or severity of sports injuries. Such measures should be based on the aetiologic factors and the mechanisms as identified in the second step. Finally, the effect of the measures must be evaluated by repeating the first step, which will lead to a time-trend analysis of injury patterns.

As seen in Table 6.2, previous research has identified many causal factors for injury. However, developing the third and fourth steps of the prevention sequence, based on the existing evidence-base, is the challenge. A recent review by Parkkari *et al.* (2001) indicated that only 16 randomised controlled trials on the prevention of sports injuries have been conducted over the past three decades. Therefore, although many risk factors have been identified, little evidence exists on the effectiveness of preventive measures. As it impossible to discuss the prevention of each injury in detail here, only general principles of acute and chronic injury prevention applicable to sport participation are given here. These are divided into three main categories: the athlete, the sport, and the risk behaviour.

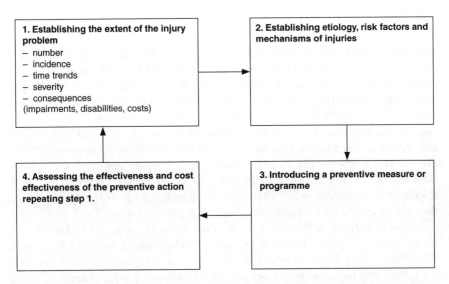

Figure 6.2   The sequence of prevention of sports injuries

The athlete

The use of braces and taping to stabilise weak or unstable joints, during the return-to-play, or rehabilitation phase is widely practised. Next to this secondary preventive application, tape and braces also have a primary preventive function (Verhagen *et al.*, 2000). However, significant controversy exists about the benefit. Taping and bracing may function more by improving proprioception and thereby stimulating earlier recruitment of supportive muscles, rather than by the actual mechanical restriction of a joint (Bahr *et al.*, 1997; Verhagen *et al.*, 2001). It is critically important to understand that no tape application, or brace can guarantee protection from either new injury, or exacerbation of a pre-existing trauma.

The use of stretching and warm-up exercises to promote suppleness and flexibility is historically believed to serve a preventive function against strain injuries to muscles and tendons. Recently, however, there is much controversy surrounding the preventive value of stretching, and in randomised studies (van Mechelen *et al.*, 1993; Pope *et al.*, 2000) found no such effect.

General and sport-specific conditioning programmes for athletes are necessary to attain successful performance and avoid injury (Zvijac & Thompson, 1996). Avoidance of overuse injuries, however, is a critical part of designing and monitoring the conditioning programme, particularly in endurance sports such as running. A common rule that may be employed to avoid overuse injuries is not to increase more than one parameter (that is, intensity, frequency, or duration) at a time.

The sport

The equipment used in sport has the potential for contributing to injury prevention. For instance, facial and head injuries in American football may be prevented through the use of properly fitted helmets and padded chin straps, which eliminate helmet rotation (Zemper, 1994). The effect of headgear on a decrease of injuries has also been shown in wrestling (Schuller *et al.*, 1989) and ice-hockey (Stuart & Smith, 1995). It is also shown that the use of improper cleats is a primary factor in lower-extremity injuries (Zemper, 1994). Preventive equipment can be individually applied depending upon sport, position and bodily dimension (Mueller *et al.*, 1996). However, equipment should always fit the conditions for which it is designed; for example, aerobic shoes should not be used for long-distance running.

In team sports an important role in injury prevention lies with the referee. In an interview study (Cattermole *et al.*, 1996) athletes believed that their injury could have been prevented if there had been tighter referee control of the game. The fact that only 8 per cent of all ice-hockey injuries are associated with a penalty, suggests that referees may allow dangerous play (Tegner & Lorentzen, 1991). Many injuries in soccer, for instance, occur during tackling and contact with the opposing player (Yde & Nielsen, 1990). To reduce injuries, referees need to keep the game under tight control, and must not allow dangerous behaviour on the field (Kibler, 1993). Coaching within the spirit, as well as within the letter, of sport laws, should be emphasised, since aggressive actions often lead to injuries in team sports (Kibler, 1993). For instance, Brust *et al.* (1992) showed that only half of the teenage ice-hockey players understood the seriousness of checking another player from behind. The coach has the power to minimise this dangerous attitude by emphasising the magnitude of the serious injury this move can inflict.

The risk behaviour

In contact sports, a debate has arisen about the introduction of preventive measures, because changes in injury patterns and mechanisms have occurred hand in hand with the introduction of protective equipment (Wilson, 1998). An example of this phenomenon was found in ice hockey, where the introduction of mandatory helmet use reduced the frequency and severity of head injuries (Reynen & Clancy, 1994; Laprade *et al.*, 1995; Murray & Livingston, 1995). However, evidence suggests that in ice hockey, neck injuries may be more frequent since the introduction of mandatory facial and head protection (Reynen & Clancy, 1994; Murray & Livingston, 1995). Furthermore, Hood (1987) identified the use of shoulder padding in American football to be primarily 'an offensive weapon', and 'not within the spirit' of the game. Looking at such findings it is noticeable that players in a variety of contact sports become more 'reckless' after the introduction of protective measures. This phenomenon is described in the literature as 'risk homeostasis' (Bouter, 1986).

The theory of risk homeostasis states that individuals maintain their 'risk behaviour' at a level they perceive as acceptable and safe. In this viewpoint, individuals adapt their behaviour to a certain level of risk they consider acceptable ('target level of risk'). This explains why the manipulation of risk factors and the introduction of preventive measures rarely completely decrease the risk for injuries. In other words, individuals compensate their risk taking behaviour under the influence of preventive measures. According to Bouter (1986), motivating individuals to decrease their 'target level of risk' is the only measure that is able to decrease the risk for injuries.

Prevention of the female triad

It is not uncommon for female athletes to train at very high intensities, to have an unhealthy diet and to perform under a great deal of stress. But why do they tend to continue these unhealthy practices? A lack of education and information about the risks for female athletes and the compulsive behaviour, often seen in training groups, might explain this (Burrows & Bird, 2000). Therefore, to identify and prevent the female triad, it is crucial to provide adequate information about the risks and consequences and to detect the triad early.

When providing education on this topic, one must realise that educating the female athlete will not be enough. Education should also be directed to the coach and especially to the parents of adolescent athletes. Topics that should be addressed, include dispelling myths regarding body weight and body fat (for example, that 'thinner is better' and 'every sport has an ideal body weight') and their relationship to performance; providing nutritional education (for example, that adequate calories should be provided to meet the energy need); and dealing with other issues of personal wellness (for example, issues related to sexuality, time management, drug and alcohol use and so on) (Sanborn *et al.*, 2000). Female athletes must also be aware of the long-term consequences of the female triad. Information should be given on the possible health consequences to fertility and osteoporosis (Burrows & Bird, 2000). An effort must be taken to persuade female athletes to change their unhealthy behaviour. As described throughout Section 3 of this text, this is not an easy task and little is known about the specific approach needed in this population.

Screening for the female triad

Early detection of the female triad (or separate parts of it) may protect female athletes from the irreversible consequences of their behaviour. In northern America, the pre-participation physical examination may be the ideal time to screen for the triad, specifically for disordered eating and amenorrhea.

However, in Europe these physicals are not mandatory for athletes and the triad may therefore stay undetected for a long period. A sports physician or family physician may also screen for the triad during acute visits for fractures, weight change, amenorrhea or disordered eating. The physician should screen for signs of disordered eating by asking the athlete about her past eating habits and by asking for a list of 'forbidden foods'. The patient's highest and lowest body weight should be ascertained, as well as whether she is happy with her current body weight (Vereeke West, 1998; Hobart & Smucker, 2000). A history of amenorrhea is another easy way to detect the triad in its earliest stages. The physician should obtain information about the menstrual history, menarche, frequency and duration of cycles and last period. The physician should be aware that there is no specific body-fat percentage below which regular periods cease. Furthermore, it is important for physicians not to discount amenorrhea as a benign consequence of intensive athletic training. This will only enforce the female athlete in her unhealthy behaviour (Hobart & Smucker, 2000).

Important aspects of the treatment of the female triad should be decreasing the training intensity, increasing the periods of rest, and regaining body weight. Although the female athlete may be unwilling to accomplish this, the at-risk athletes must be convinced – through the persistence and effort of supportive others – to adopt positive lifestyle changes. In female athletes with signs of the female triad, attention should be paid to the possible existence of osteoporosis. The physician should educate the amenorrheic patient about the possible consequences of long-term amenorrhea and the risks of irreplaceable bone loss. To obtain accurate information about the BMD, a dual energy X-ray absorptiometry (DEXA) scan can be considered. This information can be used in the consideration to start hormone therapy with the female athlete to reduce the decrease in BMD (Hobart & Smucker, 2000).

As stated earlier, it is important to provide adequate information about the risks of the female triad not only to athletes, but also to coaches and parents. They should be aware that, although disordered eating and amenorrhea are highly prevalent in female athletes performing and training at high intensities, this behaviour is unhealthy and not to be encouraged. As well, the athletes' physician must be made aware of this and attention should be paid to the early signs of the triad. Only in this manner the irreversible effect of the triad can be prevented.

Preventing sudden death in exercise

Although the absolute numbers of sudden deaths during exercise are low, screening and providing information about the possible risk is very important. The number of sudden deaths in exercise can be decreased by identifying the susceptible individuals and by persuading people to exercise in a low-risk manner.

People of all ages with congenital, acquired or degenerative heart disease can be found in health examinations and through pre-exercise examinations (Vuori, 1995; Siscovick, 1997). Although known heart defects can be an important predictor for sudden death in exercise, a large portion of these deaths occur in subjects with completely latent or sub-clinical heart disease, which cannot be detected by medical examination. Furthermore, it is known that the sensitivity of pre-exercise examination among apparently healthy people is likely to be low for sudden death during exercise (Siscovick, 1991). The predictive value of a positive exercise test for an exercise-related cardiac death was only 4 per cent. This low number is partly due to the rarity of such events (Siscovick, 1991). One of the reasons for this low sensitivity might be that heart morphology adapts to exercising vigorously. During exercise these transformations include increased heart rate, systolic blood pressure, ventricular stroke volume and increased maximum oxygen uptake (Futterman & Myerburg, 1998). These phenomena are not clearly different from the pathophysiology of cardiovascular disease, which makes it difficult to distinguish them in a pre-exercise examination. Pluim *et al.* (1998) examined the differences between the physiologically and the pathologically enlarged heart and concluded that information about diastolic function, myocardial reflectivity, family history, and the electrocardiogram can be used to classify an enlarged heart. In detecting people at risk, physicians can use this information to identify the people with a pathophysiological enlarged heart.

Providing information about the risk and the safest way to exercise is therefore of great importance. A key point in this is to detect and point out the importance of effort-related symptoms, unexplained tiredness and current febrile infections. Furthermore, attention has to be paid to the intensity of the activities. Two thirds of sudden deaths in exercise have occurred during vigorous physical activity, although all-population data indicates that only a minority of exercising people practice vigorous physical activity. As described earlier, the risk of sudden death in exercise is ten times greater for subjects with a low level of fitness, than for subjects with a high level of fitness, although the overall incidence of sudden death while exercising remains low. Participating in vigorous-intensity physical activity when not used to doing it, therefore, provides an increased risk for sudden death during this activity. In health-promotion activities, people should be encouraged to exercise in moderation to one's actual capacity and condition, and that engaging in moderate-intensity physical activity provides many health benefits as well. Sedentary people who are changing their physical activity behaviour must therefore be discouraged from starting with vigorous-intensity physical activity and encouraged to be physically active at a more sensible, moderate level.

Recommendations for future research

In this chapter we addressed different aspects of the risks of vigorous physical activity. Although a lot is known about these risks, different aspects are still under research or need further clarification. In this last section, we will discuss the gaps in the knowledge and give recommendations for future research for the three risks described.

Measures to prevent injuries do not stand by themselves. As mentioned, they form part of what is called the sequence of prevention (van Mechelen *et al.*, 1992). Preventive measures should be implemented and evaluated after the sport-specific risk factors have been identified. However, from an epidemiological standpoint, it is preferable to evaluate the effect of preventive measures by means of a randomised controlled trial (RCT). Unfortunately, only 16 RCTs on sports-injury prevention have been conducted in the past three decades (Parkkari *et al.*, 2001). Therefore, many questions regarding prevention of sports injuries remain to be answered. Further well-designed randomised studies are needed on preventive actions and devices that are in common use, such as warming up, proprioceptive training, protective equipment and education interventions.

In the case of the female triad, it was described that the prevalence in athletes is higher than in the general population. However, the different estimations of the prevalence in a female athlete population are diverse. For anorexia nervosa, for example, the reported prevalences range between 3.4 per cent and 66 per cent (Vereeke West, 1998) and the prevalence of osteoporosis among this population is unknown. Future research, therefore, should aim at retrieving more accurate information about the prevalence of the female triad and its components. Furthermore, research should be aimed at improving the methods for diagnosing and screening for the triad and at enlarging the knowledge about the irreversibility of the effects. For example, obligatory pre-physical examinations for all athletes competing in competition may be a first step in detecting the triad in its earliest stages. To prevent the triad and to be able to treat the athletes, attention should be paid to develop safe training volumes and intensities in a way that it will not effect their performance in competition. Finally, a health-behaviour-change programme must be developed for this population specifically, to convince them to change their unhealthy behaviour and to be able to effectively support them during this process.

To reduce the numbers of sudden death in exercise, a major advancement can be made in increasing the knowledge of the pathophysiological mechanisms and factors influencing them (Vuori, 1995). Furthermore, it is important to develop a risk profile. Questions that should be addressed are: 'which persons are at risk?'; 'at what time is their risk the highest?'; and, 'what are other risk factors?'. This enables caregivers to screen effectively and to inform people accurately about the risks associated with exercising vigorously. However, the low incidence of sudden death during exercise limits the ability to identify potential predictors of exercise-related sudden cardiac death.

In this chapter risks associated with vigorous physical activity and sports activities have been described. Much is known about these risks and about possible ways to minimise these risks. It remains important, however, to gather more information about both the risks involved and safe physical activity, in order to maximise the benefits and minimise the risks of physical activity.

References

American Psychiatric Association (2000) Diagnostic and Statistical Manual of Mental Disorders, Fourth Edition, Text Revision, Washington DC.

Anonymous (1996) *US Physical Activity and Health: A report of the Surgeon General.* Atlanta GA: US Department of Health and Human Services, CDC, National Centre For Disease Control and Prevention.

Bahr, R., Bahr, I.A. & Lian, Ø. (1997) A twofold reduction in the incidence of acute ankle sprains in volleyball after the introduction of an injury prevention program – a prospective study. *Scandinavian Journal of Medicine Science and Sports*, 7: 172–177.

Bouter, L.M. (1986) Spanningsbehoefte en ongevalsrisico bij sportbeoefening. *Geneeskunde en Sport*, 19(6): 205–208.

Brust, J.D., Leonard, B.J., Pheley, A. & Roberts, W.O. (1992) Children's ice hockey injuries. *American Journal of the Disabled Child*, 146: 741–747.

Burrows, M. & Bird, S. (2000) The physiology of the highly trained female endurance runner. *Sports Medicine*, 30(4): 281–300.

Cattermole, H.R., Hardy, J.R.W. & Gregg, P.J. (1996) The footballer's fracture. *British Journal of Sports Medicine*, 30: 171–175.

Ekstrand, J. & Nigg, B. (1989) Surface-related injuries in soccer. *Sports Medicine*, 8: 56–62.

Ekstrand, J. & Tropp, H. (1990) The Incidence of ankle sprains in soccer. *Foot and Ankle*, 11: 41–44.

Franklin, B.A. (1999) Exercise and cardiovascular events: A double-edged sword? *Journal of Sports Sciences*, 17: 437–442.

Futterman, L.G. & Myerburg, R. (1998) Sudden death in athletes. *Sports Medicine*, 26(5): 335–350.

Hobart, J.A. & Smucker, D.R. (2000) The female athlete triad. *American Family Physician*, 61: 3357–3364.

Hood, M. (1987) Shoulder pads. In: Hood, M. (ed.) *Preparation Performance and Patch up – Guide to Fitness Training and Injury Prevention.* Auckland: Reed publishers, pp. 25–26.

Jensen-Urstad, M. (1995) Sudden death and physical activity in athletes and non-athletes. *Scandinavian Journal of Medicine and Science in Sports*, 5: 279–284.

Jörgenson, U. (1984) Epidemiology of injuries in typical Scandinavian team sports. *British Journal of Sports Medicine*, 18: 59–63.

Keen, A.D. & Drinkwater, B.L. (1997) Irreversible bone loss in former amenorrheic athletes. *Osteoporosis International*, 4: 311.

Kibler, W.B. (1993) Injuries in adolescent and preadolescent soccer players. *Medicine and Science in Sports and Exercise*, 25: 1330–1332.

Laprade, R.F., Burnett, Q.M., Zarzour, R. & Moss, R. (1995) The Effect of the mandatory use of face masks on facial lacerations and head and neck injuries in ice hockey; a prospective study. *American Journal of Sports Medicine*, 23(6): 773–775.

Loucks, A.B. & Horvath, S.M. (1985) Athletic amenorrhoea: a review. *Medicine and Science in Sports and Exercise*, 17: 54–72.

Mosterd, W.L. (1999) Plotse dood bij sport in Nederland. *Bijblijven*, 15: 68–74.

Mueller, F., Zemper, E.D. & Peters, A. (1996) American football. In: Caine, D.J., Caine, C.G. & Lindner, K.J. (eds) *Epidemiology of Sports Injuries.* Champaign, IL: Human Kinetics, pp. 41–62.

Murray, T.M. & Livingston, L.A. (1995) Hockey helmets, face masks, and injuries behaviour. *Pediatrics*, 95(3): 419–421.

Otis, C.L., Drinkwater, B., Johnson, M., Loucks, A. & Wilmore, J. (1997) The female athlete triad. *Medicine and Science in Sports and Exercise*, 29(5): i–ix.

Parkkari, J., Kujala, U.M. & Kannus, P. (2001) Is it possible to prevent sports injuries? Review of controlled clinical trials and recommendations for future work. *Sports Medicine*, 31(14): 985–995.

Pate, R.R., Pratt, M., Blair, S.N., Haskell, W.L., Macera, C.A., Bouchard, C. *et al.* (1995) Physical activity and public health: A recommendation from the Centers for Disease Control and Prevention and the American College of Sports Medicine. *Journal of the American Medical Association*, 273: 402–407.

Petrie, T.M. (1993) Disordered eating in female collegiate gymnasts: prevalence and personality/ attitudinal correlates. *Journal of Sport and Exercise Psychology*, 15: 424.

Pluim, B.M., Vliegen, H.W., van der Laarse, A. & van der Wall, E.E. (1998) Pathologic left ventricular hypertrophy. *Cardiology*, 5: 149–468.

Pope, R.P., Herbert, R.D., Kirwan, J.D. & Graham, B.J. (2000) A randomized trial of pre-exercise stretching for prevention of lower-limb injury. *Medicine and Science in Sports and Exercise*, 32(2): 271–277.

Powell, K.E. & Blair, S.N. (1994) The public health burden of sedentary living habits: theoretical but realistic estimates. *Medicine and Science in Sports and Exercise*, 26: 851–856.

Putukian, M. (1998) The female athlete triad. *Clinics in Sports Medicine*, 17(4): 675–696.

Renström, P.A.F.H. (ed.) (1993) *Sports Injuries: Basic Principles of Prevention and Care.* Encyclopaedia of Sports Medicine Vol. IV. Blackwell Scientific Publications, Oxford.

Renström, P.A.F.H. (ed.) (1994) *Clinical Practice of Sports Injuries: Prevention and Care.* Encyclopaedia of Sports Medicine Vol. V. Blackwell Scientific Publications, Oxford.

Reynen, P.D. & Clancy, W.G. (1994) Cervical spine injury, hockey helmets, and face masks. *American Journal of Sports Medicine*, 22(2): 167–170.

Rosen, L.W. & Hough, D.O. (1988) Pathogenic weight-control behaviours of female college gymnasts. *Physician and Sportsmedicine*, 16: 141–146.

Ruwaard, D. & Kramers, P.G.N. (eds) (1997) *Volksgezondheid Toekomst Verkenning 1997: de som der delen.* Utrecht: Elsevier/De Tijdstroom.

Sanborn, C.F., Horea, M., Siemers, B.J. & Dieringer, K.I. (2000) Disordered eating and the female athlete triad. *Clinics in Sports Medicine*, 19(2): 199–213.

Schmikli, S.L., Backx, F.J.G. & Bol, E. (1995) *Sportblessures Nader Uitgediept.* Bohn Stafleu Van Loghum, Houten/Diegem.

Schuller, D.E., Dankle, S.K., Martin, M. & Strauss, R.H. (1989) Auricular injury and the use of headgear in wrestlers. *Archives of Otolaryngology Head and Neck Surgery*, 115: 714–717.

Siscovick, D.S. (1997) Exercise and its role in sudden cardiac death. *Cardiology Clinics*, 15(3): 467–472.

Siscovick, D.S., Ekelund L.G., Johnson J.L. *et al.* (1991) Sensitivity of exercise electrocardiography for acute cardiac events during moderate and strenuous physical activity. *Archives of Internal Medicine*, 151: 325–330.

Siscovick, D.S., Weiss, N.S., Fletcher, R.H. & Lasky, T. (1984) The incidence of primary cardiac arrest during vigorous exercise. *The New England Journal of Medicine*, 311(14): 874–877.

Stuart, M.J. & Smith, A. (1995) Injuries in junior A ice hockey: a three year prospective study. *American Journal of Sports Medicine*, 23: 458–461.

Tegner, Y. & Lorentzen, R. (1991). Ice hockey injuries: incidence, nature and causes. *British Journal of Sports Medicine*, 25: 87–89.

van Mechelen, W. (1992) *Aetiology and Prevention of Running Injuries [dissertation].* Amsterdam: Free University of Amsterdam.

van Mechelen, W., Hlobilm, H., Kemper, H.C., Voorn, W.J. & de Jongh, H.R. (1993) Prevention of running injuries by warm-up, cool-down, and stretching exercises. *American Journal of Sports Medicine*, 21(5): 711–719.

Verhagen, E.A., van Mechelen, W. & de Vente, W. (2000) The effect of preventive measures on the incidence of ankle sprains. *Clinical Journal of Sports Medicine*, 10: 291–316.

Verhagen, E.A., van Mechelen, W. & van der Beek, A.J. (2001) The effect of tape, braces and shoes on ankle range of motion. *Sports Medicine*, 31: 667–677.

Vereeke West, R. (1998) The female athlete triad: the triad of disordered eating, amenorrhoea and osteoporosis. *Sports Medicine*, 26(2): 63–71.

Vuori, I. (1995) Reducing the number of sudden deaths in exercise. *Scandinavian Journal of Medicine and Science in Sports*, 5: 267–268.

Vuori, I. & Fentem, P. (1995) Health, position paper. In: Vuori, I., Fentem, P., Svoboda, B., Patriksson, G., Andreff, W. & Weber, W. (eds) *The Significance of Sport for Society.* Strasburg: Council of Europe Press, pp. 11–90.

Wilson, B.D. (1998) Protective headgear in rugby union. *Sports Medicine*, 25(5): 333–337.

Wirtz, P.D., Vito, G.R. & Long, D.H. (1988) Calcaneal apophysitis associated with Ttaekwondo injuries. *Journal of the American Paediatric Medical Association*, 78: 474–475.

Yde, J. & Nielsen, A.B. (1990) Sports injuries in adolescents ball games: soccer, handball and basketball. *British Journal of Sports Medicine*, **24**: 51–55.

Zandbergen, A. (undated) *Taekwondo Blessures en Fysiotherapie*. Unpublished thesis. Twentse akademie voor fysiotherapie, Enschede.

Zemper, E. (1994) Analysis of cerebral concussion frequency with the most commonly used models of football helmets. *Journal of Athletic Training*, **29**: 44–50.

Zvijac, J. & Thompson, W. (1996) Basketball. In: Caine, D.J., Caine, C.G. & Lindner, K.J. (eds) *Epidemiology of Sports Injuries*. Champaign, IL: Human Kinetics, pp. 86–97.

SECTION III

PROMOTING PHYSICAL ACTIVITY

This third section addresses physical activity promotion. Even with the most convincing evidence that physical activity is good for health, and that it involves minimal risk, the design and implementation of methods of promoting physical activity *effectively* are likely to become dominant elements of both public-health policy and research interest. Specifically, there is a need to develop the art and the science of physical activity promotion to a higher level. There is also a need to identify, support and reward those who are best placed to do this essential work. This field of research and expertise is likely to become a specialised and critical cog in the wheel that will lead to stimulating behaviour change and sustaining the behaviour long term. It can be said with some confidence that the *outcomes* of physical activity are known and accepted. In contrast, the *processes* that will lead to either individual or population level changes in physical activity are largely unknown. There is a need to raise the status of such process issues in a medical climate where outcomes are the dominant factor.

Firstly, Woods and Mutrie explore the dominant 'counselling' models that have supported physical activity promotion at the level of the individual. In recent years, these models have undoubtedly influenced how physical activity promotion programmes are designed and delivered in primary care and other settings. This is important because programmes based on behaviour-change theory have been shown to be more effective than those that are not. Given that more than eight in ten adults visit their doctor within a five-year period, the primary-care setting has increasingly been seen as a venue for reminding inactive adults about the value of becoming more active. Taylor explores this issue, evaluating how such programmes are currently delivered, and summarising the evidence relating to their effectiveness. Harris and Fox explore similar issues for physical activity promotion in schools. Finally, noting that there are serious shortfalls in any strategy that focuses only on individual level change, Kerr and colleagues consider the potential for 'environmental' interventions to stimulate physical activity on a larger scale. They describe an innovative series of studies demonstrating that simple and cost-effective changes to the built environment can result in improvements in physical activity behaviour.

CHAPTER 7

How can we get People to become more Active? A Problem Waiting to be Solved

NANETTE MUTRIE AND CATHERINE WOODS

Chapter Contents

- Adherence to physical activity
- Levels of intervention
- Theories of exercise behaviour
- Theory of Planned Behaviour
- The Transtheoretical Model (TTM) of behaviour change
- Measurement
- Theory into practice
- Conclusions

Epidemiological data has established that sedentary lifestyles increase the incidence of 'at least 17 unhealthy conditions, almost all of which are chronic diseases or considered risk factors for chronic diseases' (Booth *et al.*, 2000, p. 774). However, despite a high proportion of individuals believing in the efficacy of physical activity for obtaining and promoting good health, sedentary behaviour is prevalent in most societies and relapse from regular physical activity is also high (Allied Dunbar National Fitness Survey, 1992; Irish Universities Nutrition Alliance, 2000). Figure 7.1 shows that two thirds of European populations are not doing sufficient activity to meet current recommendations. Yet, with little variation in fundamental beliefs by age or socio-economic status,

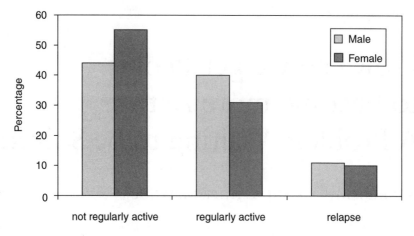

Figure 7.1   Physical activity in the European Union: percentage of males and females
Source: Kearney *et al.* (1999) *Public Health Nutrition*, **2**: 115–124

over 90 per cent of the populations in each European country believed that physical activity had many health benefits (Kearney *et al.*, 1999).

 Chapter 3 (Epidemiology) describes issues relating to how these figures may be interpreted. Chapter 8 (Primary care) discusses how physical activity may be promoted by family doctors and nurses with General Practices.

The gap between these positive beliefs and actual behaviour represents a challenge in how to increase the percentage of active people in any population. How physical activity and exercise specialists, health promoters, government or national agencies can most effectively intervene to achieve this outcome is a problem waiting to be solved. Indeed, it may be seen as one of the most pressing issues in exercise science and leaves unrealised the potential health benefits of regular activity for individuals, communities and populations.

 Chapter 11 (Biology) shows the biological responses to exercise. Chapter 12 (Anthropology) illustrates how physical activity levels can differ within and across population groups.

Adherence to physical activity

'Adherence' describes the process of initiating and maintaining physical activity or exercise. In the Natural History Model (Sallis & Hovell, 1990; Figure 7.2) exercise adherence is divided into five main categories, which offer health

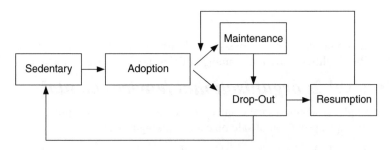

Figure 7.2 The Natural History of Exercise Model

promoters a range of different intervention 'targets'. Firstly, an inactive individual may be encouraged to adopt a physically active lifestyle. Then, once adoption is successful, maintenance of a regularly active lifestyle is the goal. However, for a variety of reasons, individuals drop out from their exercise routines. Once drop-out occurs, the individual may revert to a sedentary lifestyle, or they may restart a physically active lifestyle.

Levels of intervention

In discussing how to encourage more people to be more active, King (1994) provided an excellent framework for developing physical activity interventions that may be applied separately, or in tandem, with the different parts of the Natural History Model (Sallis & Howell, 1990). The four levels of this framework are shown in Figure 7.3. Level 1 describes how policies or legislation can influence activity levels. At this level examples include: (1) education policy to provide physical education to all pupils, (2) legal entitlement for public access to the countryside for recreation, (3) traffic-planning policy which requires cycle paths in towns, (4) making the provision of recreation facilities a legal requirement for local councils, and (5) policy documents which influence practice (for example, the Northern Ireland physical activity strategy – http://www.healthpromotionagency.org.uk – or the national quality assurance framework (NQAF) for GP Exercise Referral Schemes; Department of Health, 2001). Unfortunately, little is known about the effectiveness of Level 1 interventions. For example, the recently published NQAF for GP-referral schemes appears to be having an impact but there is no plan to evaluate how this policy might increase physical activity. Even well-intentioned policies may decrease physical activity, as happened in Australia when the wearing of cycle helmets was made compulsory (Wardlaw, 2000). The requirement for helmets suggested that cycling must be a dangerous activity and people withdrew accordingly.

- ## level 1: *legislative/policy*
  (access policies, compulsory school PE, transport policies that promote PA, facilities provision, training policies, tax incentives for activity)

- ## level 2: *organisational /environmental*
  (workplace, schools, local council initiatives, mass media approaches, prompts, provision of safe bike and walking routes)

- ## level 3: *inter-personal*
  (teaching approaches, provision of classes, peer led groups)

- ## level 4: *individual*
  (consultations, fitness assessments, written materials, postal contact, GP-referral schemes)

Figure 7. 3 Physical activity intervention levels

Source: From King, A. (1994) in Dishman, R. (ed.) *Advances in Exercise Adherence*. Human Kinetics, p. 185

Chapter 8 (Primary care) describes how this might be enacted within a general practice setting. Chapter 6 (Risks) reminds us of risks associated with physical activity. Chapter 10 (Environment) shows how environmental approaches may be developed to fit within this framework.

Level 2 of the framework focuses on how communities and organisations, such as workplaces and schools, can promote activity. For an excellent review of workplace interventions, see Dishman (1998). Increasingly, primary care is also seen as a setting where physical activity promotion can take place and an increasing number of general practices offer exercise-referral schemes (Department of Health, 2001; see Chapter 8). The World Health Authority has provided a summary of school-based interventions (http://www.who.int/hpr/archive/gshi/what.html), and Chapter 9 also provides further important insights into these issues. Higher education also has a role to play in teaching students 'transferable skills', one of which may be encouraging learning about how to lead a physically active lifestyle (Woods, Mutrie & Scott, 2002). Carney *et al.* (2000) showed that university students can transfer these adherence skills; students who were active when they graduated maintained their activity levels six months later despite the potential barriers of changing location and obtaining employment.

Chapter 9 (Schools) shows how young people can be prepared for life as a physically active student, and then as an independent adult.

Level 2 also reflects how changing the environment can help to promote physical activity. This may include using signs to encourage walking or stair use (see Chapter 10 and Chapter 11 Biddle & Mutrie, 2001), increasing the number of safe walking and cycling routes and improving countryside access. A current issue for traffic planners is to reduce levels of traffic congestion, which may in turn lead to increased physical activity. The collaboration of town planners and workplace managers may encourage active commuting to work which would increase physical activity and reduce traffic congestion (Mutrie *et al.*, in press). Mass media campaigns aimed at increasing the level of activity in a region or nation have had mixed success. In Scotland, a campaign which used television advertising to promote the message that walking was a good activity for health, created high levels of awareness of the message but little behaviour change (Wimbush *et al.*, 1997). In England, a three-year ACTIVE for LIFE campaign encouraged 'active living' (Hillsdon *et al.*, 2001) and was evaluated by three interviews with over 3000 participants. Small increases were seen in the proportion of people who knew about the active-living message, but no increases were observed in the numbers meeting the health-related activity guidelines. This evidence suggests that mass-media interventions, as currently designed, do not have significant impacts on population behaviour, though they may be important for increasing awareness. Supplementing these interventions with local support and reinforcement may lead to behaviour change, although this remains a challenge for future campaigns.

Level 3 of this model is concerned with how leaders, teachers and programme providers can create the most appropriate intra- and inter-personal climates to encourage groups of people to increase or maintain physical activity. The provision of exercise classes in private and public leisure centres is a common Level 3 intervention. Access to these centres and the classes offered there increase the choice of exercise options from aerobics to strengthening, and may be complemented by being offered in a wide range of timings and styles. However, there is still a need to encourage adherence even when this choice is available. Central to this concept of 'climate' is the way in which class leaders interact with and provide encouragement to participants. The class leader must create a positive motivational climate to foster enjoyment and hence adherence. Research conducted in physical education classes (Papaioannou & Goudas, 1999), but not yet explored in physical activity or exercise settings, suggests that positive motivation is most likely to stem from rewarding and emphasising skill mastery, personal improvement and effort (task involvement), rather than encouraging comparison with other people and competition (ego involvement).

Within the 'choice' framework it may also be important to offer options for exercising alone. Lack of time, money, confidence or inclination to attend class-based programmes and lack of class availability will all restrict the potential of class-based approaches for sustaining high levels of regular involvement in physical activities. Alternatives such as home-based programmes have been shown to be successful in creating regular activity (King *et al.*, 1991). In the UK, Mutrie *et al.* (1994) compared adherence rates over six months for participants aged over 55 in home-based and class-based exercise programmes. At the six-month follow-up, 66 per cent of the home-based and 71 per cent of the class-based participants were averaging 60 minutes of exercise a week. This high level of programme impact was surprising, since the class-based group was supported by the teacher and other class members, whereas the home-based group exercised on their own without supervision. It was concluded that home-based exercise programmes could successfully promote increased activity in this age group. Other interpersonal approaches include creating local walking groups led by peers, or buddy systems that encourage participation and that introduce people to new physical activity opportunities.

Level 4 in King's (1994) model refers to interventions aimed at individuals. Individual-level interventions include provision of fitness assessments, individual consultations, telephone contact or written interventions. Woods *et al.* (2002) used a pre-post randomised control design to investigate the effectiveness of a self-instructional intervention for helping sedentary young adults (mean age 19 years SD 4.5) to initiate physical activity. Participants were randomly assigned to either a control group (no intervention) or an experimental group (physical activity intervention). The intervention was personally focused and delivered by post. Examples of strategies suggested to the intervention group included: (1) 'read the materials that they received in the post', (2) 'become aware of how physical activity was normal in their university environment', and (3) 'make a commitment to become more active through small changes initially, and build from there'. Six months after baseline (post intervention), significantly more people in the experimental group (80 per cent), in comparison to the control group (68 per cent), were more ready to increase, or already had increased, their exercise involvement compared to baseline ($p < 0.05$).

When considering the public-health implications of King's model, Level 1 and Level 2 interventions must be further investigated and understood since they are likely to influence greater numbers of the population than Levels 3 and 4. In addition, it is clear that environmental support for activity (such as safe walking and cycling routes or sports facilities) must be in place before people can consider using them. However, to effect change at all levels there is a need to develop a knowledge and understanding of what factors – either individually or in combination – determine exercise avoidance, adoption and/or adherence. The next section of this chapter provides some guidance about theories of behaviour change that can be applied to physical activity and exercise.

Chapter 10 (Environment) shows how environmental interventions can help individuals and/or groups to become physically active.

Theories of exercise behaviour

Theories of physical activity and exercise behaviour help to develop under-standing of behaviour change in physical activity. They also allow researchers to formulate and test hypotheses and to examine the efficacy of possible explanatory mechanisms for exercise adoption and adherence. This, in turn, helps physical activity promoters, even though there is no single theory that thoroughly explains physical activity or exercise behaviour, or confirms how best to intervene. Some progress has been made in recent years in terms of understanding physical activity behaviour from a theoretical perspective (Marcus *et al.*, 1996; Biddle & Nigg, 2000), but there is still a need to develop a comprehensive theory of exercise-behaviour change that informs the design of interventions. In the UK, the recent publication of National Service Framework documents underlines the growing con-cern for effective delivery of evidence-based programmes (Chapman *et al.*, 2001).

Exercise psychology has borrowed theories of behaviour change from social-cognitive, behavioural and health psychology. These theories have then been adapted for an exercise application. The function of this chapter is not to explain all of the exercise-behaviour theories (for a more detailed account of these theories see Dishman (1994a); Marcus *et al.* (1996); Biddle & Nigg (2000); Biddle & Mutrie (2001)). Rather, we will focus on two key theories of exercise behaviour that show promise. These are the Theory of Planned Behaviour (TPB) (Ajzen, 1988) and the Transtheoretical Model of Behaviour Change (TTM) (Prochaska & DiClemente, 1983). During the 1990s these theories were more frequently cited than other exercise theories (for example, Self-Determination Theory, or Protection Motivation Theory). Both theories have also received substantial support from research investigations that explored their usefulness in understanding exercise adoption and/or adherence. These themes justify their close consideration.

From the outset it should be emphasised that these two theories focus on the individual, and do not account for an environmental perspective. Other approaches, like the ecological model (Sallis & Owen, 1999), take a broader view to understanding behaviour change in physical activity. In these approaches the individual is one component part of a complex interaction between person and environment. For a more extensive review of this concept see Chapter 10.

Theory of Planned Behaviour

This theory emerged from the Theory of Reasoned Action (TRA) (Ajzen & Fishbein, 1980). According to the TRA, whether a person becomes involved in physical activity or not can be predicted by their *intentions* toward physical activity. In turn, intention is based on two factors: (1) personal attitude to physical activity, and (2) the influence of social norms towards getting involved in physical activity. *Attitude*, which carries an emotional component, is a function of an individual's belief about physical activity (good, bad, enjoyable and so on) and how they perceive the expected outcomes of adopting this behaviour (the pros and cons). An individual's perception of what significant others (for example, parent, teacher, sibling) expect them to do and their motivation to comply is described as the *subjective social norm*.

Godin (1994) reviewed 12 studies that investigated the relationship between intention to exercise and exercise behaviour. He concluded that approximately 30 per cent of the statistical variance in exercise behaviour (that is, participation versus non-participation) could be predicted from intention alone. The attitudinal variable has been found to have a much greater influence than the social norm variable on predicting variance in intention to exercise (Hausenblas *et al.*, 1997). Example One shows how elements of the TRA/TPB can combine to influence physical activity behaviour.

Example One: The TRA/TPB in practice

Anna is an exerciser; she enjoys attending the local step-aerobics class regularly. It is a good opportunity to meet her friends and she likes being fit and active. However, at the last minute her babysitter phones to cancel. Anna has two young children and there is no crèche facility at the local gym. Anna has to phone her friend to say she cannot make it.

COMMENTARY: According to the TRA, Anna's attitude, beliefs and social norm all contributed to a positive intention to become more active. However, something outside of Anna's control – the availability of a childminder – prevented her from exercising on this particular occasion. This variable was not accounted for in the TRA, but is considered in the subsequent development of the TRA, the Theory of Planned Behaviour.

Ajzen (1988) recognised the importance of examining behaviours that may not entirely be under an individual's control. To account for this, he developed the TRA into the TPB (Figure 7.4). The TPB contains an additional variable – perceived behavioural control, in which there is a continuum of control which applies to choices about physical activity involvement, as shown in Anna's story (Example One). Perceived behavioural control is defined by Ajzen (1988, p. 132) as 'the perceived ease or difficulty of performing the behaviour'. What an individual perceives as their level of behavioural control will be a function of their previous experience of physical activity, as well as their anticipated barriers for becoming more active or maintaining a regularly active lifestyle. The opportunities, the required resources or skills, and whether or not control of these variables is possible will influence an individual's confidence. In summary, according to the TPB, perceived behavioural control as well as the attitudinal and normative variables can influence intention – and in turn can influence behaviour.

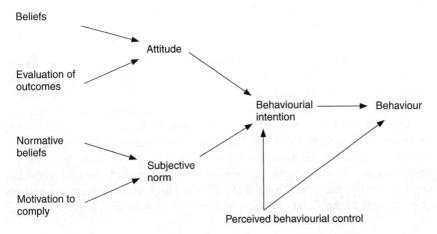

Figure 7.4 The Theory of Planned Behaviour (Ajzen, 1988)

Theory of Planned Behaviour strengths and weaknesses

Support for the TPB has been evidenced by a number of researchers (Godin, 1994; Godin & Kok, 1996; Hausenblas *et al.*, 1997). Godin & Kok (1996) found that intention and perceived behavioural control explained approximately 36 per cent of the statistical variance in exercise behaviour, though with the addition of the perceived behavioural-control variable, the TPB predicted an average of 8 per cent extra variance in exercise intention when compared to TRA. Godin comments that 'the usefulness of the theory of planned behaviour in exercise seems to be to further understand the formation of intention because, in addition to the attitudinal and normative components, perceived limitations to exercise are also considered' (1994, p. 1393). Thus, the TRA and the TPB provide physical activity promoters with clear elements around which they can build programmes that build exercise intentions.

However, most of the TRA and TPB studies reviewed were based on the ACSM (American College of Sports Medicine, 1990) 'vigorous continuous' message for physical activity, which focused on 3×20 minutes of sustained fitness training. Now the predictive capacity of the TPB needs to be examined in relation to the more contemporary 'moderate accumulative' message (CDC/ACSM, 1995; Pate *et al.*, 1995), which advocates accumulating 30 minutes of physical activity on five or more days a week. Further, researchers will also need to explore whether the relationships between the variables are unidirectional for this style of physical activity. This has been one consistent criticism of the model. There will also be a need to consider the variables that could influence social norm, and how past experiences of participation influence subsequent physical activity.

The Transtheoretical Model (TTM) of behaviour change

The TTM is an integrative and comprehensive model of behaviour change drawn from all major theories of psychotherapy (Prochaska & Norcross, 1999). Originating in research into negative addictive behaviours such as smoking, the model was used to explore how self-changers made successful changes without professional intervention (Prochaska & DiClemente, 1983; Prochaska & Norcross, 1999). It has been cited as one of the most important theoretical health-promotion developments of the 1990s (Samuelson, 1997), has been used in many studies of individual behaviour, and also in studies that compare behaviours (Prochaska *et al.*, 1994). There are four main dimensions or constructs in the TTM and each of these will now be explained.

Processes of change

The processes of change dimension describes 'how' an individual changes their behaviour. The processes of change include cognitive, affective, evaluative and behavioural strategies that an individual may use to modify a problem behaviour. Ten processes of change represent two underlying constructs: the experiential (thinking) and the behavioural (doing) processes (Prochaska *et al.*, 1988). Table 7.1 defines each of the ten processes of change as they have been conceptualised within physical activity.

Table 7.1   The processes of change as they apply to physical activity

Process	Definition
Experiential Processes	
C/raising	Undertaken by the individual to find out more about physical activity
Dramatic relief	Emotional experiences associated with change
Environmental re-evaluation	Understanding how inactivity affects the physical/social environments
Self-re-evaluation	Emotional and cognitive reappraisal of values by the individual with respect to inactivity
Social liberation	Awareness and acceptance of social changes encouraging active lifestyles
Behavioural Processes	
C/conditioning	Substitution of physical activity for sedentary behaviour
H/relationships	Seeking out social support to help initiate and maintain activity
R/management	Using rewards to encourage or maintain behaviour changes
Self-liberation	Choosing and making a commitment to change, believing in one's ability to change/control behaviours
Stimulus control	Avoiding or controlling stimuli and other causes that support inactivity

C/raising – Consciousness raising, C/conditioning – Counter conditioning, H/relationships – Helping relationships and R/management – Reinforcement management.

The Stages of Change (SOC)

The SOC represent the temporal dimension of the TTM; stages identify the 'when' element of behaviour change. Although there are debates about precise definitions, there are essentially five stages of exercise-behaviour change. These are

1. precontemplation (sedentary individuals who have no intention of changing their behaviour),
2. contemplation (sedentary individuals and intention to become more active),
3. preparation (irregularly active and intention to become more regularly active),
4. action (regular physical activity for the past six months), and
5. maintenance (regularly physically active for longer than six months).

Individuals are thought to move through the SOC at different rates. Whereas the time to progress through the stages is variable, the 'set of tasks' which have to be accomplished at each SOC are less variable (Prochaska & Norcross, 1999). Originally, progression through the stages was conceived as linear, as individuals were thought to progress from one stage to another in a simple discrete fashion (Prochaska *et al.*, 1992). However, linear progression – though possible – has been identified as rare (Prochaska & Norcross, 1999). This has led to the TTM being conceptualised into a spiral pattern (Figure 7.5).

In this spiral pattern, people in each stage can reflect elements of both stability and change depending on the individual. For example, individuals progress through the SOC at different rates, with some individuals remaining in certain stages while others relapse to earlier stages. People who relapse may recycle within the stages, or for a variety of reasons, for example, guilt or embarrassment, may return to precontemplation. A large number of relapsers recycle back to contemplation or to preparation (Prochaska & Norcross, 1999), though the

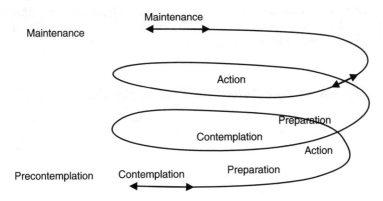

Figure 7.5   A Spiral Model depicting progression or regression through the Stages of Exercise Behaviour Change

spiral model suggests that most relapsers do not revolve endlessly, nor do they regress into the stages with least potential for change. Rather, as a result of their recycling through the stages, relapsers may learn from their mistakes and be more successful in subsequent change efforts (DiClemente *et al.*, 1991).

Self-efficacy

Self-efficacy is a central concept within the TTM. It implies that if a person feels confident in their ability to perform a desired behaviour, within a specific setting, then they are more likely to engage in that activity (Bandura, 1977, 1986). Self-efficacy is developed through past performance, vicarious experience (that is, learning from others), verbal persuasion (reinforcement) and physiological feedback (Bandura, 1986; King *et al.*, 1992). Therefore, feeling confident about successfully adopting and maintaining a regular exercise routine, and believing in the benefits of being regularly active, increases the likelihood of an individual being regularly active, compared to an individual who does not feel confident, and does not accept physical activity as a 'normal' behavioural option. Bandura (1986) noted that highly self-efficacious individuals tend to take on more challenging tasks, expend more effort, and persist longer in the face of obstacles, barriers and aversive or stressful stimuli.

Exercise-specific self-efficacy is directly linked to SOC, though causality has not been confirmed. Cross-sectional data shows that the most efficacious individuals are most likely to be regularly active, and vice versa. Thus, precontemplators have reported lower self-efficacy scores than maintainers (Bock *et al.*, 1998).

Decisional balance

In contemporary TTM studies, decision-making (Janis & Mann, 1977) reflects the balance of the co-existing pros and the cons for changing (Marcus *et al.*, 1992), and their use is systematically arranged with SOC in a wide range of health behaviours (Prochaska *et al.*, 1994). Specifically, as progress through SOC takes place there is an increase in the evaluation of the benefits (pros) over the barriers (cons) of regular activity.

Example Two: The TTM in practice

Peter until recently was in the precontemplation stage of exercise behaviour. He is currently recovering from his first myocardial infarction (MI); this was mild but completely unexpected. When he was in hospital Peter read that a physically active lifestyle has potential health benefits for him. Peter is thinking seriously about becoming more active, putting him in the contemplation stage. However, he feels scared that he could 'over do' things and he does not see himself as 'the sporty type'. His exercise self-efficacy is low, and currently his Cons for changing outweigh his Pros on a decisional-balance scale. On recommendation from his GP, Peter approaches an exercise consultant for advice.

According to the TTM, the shock of having an MI is linked to a cognitive-change process (dramatic relief) that prompted Peter to change so that he became serious about adopting a more physically active lifestyle. During the initial stages of change Peter will need to identify and then weigh up the personal Pros and Cons to him of becoming more active, to establish ways of improving his exercise self-efficacy and to increase his use of the experiential processes of change. These include consciousness raising (for example, read more about how to initiate a physically active lifestyle) and self-re-evaluation (for example, evaluating 'what's in it for me?').

TTM strengths and weaknesses

The TTM is supported by extensive research in physical activity and exercise, most of which has been completed in the 1990s. This suggests that much of what is known is likely to require replication, and as a result will almost certainly be refined and improved. As a theoretical model the TTM helps to understand how physical activity and exercise are initiated, adopted and sustained. Because it has a temporal dimension, the TTM has mapped out when shifts in attitudes, intentions and behaviours are most likely to occur. This has advanced our understanding of how to target and recruit different groups depending on how ready they are to change, and it has positively affected retention rates. The model may also now be further developed to consider changing multiple risk behaviours rather than tackling them separately (Herrick *et al.*, 1997; LaForge *et al.*, 1999).

However, as with all models, the TTM has its problems. First, the SOC component of the TTM describes a simple, categorical relationship between intention and behaviour. Behavioural intention is central to understanding when an individual is likely to change from leading a sedentary lifestyle to becoming more physically active. This readiness to change has been central to the design, delivery and evaluation of stage-matched interventions. However, compared with other models, such as TPB, the TTM does not give close attention to behavioural intention, and this implies that there is still scope for the further development of the model. Second, the TTM advocates individual responsibility for behaviour change. The TTM was designed to help clarify the concept of intentional behaviour change, and it does not examine societal, developmental or imposed change. Third, all stage models have an inherent ethical issue (Oldenburg *et al.*, 1999), which revolves around the notion of offering specific treatment to individuals in one stage, but not to those in other stages. Even though it may be evidence-based, intentionally *not* advising sedentary patients to exercise – because the TTM shows that they lack change potential – may be seen as unethical. However, finite resources have to be used to target all individuals. This model identifies individuals in the 'hard-to-reach group' and provides an approach for targeting limited resources in an effective and efficient manner. Future qualitative research needs to explore the experiences of precontemplators are targeted within health-promotion interventions.

Chapter 8 (Primary care) describes how approaches used within General Practices can help to target individuals or groups.

The debate about the nature of the TTM is well-documented (Davidson, 1992; Bandura, 1997, 1998; Weinstein *et al.*, 1998; Rollnick *et al.*, 1999). Bandura (1997) suggested that the TTM is at best a theoretical, rather than a transtheoretical model, because it is essentially eclectic through its integration of diverse systems of psychotherapy, such as psychoanalysis and humanism. The assumption that successful self-changers use processes that some theorists consider incompatible has yet to be proven and may be best explored in longitudinal studies of change, or in naturalistic studies of change as it happens.

In contrast, TTM proponents support the view that apparently incompatible processes from competing theories can be integrated in the change process and applied at appropriate stages. In Example Two, Peter could benefit from the powerful effects of planning the first steps he will take (also known as implementation intentions) as he moves into the preparation stage for his newly active lifestyle (Gollwitzer, 1999). Successful integration of perspectives from a wide range of theoretical perspectives may have important practical value, and a new generation of studies will integrate these perspectives in the search for the most powerful factors in initiating and sustaining change (for example, Courneya & Bobick, 2000; Courneya *et al.*, 2001).

The TTM has allowed researchers to identify and work with sedentary populations, and to explore how change occurs, or less often to investigate why it does not (McKenna & Francis, in press). Distinctive use of the processes of change has also been identified across the SOC (Prochaska & DiClemente, 1983; Marcus & Simkin, 1993; Marcus *et al.*, 1996). This suggested that in helping someone to modify a behaviour, once SOC is established then the processes of change most applicable to that SOC would be used to design an intervention. This provides the exercise consultant with an effective way of helping an individual to adopt a physically active lifestyle. Research has begun to demonstrate that an integration of the stages and processes of change can provide a useful guide for physical activity interventions (Marcus *et al.*, 1998). Yet, more longitudinal research is needed to determine the exact nature of the interaction between the stages and processes of change, such as that recently undertaken by Plotnikoff *et al.* (2001). This needs to be undertaken both inside and outside formal exercise interventions. Research also needs to address the question of why people do not change their exercise behaviour and some people do, despite being exposed to the most (evidence-based) powerful behaviour-change interventions. An on-going research problem is that we still do not fully understand why people opt not to change from being inactive, or how they sustain positive change (Muehrer, 2000; Rothman, 2000).

Measurement

The core components of the TPB and the TTM are typically measured through self-report instruments. Many of the physical activity-assessment instruments were adapted from those developed for other health behaviours (for example, Prochaska *et al.*, 1988). Measuring instruments comprise of a range of ordered categorical, true/false, bipolar and Likert scales. Table 7.2 provides examples of measurement for the TPB.

Transtheoretical model of behaviour change

1. It is normally recommended to use a five-point ordered categorical measure as an accurate and expedient method of assessing exercise SOC (Mutrie & Caddell, 1994; Cardinal, 1995a,b; Cardinal, 1997b; Richards *et al.*, 1997). The measure would include a clear definition of each SOC, a complete definition of physical activity including reference to frequency (how often), intensity (how hard) duration of the activity (how long), and examples of activities. Each of these increase the accuracy with which respondents classify themselves into the stages. The respondent should select what they think is the most appropriate SOC for them (Mutrie & Caddell, 1994), and under these conditions the Kappa index of reliability over a two-week period was 0.78 (Marcus *et al.*, 1992).

Table 7.2 Examples of measurement items for the components of the Theory of Planned Behaviour

Variable (Authors)	Scale	Example of measurement item	Cronbach's Alpha
Attitude (Courneya & Bobick, 2000)	7-point bipolar scale Instrument (for example, useful–useless, harmful–beneficial) Affective (for example, enjoyable–unenjoyable, boring–interesting)	'For me to participate in regular exercise is…'	0.81
Subjective Social Norm (Courneya *et al.*, 1999)	3 items 7-point Likert scale from 1 (strongly disagree) to 7 (strongly agree)	'Most people who are important to me think I should participate in regular physical exercise'	0.81
Perceived Behavioural Control (Courneya *et al.*, 1999)	5 items 7-point Likert scale ranging from 1 (very little control) to 7 (complete control).	'How much control do you have over participating in regular exercise?'	0.83
Behavioural Intention (Courneya *et al.*, 2000)	3 items 7-point Likert scale from 1 (strongly disagree) to 7 (strongly agree)	'My goal is to participate in physical exercise at least three times per week, every week'	0.83

Its significant association with the Seven Day Recall Physical Activity Questionnaire (Marcus & Simkin, 1993) demonstrated the concurrent validity of the SOC measure.

2. Processes of change can be assessed using the questionnaire developed by Marcus *et al.* (1992). A five-point Likert scale, never (1) to frequently (5), allows individuals to rate how frequently they used each process of change during the previous month. The processes are each scored in the range 4–20, after combining the responses to four items. Marcus *et al.* (1992) have demonstrated good reliability and validity for this measure. However, a number of authors, such as Plotnikoff *et al.* (2000); Rosen (2000); Mutrie *et al.* (in press); McKenna and Francis (in press), have recently suggested that the relationship of the processes with the stages may differ for physical activity as compared to other behaviours. Indeed, the relationship may even differ across physical activity modes (Miilun-palo *et al.*, 2000). Woods (unpublished PhD thesis) highlighted the import-ant difference between frequency-of-use versus the importance an individual may attach to using a particular process. More fully explored, these issues will improve our understanding of behaviour change in physical activity.

3. Exercise self-efficacy and exercise decisional balance are both measured using the short Likert-based measures developed by Marcus and Owen (1992). Good validity and reliability for both of these measures has been demonstrated (Cardinal, 1997a). The self-efficacy items request respond-ents to indicate how confident they feel (one – not at all confident to seven – extremely confident) in their ability to exercise in different circum-stances, for example, 'When I am tired' or 'When it is raining or snowing'. The decisional balance (Marcus & Simkin, 1993; Marcus *et al.*, 1994; Wyse *et al.*, 1995; Cardinal *et al.*, 1998) measure asks respondents to indicate how important (one – not at all important to seven – extremely important) statements such as 'I would be healthier if I exercise regularly' are for them. A separate summative score is achieved for each of the Cons and the Pros subscales, although because they are based on different numbers of contributing items, standardisation into T-scores is often necessary.

Theory into practice

In this section we offer a simple acronym 'ACTIVE' to assist individuals to adopt and adhere to a physically active lifestyle. This acronym is shown in Example Three, and is based on basic principles of behaviour change and on current physical activity recommendations. In addition, two case studies are offered to illustrate the theories of behaviour change in practice for both clinical and non-clinical settings.

Putting theory into practice: A simple acronym for increasing adherence – ACTIVE

A – Add: Total all bouts of physical activity each day, 'Some is better than none.'

C – Confidence: Chose an activity that you feel confident that you can do.

T – Time: Add minutes to your daily routine gradually, aim for 30 minutes or more each day.

I – Intensity: Work a pace that you find comfortable and build your effort gradually.

V – Variety: Aerobic activities include walking, gardening, and physically demanding housework. Be active on your own, with friends, in a group. Muscular endurance, strength and flexibility are also important and can add variety to your routine.

E – Enjoyment: If you don't like an activity, don't do it! Choose an activity that you enjoy.

The primary purpose of an intervention is to change behaviour, in this case physical activity behaviour. To do this, the strategies that modify human behaviour from the norm of sedentariness to being regularly physically active need to be identified, studied and targeted efficiently. This section will give an example of a theoretically based intervention study.

Case Study 1 General Population

The *Project Active* intervention study (Dunn *et al.*, 1999) recruited sedentary adults (N = 235, mean age = 45 (range 35–60), 56 per cent female) from a local community sample and then randomised participants into one of two intervention arms. In the lifestyle physical activity programme staff promoted the lifestyle activity message – accumulate at least 30 minutes of moderate intensity physical activity most days of the week (CDC/ACSM, 1995; Department of Health, 2001). In the structured traditional exercise programme, participants were encouraged to exercise 3–5 days a week, exercise intensity of 50–85 per cent of maximal aerobic power and duration of 20–60 minutes an exercise session (ACSM, 1990). Data was collected at baseline, 6 months, 24 months. Both groups received six months of intensive, plus a further 18 months of maintenance support over the two-year trial. In the first six months, people in the structured-exercise group were provided with supervised exercise sessions five days a week for six months in a local fitness centre. Participants were asked to attend at least three supervised sessions and gradually increase their sessions to five a week. In contrast, the lifestyle group received a stage-matched intervention designed using cognitive and behavioural change strategies based on the TTM. They met in small groups for an hour, one night a week for the first 16 weeks and then with decreasing frequency during weeks 17–24. Participants learned strategies to help them maintain an active lifestyle.

Case Study 1 (*Cont'd*)

Both intervention groups produced significant and comparable beneficial changes in physical activity, cardio-respiratory fitness, blood pressure and percentage body fat at 24 months. The conclusion was that a stage-based lifestyle approach to increasing physical activity in sedentary populations is as effective over 24 months as more traditional structured-exercise approaches.

Case Study 2 Clinical Population

Steptoe *et al.* (2000) used the TTM to effect behaviour change within a clinical sample. Adults with one or more modifiable cardiovascular disease risk factors were chosen as participants. Almost 2000 subjects were recruited from 20 general practices. Fifty-four per cent of the subjects were female. Participants were randomly assigned into either an experimental or a control group. Data was collected at baseline, 4 and 12 months. The intervention group received three behavioural counselling sessions (20-minutes duration), together with follow-up phone calls. These were aimed at reducing fat intake and smoking and increasing physical activity, and were carried out by a practice nurse. Seventy per cent of patients completed the four-month assessment, 60 per cent completed that at 12 months, and 883 completed the study. Targets for physical activity were based on the traditional structured exercise message (frequency of 3–5 days a week, exercise intensity of 50–85 per cent of maximal aerobic power and duration of 20–60 minutes per each exercise session – ACSM, 1990). Within this framework the participants chose the activities to match their preferences. The intervention group showed greater reductions in dietary fat, smoking cessation and increased amounts of physical activity than the control group at both measurements (4 and 12 months).

Some caution is required in interpreting many of the intervention studies in this area. Many samples have been self-selected which can introduce socially desirable responses. Most studies also rely on self-reported physical activity, and these devices are affected by over-reporting the minutes of actual activity (Marcus *et al.*, 1994; Lowther *et al.*, 1999), and compared with objective devices, these invariably demonstrate low concurrent validity. Until unobtrusive measurement devices are available cheaply (see Cooper, Chapter 5), population-based interventions are likely to continue to rely on self-report.

 Chapter 5 (Measurement) describes the scientific issues surrounding accurate measurement of physical activity.

Conclusions

Physical activity is a complex and dynamic behaviour. Individuals change their intention, behaviour, attitude, and their reasons for exercising many times before a stable behaviour can be established. Further studies of individual theories will help to improve understanding of their relevance to positive physical activity change, both in interventions and through self-change. Studies that combine theoretical perspectives will help to identify the most powerful factors in initiating and sustaining change. With a better understanding of how these elements are used in effective change attempts, researchers and practitioners will be closer to the solutions of how to get more people more active.

References

Ajzen, I. (1988) *Attitudes, Personality and Behaviour*. Milton Keynes: Open University Press.

Ajzen, I. & Fishbein, M. (1980) Understanding attitudes and predicting social behaviour. Englewood Cliffs, NJ: Prentice-Hall.

Allied Dunbar National Fitness Survey (1992) Allied Dunbar National Fitness Survey: A summary of the major findings and messages from the Allied Dunbar National Fitness Survey (Rep. No. 1). London: Allied Dunbar, HEA & Sports Council.

American College of Sports Medicine (1990) The recommended quantity and quality of exercise for developing and maintaining cardiorespiratory and muscular fitness in healthy adults. *Medicine and Science in Sports and Exercise*, 2: 265–274.

Bandura, A. (1977) Self-efficacy: toward a unifying theory of behavioural change. *Psychological Review*, **84**: 191–215.

Bandura, A. (1986) Social foundations of thought and action: a social cognitive theory. Englewood Cliffs, NJ: Prentice-Hall.

Bandura, A. (1997) The anatomy of stages of change. *American Journal of Health Promotion*, **12**: 8–10.

Biddle, S. & Mutrie, N. (2001) *Psychology of Physical Activity: Determinants, Well-being and Interventions. (2 ed.)* London: Routledge.

Biddle, S. & Nigg, C.R. (2000) Theories of exercise behaviour. *International Journal of Psychology*, **31**: 290–304.

Bock, B.C., Marcus, B.H., Rossi, J.S. & Redding, C.A. (1998) Motivational readiness for change: diet, exercise and smoking. *American Journal of Health Behaviour*, **22**: 248–258.

Booth, F., Gordon, S., Carlson, C. & Hamilton, M. (2000) Waging war on modern chronic diseases: primary prevention through exercise biology. *Journal of Applied Physiology*, **88**: 774–787.

Cardinal, B.J. (1995a) Behavioural and biometric comparisons of the preparation, action and maintenance stages of exercise. *Wellness Perspectives: Research, Theory, and Practice*, **11**: 36–43.

Cardinal, B.J. (1995b) The stages of exercise scale and stages of exercise behaviour in female adults. *Journal of Sports Medicine and Physical Fitness*, **35**: 87–92.

Cardinal, B.J. (1997a) Construct validity of stages of change for exercise behaviour. *American Journal of Health Promotion*, **12**: 68–74.

Cardinal, B.J. (1997b) Predicting exercise behaviour using components of the transtheoretical model of behaviour change. *Journal of Sport Behaviour*, **20**: 272–283.

Cardinal, B.J., Engels, H.J. & Zhu, W. (1998) Application of the transtheoretical model of behaviour change to preadolescents' physical activity and exercise behaviour. *Pediatric Exercise Science*, **10**: 69–80.

Carney, C., Mutrie, N. & McNeish, S. (2000) The transition from University and its effect on physical activity patterns. *International Journal of Health Promotion and Education*, **38**: 113–118.

Chapman, G., Adam, S. & Stockford, D. (2001) National Service Frameworks; promoting the public health. *Journal of Epidemiology and Community Health*, **55**: 373–374.

Courneya, K.S. & Bobick, T. (2000) Integrating the theory of planned behaviour with the processes and stages of change in the exercise domain. *Psychology of Sport and Exercise*, **1**: 41–56.

Courneya, K.S., Bobick, T. & Schinke, R. (1999) Does the theory of planned behaviour mediate the relation between personality and exercise behaviour? *Basic and Applied Social Psychology*, **21**: 317.

Courneya, K.S., Plotnikoff, R.C., Hotz, S.B. & Birkett, N.J. (2001) Predicting exercise stage transitions over two consecutive 6-month periods: A test of the theory of planned behaviour in a population-based sample. *British Journal of Health Psychology*, 6: 135–150.

Davidson, R. (1992) Prochaska and DiClemente's model of change: A case study. *British Journal of Addiction*, 87: 821–822.

Department of Health (2001) *Exercise Referral Systems: A National Quality Assurance Framework.* London: Department of Health.

DiClemente, C.C., Prochaska, J.O., Fairhurst, S.K., Velicer, W.F., Velasquez, M.M. & Rossi, J.S. (1991) The process of smoking cessation: an analysis of precontemplation, contemplation, and preparation stages of change. *Journal of Consulting and Clinical Psychology*, 59: 295–304.

Dishman, R.K. (1994) *Advances in Exercise Adherence.* Champaign, IL: Human Kinetics.

Dishman, R.K. (1994a) The measurement conundrum in exercise adherence research. *Medicine and Science in Sports and Exercise*, 26: 1382–1390.

Dishman, R.K., Oldenburg, B., O'Neal, H. & Shephard, R.J. (1998) Worksite physical activity interventions. *American Journal of Preventive Medicine*, 15: 344–361.

Dunn, A.L., Marcus, B.H., Kampert, J.B., Garcia, M.E., Kohl, H.W. & Blair, S.N. (1999) Comparison of lifestyle and structured interventions to increase physical activity and cardio-respiratory fitness. *Journal of the American Medical Association*, 281: 327–334.

Godin, G. (1994) Theories of reasoned action and planned behaviour: usefulness for exercise promotion. *Medicine and Science in Sports and Exercise*, 26: 1391–1394.

Godin, G. & Kok, G. (1996) The theory of planned behaviour: A review of its applications to health-related behaviours. *American Journal of Health Promotion*, 11: 87–98.

Gollwitzer, P.M. (1999) Implementation intentions: strong effects of simple plans, *American Psychologist*, 54: 493–503.

Hausenblas, H., Carron, A. & Mack, D. (1997) Application of the theories of reasoned action and planned behaviour: A meta-analysis. *Journal of Sport and Exercise Psychology*, 19: 36–51.

Herrick, A.B., Stone, W.J. & Mettler, M.M. (1997) Stages of change, decisional balance, and self-efficacy across four health behaviours in a worksite environment. *American Journal of Health Promotion*, 12: 49–56.

Hillsdon, M., Cavill, N., Nanchahal, K., Diamond, A. & White, I.R. (2001) National level promotion of physical activity: results from England's ACTIVE for LIFE campaign. *Journal of Epidemiology and Community Health*, 155: 755–761.

Irish Universities Nutrition Alliance (2000) Results of a survey on consumer attitudes to physical activity, body-weight and health in a nationally representative sample of Irish adults. Dublin: Trinity College.

Janis, I.L. & Mann, L. (1977) *Decision Making: A Psychological Analysis of Conflict, Choice and Commitment.* New York: Collier Macmillan.

Kearney, J.M., de Graff, C., Damkjaer, S. & Magnus Engstrom, L. (1999) Stages of change towards physical activity in a nationally representative sample in the European Union. *Public Health Nutrition*, 2: 115–124.

King, A.C. (1994) Clinical and community interventions to promote and support physical activity participation. In: Dishman, R.K. (ed.) *Advances in Exercise Adherence*, Champaign, IL: Human Kinetics, pp. 183–212.

King, A.C., Blair, S.N., Bild, D.E., Dishman, R.K., Dubbert, P.M., Marcus, B.H., Oldridge, N.B., Paffenbarger, R.S., Powell, K.E. & Yeager, K.K. (1992) Determinants of physical activity and interventions in adults. *Medicine and Science in Sports and Exercise*, 24: S221–S235.

King, A.C., Haskell, W.L., Taylor, B., Kraemer, H.C. & DeBusk, R.F. (1991) Group vs. home-based exercise training in healthy older men and women. *Journal of the American Medical Association*, 266: 1535–1542.

LaForge, R.G., Velicer, W.F., Richmond, R.L. & Owen, N. (1999) Stage distribution for five health behaviours in the United States and Australia. *Preventive Medicine*, 28: 61–74.

Lowther, M., Mutrie, N., Loughlan, C. & McFarlane, C. (1999) Development of a Scottish physical activity questionnaire: a tool for use in physical activity interventions. *British Journal of Sports Medicine*, 33: 244–249.

McKenna, J. & Francis C. (in press) Exercise contemplators; unravelling the processes of change. *Health Education.*

Marcus, B.H., Eaton, C.A., Rossi, J.S. & Harlow, L.L. (1994) Self-efficacy, decision-making, and stages of change: an integrative model of physical exercise. *Journal of Applied Social Psychology,* **24**: 489–508.

Marcus, B.H., Emmons, K.M. & Simkin-Silverman, L. (1998) Evaluation of motivationally tailored vs. standard self-help physical activity interventions at the workplace. *American Journal of Health Promotion,* **12**: 246–253.

Marcus, B.H., King, A.C., Pinto, B.M. & Bock, B.C. (1996) Theories and techniques for promoting physical activity behaviours. *Sports Medicine,* **22**: 321–331.

Marcus, B.H. & Owen, N. (1992) Motivational readiness, self-efficacy and decision-making for exercise. *Journal of Applied Social Psychology,* **1**: 3–16.

Marcus, B.H., Pinto, B.M., Simkin, L.R., Audrain, J.E. & Taylor, E.R. (1994) Application of theoretical models to exercise behaviour among employed women. *American Journal of Health Promotion,* **9**: 49–55.

Marcus, B.H., Rakowski, W. & Rossi, J.S. (1992) Assessing motivational readiness and decision making for exercise. *Health Psychology,* **11**: 257–261.

Marcus, B.H., Rossi, J.S., Selby, V.C., Niaura, R.S. & Abrams, D.B. (1992) The stages and processes of exercise adoption and maintenance in a worksite sample. *Health Psychology,* **11**: 386–395.

Marcus, B.H. & Simkin, L.R. (1993) The stages of exercise behaviour. *Journal of Sports Medicine and Physical Fitness,* **33**: 83–88.

Marcus, B.H., Selby, V.C., Niaura, R.S. & Rossi, J.S. (1992) Self-efficacy and the stages of exercise behaviour change. *Research Quarterly for Exercise and Sport,* **63**: 60–66.

Marcus, B.H., Simkin, L.R., Rossi, J.S. & Pinto, B.M. (1996) Longitudinal shifts in employees' stages and processes of exercise behaviour change. *American Journal of Health Promotion,* **10**: 195–200.

Miilunpalo, S., Nupponen, R., Laitakari, J., Marttila, J. & Paronen, O. (2000) Stages of change in two modes of health-enhancing physical activity: Methodological aspects and promotional implications. *Health Education Research: Theory and Practice,* **15**: 435–448.

Muehrer, P. (2000) Research on adherence, behaviour change, and mental health: a workshop overview. *Health Psychology,* **19**: 304–307.

Mutrie, N. & Caddell, C. (1994) Stages of exercise behaviour change in corporate employees. *Journal of Sports Sciences,* **12**: 202–203.

Mutrie, N., Blamey, A., Davison, R. & Kelly, M. (1994) Adherence to home-based and class-based exercise programmes for older adults. Proceedings of the 10th Commonwealth Games Scientific Congress Vancouver, Canada, August 9–14, pp. 262–265.

Mutrie, N., Carney, C., Blamey, A., Crawford, F., Aitchison, T. & Whitelaw, A. (2002) "Walk in to Work Out": A randomised controlled trial of a self-help intervention to promote active commuting. *Journal of Epidemiology and Community Health,* **56**: 407–412.

Oldenburg, B., Glanz, K. & Ffrench, M. (1999) The application of staging models to the understanding of health behaviour change and the promotion of health. *Psychology and Health,* **14**: 503–516.

Papaioannou, A. & Goudas, M. (1999) Motivational climate of the physical education class. In: Vanden Auweele, Y., Bakker, F., Biddle, S., Durand, M. & Seiler, R. (eds) *Psychology for Physical Educators.* Champaign, Il: Human Kinetics, pp. 51–68.

Pate, R.R., Pratt, M., Blair, S.N., Haskell, W.L., Macera, C.A., Bouchard, C. *et al.* (1995) Physical activity and public health: a recommendation from the centres for disease control and prevention and the American college of sports medicine. *Journal of the American Medical Association,* **273**: 402–407.

Plotnikoff, R.C., Hotz, S.B., Birkett, N.J. & Courneya, K.S. (2001) Exercise and the transtheoretical model: A longitudinal test of a population sample. *Preventive Medicine,* **33**: 441–452.

Prochaska, J.O. & DiClemente, C.C. (1983) Stages and processes of self-change of smoking : Toward an integrative model of change. *Journal of Consulting and Clinical Psychology,* **51**: 390–395.

Prochaska, J.O., DiClemente, C.C. & Norcross, J.C. (1992) In search of how people change. *American Psychologist*, **47**: 1102–1114.

Prochaska, J.O. & Norcross, J.C. (eds) (1999) Comparative conclusions: toward a transtheoretical therapy. In: *Systems of Psychotherapy: A Transtheoretical Analysis* (4 edn) Pacific Grove, CA: Brooks/Cole Publishing Company, pp. 487–528.

Prochaska, J.O., Velicer, W.F., DiClemente, C.C. & Fava, J. (1988) Measuring processes of change: application to the cessation of smoking. *Journal of Consulting and Clinical Psychology*, **56**: 520–528.

Prochaska, J.O., Velicer, W.F., Rossi, J.S., Goldstein, M.G., Marcus, B.H., Rakowski, W., Fiore, C., Harlow, L.L., Redding, C.A., Rosenbloom, D. & Rossi, R.R. (1994) Stages of change and decisional balance for 12 problem behaviours. *Health Psychology*, **13**: 39–46.

Richards, R.G., Velicer, W.F., Prochaska, J.O., Rossi, J.S. & Marcus, B.H. (1997) What makes a good staging algorithm: examples from regular exercise. *American Journal of Health Promotion*, **12**: 57–66.

Rollnick, S., Mason, P. & Butler, C. (1999) *Health Behaviour Change a Guide for Practitioners*. London: Churchill Livingston.

Rosen, C. (2000) Is the sequencing of change processes by stage consistent across health behaviours? A meta-analysis. *Health Psychology*, **19**: 593–604.

Rothman, A.J. (2000) Toward a theory-based analysis of behavioural maintenance. *Health Psychology*, **19**: (Suppl.) 64–69.

Sallis, J. & Owen, N. (1999) *Physical Activity and Behavioural Medicine*. London: Sage Publications.

Sallis, J.F. & Hovell, M.F. (1990) Determinants of exercise behaviour. *Exercises and Sports Sciences Reviews*, **18**: 307–330.

Samuelson, M. (1997) Changing unhealthy lifestyle: who's ready . . . who's not? An argument in support of the stages of change component of the transtheoretical model. *American Journal of Health Promotion*, **12**: 13.

Steptoe, A., Doherty, S., Rink, E., Kerry, S., Kendrick, T. & Hilton, S. (2000) Behavioural counselling in general practice for the promotion of healthy behaviour among adults at increased risk of coronary heart disease. *British Medical Journal*, **319**: 943–948.

Wardlaw, M.J. (2000) Three lessons for a better cycling future. *British Medical Journal*, **321**: 1582–1585.

Weinstein, N.D., Rothman, A.J. & Sutton, S.R. (1998) Stage theories of health behaviour: Conceptual and methodological issues. *Health Psychology*, **17**: 290–299.

Woods, C.B. Exercise behaviour change in a young adult population: A qualitative and quantitative study. Unpublished PhD thesis, University of Glasgow, Scotland.

Woods, C.B., Mutrie, N. & Scott, M. (2002) A transtheoretical model based intervention designed to help sedentary young adults become active. *Health Education Research: Theory and Practice*, **17(4)**, 451–460.

Wimbush, E., Macgregor, A. & Fraser, E. (1997) Impacts of a mass media campaign on walking in Scotland. *Health Promotion International*, **13**: 45–53.

Wyse, J., Mercer, T., Ashford, B., Buxton, K. & Gleeson, N. (1995) Evidence for the validity and utility of the stages of exercise behaviour change scale in young adults. *Health Education Research*, **10**: 365–377.

CHAPTER 8

The role of Primary Care in Promoting Physical Activity

ADRIAN TAYLOR

There is now substantial evidence that regular physical activity is beneficial for health, well-being and quality of life (Bouchard *et al.*, 1994; Pate *et al.*, 1995; US Department of Health and Human Services, 1996; Van Tulder *et al.*, 1997; ACSM, 1998; Campbell *et al.*, 1998; Abenhaim *et al.*, 2000; Batty & Thune, 2000; Biddle *et al.*, 2000; Department of Health, 2000a, 2000b, 2001a; McMurdo *et al.*, 2000; Blair & Jackson, 2001). Despite this accumulation of knowledge, levels of inactivity and associated health problems are increasing (Department of Health, 2000c; National Audit Office, 2001) throughout industrialised nations and the trend is expected to continue. The challenge is therefore to facilitate and encourage more physically active lifestyles.

Most importantly, in the past 20 years, epidemiologists, public-health consultants, health-promotion specialists, exercise scientists and social scientists have begun to investigate what factors influence exercise adherence

(Dishman, 1994; Sallis & Owen, 1999) and what interventions are most effective in increasing physical activity. It has become clear that it is necessary to promote physical activity at a variety of levels (for example, at population, community and individual level), in a variety of settings (for example, schools, workplace, primary and secondary health care, and so on) and in partnership with a variety of agencies (HDA, 2000). For example, the efforts of one general practitioner (GP) who is keen to promote physical activity to his or her patients may have little impact on the health and well-being of a whole community. Physical activity promotion must therefore be guided by a policy-driven infrastructure that supports evidence-based interventions. Efforts have focused on understanding the psychological processes that explain why individuals are active or not. Increasingly, we are learning more about how important others can be in reinforcing behavioural change, and also, how environments or settings can be designed to facilitate physically active options.

 Chapter 10 (Environment) shows how environmental development can be an important element of policy.

One setting where increases in physical activity may be facilitated is in primary health care (PHC): that is where patients initially come into contact with health-care services (with the exception of accident and emergency departments in hospital settings). Over 70 per cent of the population in the UK visit their GP at least once a year and almost 95 per cent do so over a three-year period (OPCS, 1995). Given the high contact rate, and the high esteem generally attached to GPs and health professionals working in PHC, particularly among older people, one may speculate that an opportunity exists for the promotion of physical activity. Increasingly, health and exercise professionals, and exercise scientists, are finding themselves working within or in partnership with the primary health-care team (Department of Health, 2001b). This chapter will offer new ideas for career opportunities and open new areas of work for existing practitioners, founded on the most current evidence for effective interventions.

The chapter will address three main questions, namely:

1. What approaches have been used in association with primary health care to promote physical activity?
2. Can interventions delivered in association with primary health care increase levels of physical activity?
3. What do we need to know to make PHC interventions more effective?

In order to answer these questions it is important to provide a framework in which to systematically consider these questions. Figure 8.1 shows a model for promoting physical activity in primary care that will be used throughout the chapter.

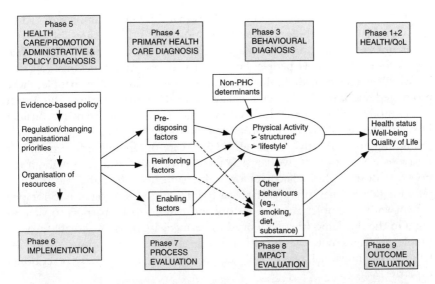

Figure 8.1 A framework for promoting physical activity in primary care

This has a foundation in the PRECEDE-PROCEED health promotion model described by Green & Kreuter (1991). The 9-Phase Model provides a useful tool to develop, implement and evaluate policy which can drive interventions to maximum effectiveness using a whole-systems approach. In considering Phases 1–4 a diagnosis of why and how physical activity is promoted through PHC will be considered, then through Phases 7–9 the potential of interventions to increase levels of physical activity will be considered.

Phases 1 and 2: health and quality-of-life diagnosis

Green and Kreuter differentiated between quality of life (Phase 2) and health status (Phase 1). This differentiation is not important here and so they will be treated together. The consideration in these phases is to understand the health status of the patients on a GP's list or local community. For example, there may be localised data on the incidence rates and prevalence of disease, health indicators and quality of life among communities and possibly within primary-care groups. The strength of evidence for the effects of physical activity as a protective behaviour and as part of a therapeutic regimen varies for different dimensions of health, well-being and quality of life. Also, the dose-response relationship between physical activity and health, well-being and quality of life varies. Increasingly, we know more about the effects of varying frequency, intensity, duration and type of activity on health outcomes and this differentiated evidence is essential to accumulate and present to policy makers. It is beyond the scope of this chapter to explore these links, other than to restate the current consensus that CHD risk can be reduced by an accumulation of three 10-minute sessions, two 15-minute sessions, or 30 minutes of continuous moderate intensity activity a day on at least five days a week for the least active people. For people with restricted functional capacity, a lower dose may provide health benefits. For moderately active people, more prolonged and intensive exercise will also provide health benefits. This aspect of the model will not be considered in detail but it is important to consider just what 'dose' of exercise is promoted and how this impacts on effectively promoting physical activity through primary-care-originating interventions. It is easy to see how a PHC worker may be sceptical and/or uncertain about the necessary dose of physical activity for health gain. Also, the public-health message for dosage may not translate easily into a specific programme for one patient with a complex medical history and psycho-social barriers to exercising. On the one hand, there is a need to de-medicise physical activity through simple messages but, on the other hand, exercise prescriptions should be tailored to individual needs and require considerable exercise-practitioner expertise.

Phase 3: behavioural diagnosis

The literature has started to differentiate between structured (or facility-based) and lifestyle (or free-living, home-based) forms of physical activity. PHC has a role in promoting both but may effectively do this in different ways through targeted interventions. There is little doubt that levels of inactivity (occupational, household, commuter and leisure-time) are increasing. However, the key question here is what is known about the levels of activity among the patients of primary-care practices. Is information recorded and if so what measures are used? Are those measures collected for a particular purpose? Other lifestyle behaviours are more likely to be recorded (for example, smoking) because they have fewer dimensions than multi-faceted sport, exercise, physical activity and fitness. Within a primary care group/ trust, the recording of physical activity data may vary considerably, from none to a relatively sophisticated tool to assess different dimensions of activity frequency, intensity, duration and type. Documenting the relative levels of physical activity (compared with national norms or national guidelines), in a community or on a primary-care patient list, should be an essential starting point to designing a physical activity intervention in the primary-care setting. Once levels of physical activity are known, the challenge is to understand what are the determinants (within the control of the PHC team) that influence those levels, for the purposes of designing an intervention. Obviously non-PHC factors (such as safe community facilities, weather, poverty, and so on) can have an enormous impact on physical activity levels, and PHC interventions are just one piece of the overall picture. Undoubtedly, there is a challenge to develop valid and reliable tools to assess levels of physical activity within primary-care settings (and elsewhere). Time for the administration of these tools is critical, with the quality of data declining with less intense questioning. For further information on measurement of physical activity the reader is directed to a special edition of *Research Quarterly*, 2000, volume 71, supplement to issue 2, with 19 papers on different aspects of measurement. Within the PRECEDE-PROCEED framework, the PHC diagnosis has three key dimensions, namely: pre-disposing, reinforcing and enabling factors which are expected to influence behaviour and these will now be considered.

 Chapter 5 (Measurement) illustrates the importance of acting on accurate physical activity data. Chapter 10 (Environment) shows how infrastructure can pre-dispose, reinforce or enable physical activity.

Phase 4: primary health care diagnosis

Pre-disposing factors are those that a patient brings to the primary-care setting, in the form of patient knowledge, attitudes, beliefs, and values about the role of lifestyle/physical activity in the promotion of health, and also expectations of the PHC worker and the GPs' role in promoting health. Social, economic and medical/health status can also be included as a pre-disposing factor for being physically active. *Reinforcing factors* are those that the PHC worker brings to the consultation with a patient. These may be an overt demonstration by the PHC worker of their personal lifestyle (for example, cycling shoes in the corner of the room, a smoky odour or appearing overweight), or asking and advising patients about physical activity when appropriate and expressing affirmative beliefs about the positive role of physical activity. *Enabling factors* in any PHC setting may include availability of resources, referrals, rules or protocol, and service structures. For example, a patient may or may not have access to the following: written information about how to access opportunities to exercise; a lifestyle consultation with a trained counsellor or health screening; a place to leave cycles outside a surgery; an opportunity to join volunteer-led walks from the surgery (or elsewhere); or access to an exercise-referral scheme at a local leisure facility. There will inevitably be overlap between counselling, advice giving and health screening as interventions in the PHC setting. However, in the interests of consistency and clarity within this chapter, the act of counselling (for example, cognitive-behavioural approaches) aimed at changing modifiable pre-disposing factors will be considered. Advice giving will be considered as something that the PHC worker does as a reinforcing factor, and health screening, giving a written prescription and exercise referral, as enabling factors.

A PHC diagnosis: pre-disposing factors

Efforts to promote physical activity have largely focused on cognitive behavioural strategies, founded in the health and exercise psychology literature. The influence of beliefs and attitudes on physical activity have been demonstrated through a number of theoretical perspectives, including Social Cognitive Theory, the Health Belief Model, the Theory of Reasoned Action, the Theory of Planned Behaviour and others (see Smith, 1998; Bull, 1999; Biddle & Mutrie, 2001). More recently, the Transtheoretical Model (Prochaska & DiClemente, 1983) has been adopted to help understand the processes of change in physical activity adoption and maintenance. The important thing to appreciate though is that, it is likely that theory-based interventions to modify patient beliefs will probably have some impact on behaviour (Pinto *et al.*, 1998a). Psychological theories have typically predicted, at best, 30 per cent of variability in exercise behaviour (Biddle & Mutrie, 2001). Such interventions in the PHC setting will be reviewed in Phase 7, process evaluation.

 Chapter 7 (Inactivity) details other theories of behaviour change.

Recent interest has focused on ecological factors, including social, economic and geographic determinants of physical activity (Chinn *et al.*, 1999; Sallis & Owen, 1999; Grzywacz & Marks, 2001). Patient perceptions of the pros and cons of an active lifestyle, the available options for physical activity and the likelihood of changing behaviour will all be moderated by the ecological variables within the vicinity of the PHC setting. Within the diagnosis of pre-disposing factors it is therefore critical to understand the meaning of physical activity at an individual and community level.

A PHC diagnosis: reinforcing factors

The role of the PHC professional, as a reinforcer for increasing patient physical activity, has been examined less. Calnan & Williams (1993) reported a generally low-status for health-promotion activity among GPs in the UK. In the US, fewer than 50 per cent of patients were routinely asked by their GP about their exercise habits (Henry *et al.*, 1987) though a variation from 15–84 per cent has been reported (Pender *et al.*, 1994; Walsh *et al.*, 1999; Nawaz *et al.*, 2000) with very few spending more than three to five minutes engaged in promoting physical activity. A recent observational study of 4215 patient consultations in the US revealed that exercise counselling took place in 22.3 per cent of the visits, with a mean time of 0.78 minutes (range 0.33–6.0 minutes) (Podl *et al.*, 1999). A random telephone survey of 793 Israel residents revealed that of those visiting a GP in the past three months, 22 per cent, 16 per cent and 7 per cent has been assessed, advised and assisted, respectively, regarding physical activity by a health care provider (Epel & Ziva Regev, 2000). In both the Podl and the Epel studies, patients with chronic disease were more likely to receive counselling, and it was most frequently associated with weight management. In the UK, Taylor (1994) reported that in a sample of 310 over 35-year-olds, of whom 52 per cent had done no moderate or vigorous intensity activity in the previous week, only 13 per cent claimed to have been advised to exercise more by their GP.

Lawlor *et al.* (2000) concluded from a survey of GPs' attitudes towards promoting physical activity to all inactive patients (rather than just those with poor-health status or high risk) that it would take large amounts of resources to convince GPs to adopt such an approach. Nevertheless, a growing interest in promoting physical activity in PHC has occurred (Harris *et al.*, 1989; Biddle *et al.*, 1994; Pender *et al.*, 1994; Fox *et al.*, 1997; Patrick *et al.*, 1997; Riddoch *et al.*, 1998; Simons-Morton *et al.*, 1998; Sallis & Owen, 1999; Taylor, 1999; Department of Health, 2001b).

A variety of barriers exist for those working in PHC, particularly general practitioners, which appear to influence the decision to promote physical activity (Henry *et al.*, 1987; Williford *et al.*, 1992; Bull *et al.*, 1995; Harsha *et al.*, 1996; Long *et al.*, 1996; Swinburn *et al.*, 1997; Dupen *et al.*, 1999; Steptoe *et al.*, 1999; Walsh *et al.*, 1999). Perhaps the most consistently reported has been that of time, within average GP-patient consultations of seven to 15 minutes. Clearly, time costs money. In addition to financial issues, prioritising attempts to influence a patient's lifestyle has several other important determinants, including the moral views of the practitioner (for example, 'it is the patient's decision to live how they wish'), and socio-economic perceptions (for example, 'it isn't worth trying to change an old person's lifestyle'). A multi-dimensional examination of the determinants of why a member of the PHC team will or will not focus on health and exercise promotion is clearly important and a range of characteristics associated with the health professional and also the patient have been identified.

Findings from a study of practice nurses by McDowell *et al.* (1997) and of nurses and GPs by McKenna *et al.* (1998) supported a review by Pender *et al.* (1994) which suggested that those PHC workers who exercised and held more positive attitudes towards exercise were up to four times more proactive in raising issues concerned with physical activity. In addition to personal habits, a PHC professional's self-efficacy, with respect to counselling patients, may also be an important determinant of exercise promotion activity (Williford *et al.*, 1992; Steptoe *et al.*, 1999; Walsh *et al.*, 1999). In addition, GPs with a low belief in their own effectiveness when exercise counselling (outcome expectancy) limited the use of counselling (Mullen & Tabak, 1989; Bull *et al.*, 1997; Steptoe *et al.*, 1999). Walsh *et al.* (1999) also reported that older physicians were more likely to advise patients to exercise more.

GPs are less likely to advise patients to increase physical activity than other health behaviours (Mullen & Tabak, 1989; Steptoe & Wardle, 1994; Long *et al.*, 1996). Despite national campaigns, there is still a surprising lack of knowledge among GPs about the simpler messages within current guidelines to accumulate 30 minutes of moderate-intensity activity such as walking, on at least five days a week (Gould *et al.*, 1995). Steptoe & Wardle (1994) also reported differences between countries within Europe, with health professionals in the UK and Ireland less likely to endorse lifestyle-disease links than those from other countries.

A PHC diagnosis: enabling factors

The shifting emphasis towards greater health promotion activity (Williams *et al.*, 1993; Department of Health, 2000a,b, 2001a,b; HDA, 2000) is leading to a change in roles and team membership within PHC. While GPs remain central to the initial diagnostic process and gatekeeper to some health-promotion interventions and secondary health care, their opportunistic advice-giving role in promoting health may be somewhat limited (Williams *et al.*, 1993; Stott *et al.*, 1994). Other PHC professionals (such as practice nurses, health visitors, and specialist counsellors) may play a more effective role in behaviour change, with appropriate training and time to work with patients (McDowell *et al.*, 1997). The process of referral to another PHC professional or 'allied health professional' within a PHC setting is considered an enabling factor and the effectiveness of such a strategy will be considered later.

Relatively little has been written on the impact of changing other enabling factors in PHC on structured or lifestyle physical activity, although several recent studies have focused on giving written advice to patients (Swinburn *et al.*, 1998; Smith *et al.*, 2000). Similarly, providing a place to leave cycles outside a surgery may be a small but effective part of an overall strategy to change social norms. In the UK, the national Walking the Way to Health initiative (British Heart Foundation/Countryside Agency, 2001) has linked into PHC in a number of places. A co-ordinated network of trained volunteer walk leaders is emerging through lottery money and private sponsorship. The extent to which volunteers can offer appropriate skills for motivating inactive patients with known disease risk factors and health problems remains to be seen. Urban environments and the weather may also serve as barriers to regular walking.

 Chapter 10 (Environment) provides evidence of how the environment can act as an important enabling factor for living actively.

Fox *et al.* (1997) identified only a few schemes in the UK in which exercise sessions took place within a PHC setting. In these circumstances there was an opportunity to run classes for groups with specific needs, though the environment may not have encouraged social interaction and community integration, often observed in leisure centres. In contrast, patients referred to leisure centres are usually limited to attending only during off-peak hours and, even then, they compete for space with non-referred patients. Leisure centres with swimming pools and other facilities do have the opportunity to run sessions in groups and offer a choice of activity, but this requires greater organisation. The challenge for exercise leaders is to develop programmes and interventions that enable patients to become independently active through structured, supportive sessions which promote lifestyle or free-living activity which may be more sustainable with low cost and high convenience. A National Quality Assurance Framework (NQAF) was launched in the UK to guide best practice and best value from exercise referral schemes (Department of Health, 2001b). The effectiveness of such schemes will be considered later.

 Chapter 7 (Inactivity) describes how theoretical ideas can be converted into practical support for inactive people.

Despite the rapidly growing popularity of exercise-referral schemes, Fox *et al.* (1997) noted that leisure-centre-based schemes could have only very limited impact on public health since no scheme involved more than one per cent of a PHC caseload. However, Taylor (1999) speculated that such an intervention has a multiplier effect through referred patients advocating exercise in the community to friends and relatives. Hardcastle & Taylor (2001) have since found evidence of this through extensive interviews with referred patients.

Phase 5: health care/promotion administrative and policy diagnosis

Following a Health/Quality of Life, Behavioural and PHC Diagnosis it is necessary to consider whether policies exist for promoting physical activity within PHC structures. In the UK, by April 2002, it is expected that every Health Authority (HA) will have in place a strategy for promoting physical activity. This governance has emerged from the National Service Framework for Department of Health (2000a). Previously, promoting physical activity through PHC has been rather hit and miss; some health authorities have been more progressive than others. Such enforced national policy change may force a re-organisation of resources and a diagnostic consideration of what is being done to promote physical activity through PHC.

Following a review by Riddoch *et al.* (1998) the need to guide evidence-based practice in exercise-referral schemes became evident. The NQAF provides the guidelines for local policy-makers to develop schemes that involve everyone, from those working in the health-care practice to the exercise practitioner, within a whole system approach. Clarifying the processes for PHC professionals and establishing the level of expertise among exercise practitioners for GPs to confidently refer patients may well lead to new resources being directed towards such an intervention. It is likely that many schemes will play a significant part in the Health Authority's plans to promote physical activity.

Phase 6: implementation of policy

The framework described in this chapter has a strength in being systematic. It is likely that an effective policy to promote physical activity through PHC will be multi-faceted and based on a systematic diagnosis. The NQAF (Department of Health, 2001b) provides the basis for a co-ordinated approach to promoting physical activity involving both PHC and exercise professionals. The simple opportunistic referral of patients to a community leisure centre (that is, changing an enabling factor) is unlikely to be optimally effective. It requires the GP or PHC professional to consider all the factors considered in the PHC diagnosis (pre-disposing and reinforcing) discussed above. This will require training of all those involved in the referral process, development of appropriate referral materials, and feedback mechanisms to ensure the GP is informed of, and can act upon, changing patient circumstances and health status.

Referral to a structured exercise programme is just one approach. In the next part of the chapter, the focus will be on evidence for the effectiveness of different interventions to change pre-disposing, reinforcing and enabling factors (Process Evaluation), designed to increase patient levels of physical activity (Impact Evaluation) and health status, well-being and quality of life (Outcome Evaluation).

Phase 7: process evaluation

Within the discussion earlier on Phase-4 diagnosis, interventions involving counselling, advice and use of materials were considered. For the purposes of this chapter, this section will again focus on these under the headings of pre-disposing, reinforcing and enabling, respectively, for the purposes of organisation. There is a caveat that in practice it may be difficult to differentiate between these approaches or that they may all occur within the same intervention.

Effectiveness of strategies to influence pre-disposing factors

In Phase 4, reference was made to a major focus on the cognitive determinants of exercise behaviour. Relatively fewer studies have focused on manipulating these variables through interventions to determine if behaviour changes occur, and only a handful of such studies have taken place in the PHC setting. Two features distinguish this research. Firstly, they may attempt to increase the counselling skills and counselling behaviour of PHC workers; and, secondly, observe the effectiveness of such counselling on patient behaviour.

A significant initiative has emerged in the USA which involves a carefully designed exercise counselling strategy in PHC (Patrick *et al.*, 1994a,b). Physician-based Assessment and Counselling for Exercise (PACE) attempts to focus the practitioner on specific behaviour-change strategies using a simple client-centred approach, which takes only three to five minutes of interaction, in order to overcome many of the barriers previously highlighted. Prior to the consultation, a patient completes a brief assessment form (taking less than one minute) to identify 'stage of readiness to change' (Prochaska & DiClemente, 1983; Marcus *et al.*, 1992) and the PAR-Q (Shephard, 1988). The practitioner then negotiates behaviour change by systematically exploring perceived barriers to, and benefits from, exercise, support from family and friends, and self-efficacy towards exercising. Three specific counselling protocols are used, matched to the stages of change (that is, pre-contemplators, contemplators, and actives). At the end of the consultation patients may be given a prescription for exercise and a booklet on physical activity. This is followed by inexpensive brief communication by phone and/or post card.

In a study of the effectiveness of training practitioners to conduct physical activity counselling, four American physicians were selected to receive training (Marcus *et al.*, 1997). Prior to this, 25 patients (control group) were asked about their physicians' exercise-advice giving/counselling. After a two-hour training session on using PACE with these physicians, a further 19 patients (experimental group) were asked about exercise-related physician counselling. Comparisons between the groups revealed that all patients in the experimental group had been spoken to about exercise and two-thirds had been given a prescription and written materials, whereas 32 per cent of the controls had been spoken to about exercise and none had been given a prescription or written materials. Practitioners confirmed the acceptability of the intervention and reported a considerable increase in their counselling self-efficacy. The average time spent counselling was five minutes and was described as relatively brief. However, even this would serve as a significant barrier in the UK where average NHS consultations are only seven minutes. It may also be difficult to entice GPs to attend a two-hour training session, unless clear policy existed within a PHC structure.

In a much larger study, at ten locations across the USA with a diverse range of patients, the acceptability of Project PACE was assessed (Long *et al.*, 1996). Once again, this involved an evaluation of: a training programme, the PACE programme and materials, and 107 patients' perceptions of PACE. There were notable improvements in knowledge about physical activity, perceived counselling ability (self-efficacy), and use of exercise counselling by the physicians.

Albright *et al.* (2000) examined adherence among health-care providers to the Activity Counselling Trial (ACT) protocol for delivering initial 'physician' advice on physical activity. Fifty-four physicians or physician assistants from 11 primary-care practices were trained to integrate three to four minutes of initial physical activity advice into the routine office visits of sedentary patients, aged 35–75 years, with no acute or serious chronic conditions. This advice included assessment of current physical activities, advising the patient about an appropriate physical activity goal, and referring the patient to the health educator. Ninety-nine percent of patients received the initial physician advice about physical activity. Eighty-three percent of the providers spent less than six minutes, and 46 per cent spent the recommended three to four minutes providing advice. Their response to the ACT advice protocol was positive and participation in the study was viewed as beneficial. Again, even this small time investment would severely disrupt the normal working practice within the NHS in the UK if it was delivered by GPs. Brief counselling may, however, be a fruitful approach if delivered by trained exercise counsellors (who could be practice nurses, other health professionals or exercise practitioners). The successful outcomes from this trial are discussed later.

In a UK study of the effects of stage-based materials and verbal counselling by practice nurses (compared with just materials, non-staged materials with counselling, and normal advice giving) Naylor *et al.* (1999) reported a significant change in patients' readiness to change after 24 weeks, but no effect on self-efficacy or self-reported physical activity.

Effect of strategies to influence reinforcing factors

There have been few studies designed to test the effectiveness of strategies to influence advice giving, among PHC workers. In one such study, Lewis & Lynch (1993) described research in which normative advice giving was monitored, followed by a period during which intervention doctors (trained to give a 2–3 minute protocol of advice on exercise) and control doctors (not trained) were compared. The simple protocol involved three steps of patient interaction, 'ASK', 'ASSESS', and 'ADVISE'. Training about the protocol involved just 15 minutes. Doctors in the intervention group increased advice giving from 21–80 per cent while those in the control group increased from 30–40 per cent.

Pinto *et al.* (1998b) reported findings from the Physically Active for Life (PAL) project involving a randomised study of the effects of brief physician counselling plus follow-up on physical activity behaviours in older adults. Physicians favourably endorsed a one-hour training session and support materials to promote physical activity. Comparisons between a group receiving the training and a control group showed significant improvements in confidence for counselling, but no significant changes in physician reports of exercise counselling. Pre-disposing (or mediating) factors among patients (that is, decisional balance, self-efficacy and behavioural processes) were enhanced at six weeks, but not at eight months (Pinto *et al.*, 2001).

Effect of strategies to influence enabling factors

The use of written materials has been considered in a variety of studies (Marcus *et al.*, 1998). Traditionally this may have involved standard leaflets about desirable frequency, intensity, duration and type of exercise. It is of interest to note that there may be differences in effectiveness of materials that promote three vigorous sessions of exercise a week, as opposed to at least five days of accumulated moderate intensity physical activity. Some of these have been tailored or matched to the stage of readiness to change (for example, Naylor *et al.*, 1999) or to some other characteristic of the individual (or predisposing factor).

 Chapter 7 (Inactivity) shows how theoretical ideas can be 'tailored' to offer practical support for people trying to become more active.

The PACE materials (Patrick *et al.*, 1994a,b; Norris *et al.*, 2000) were rated highly, although a major barrier to their use was identified as a lack of staff support (Long *et al.*, 1996). The researchers examined this organisational aspect in more detail and revealed that office staff, in practices where the PACE programme worked effectively, were instrumental in ensuring that physicians engaged in exercise counselling. In particular, office staff ensured that forms were kept in convenient places and had clear responsibilities for handing out PACE forms, and completed protocols were consistently placed in patient records. It was concluded that for successful implementation of the PACE programme, training of office staff was essential.

One concern raised by GPs about giving out written materials to enable patients to be guided into more physical activity is one of time. One may expect that standardising such material can remove this barrier to some extent.

Swinburn *et al.* (1997) and Gribben *et al.* (2000) reported general acceptance by the GP of a 'Green Prescription' pack, although their use required some training and up to five minutes of GP time to administer the pack to the patient. A survey mailed to 433 GPs resulted in a 73 per cent response rate, of whom 65 per cent reported having written a Green Prescription (Smith *et al.*, 2000). Achieving an optimal balance between offering over-simplistic advice and a specific written 'prescription' was a challenge. To reduce the time and make the materials more tailored for individual patients, some GPs requested a computerised version of the Green Prescription pack.

The issue of specificity of the prescription and the competencies needed to fulfil this role were considered in the NQAF for Exercise Referral Systems (Department of Health, 2001b). The words, 'advise', 'refer' and 'prescribe' have been used interchangeably in the physical activity promotion literature and, in practice, but the NQAF attempts to clarify this, for medico-legal reasons. We suggested that advice should always be given by a PHC worker, where appropriate, for a patient to increase physical activity. However, a GP or PHC professional is not normally in an ideal position to prescribe a tailored exercise programme, due to time and training limitations. The NQAF therefore advocates that a patient be referred to an exercise professional, who may then develop a specific exercise prescription or provide exercise counselling. This concept is at odds with the 'Green Prescription' intervention, though in reality this prescription largely involved fairly general advise about walking (personal communication with Boyd Swinburn, 1996).

As a process evaluation, there has undoubtedly been a rapid growth of GP exercise-referral schemes (Fox *et al.*, 1997; Riddoch *et al.*, 1998). One of several training providers has reported that almost 500 staff have attended a GP exercise referral training programme between 1999 and 2001 (personal communication, Gayton Group, 2001). With the launch of the NQAF, this may serve as a catalyst for even more schemes. Riddoch *et al.* (1998), Singh (1997), and Smith *et al.* (1996) reported that the schemes were generally popular with patients (who attended), GPs and practice nurses, as a way to enable patients to become more active. Many schemes have not required GPs to keep a record of the patients referred to an exercise programme, so it has been difficult to determine take-up rates. In a study by Taylor *et al.* (1998), only 13 per cent did not arrive at the leisure centre for their first appointment. In contrast, Lord & Green (1995) reported that 40 per cent of those given prescriptions did not attend an initial consultation at the health centre and initial attendance at the 15 activity centres was lower. Davey & Cochrane (1998), and Cochrane & Davey (1998) reported difficulty in recruitment to a community-based, multi-centre programme in an area of high social deprivation. Only 20 per cent ($n=600$) of those recommended to attend one session a week responded. It is very likely that the recruitment strategy into such schemes will influence patient responses (King *et al.*, 1994; Fielder *et al.*, 1995; Harland *et al.*, 1997; Margitic *et al.*, 1999).

In a recent study in the UK, Stevens *et al.* (1998) conducted a randomised controlled trial to compare the effects of a GP sending an invitation to patients (45–74-year-olds) to visit an 'exercise development officer' at a leisure centre, as opposed to mailing information about local leisure centres. Of the 126 (35 per cent) in the invitation group who attended the first consultation, 91 returned for a follow-up session with the exercise officer, after a ten-week personalised exercise programme. Clearly, patients who have the least interest in changing behaviour will require careful consideration if the uptake of interventions designed to change enabling factors is to be satisfactory.

Finally, despite evidence that social support is valuable for adopting and maintaining exercise (Hardcastle & Taylor, 2001), no interventions in PHC appeared to have specifically looked at the acceptability of developing this as an intervention in primary care. There are many volunteer-led walking groups based at PHC settings emerging in the UK, but to date little evidence exists on their acceptability and effectiveness. Their growing number suggests acceptance, but this approach may work only for specific individuals who are already active and/or gregarious.

Phase 8: impact evaluation

It is important to consider how factors expected to influence behaviour change respond to different strategies, but from a public-health perspective the bottom line is: does the intervention lead to long-term increases in physical activity sufficient to promote improved health? This section will begin with reference to the findings of several reviews that have attempted to address this question, followed by a discussion of the findings of some recent rigorous studies.

Reviews

Harris *et al.* (1989) reviewed the evidence for the effectiveness of exercise counselling in PHC on change in physical activity and concluded that little evidence existed. The few studies had a variety of methodological limitations which made interpretation difficult. More recently, Hillsdon & Thorogood (1996), and Hillsdon *et al.* (1995), in a review of randomised controlled trials to specifically evaluate free-living exercise promotion schemes, reported no studies in which the intervention was PHC-based. In contrast, Eaton & Menard (1998) conducted a systematic review of eight clinical trials in which the efficacy of primary care office-based exercise promotion was investigated. Again, they concluded that most studies had significant methodological limitations, and there was little evidence that the interventions led to any long-term change in physical activity. Simons-Morton *et al.* (1998) reviewed the effects of 12 primary prevention studies of physical activity counselling in health-care settings (including three medical clinics which may not normally be classified as PHC settings). Half the studies reviewed reported a theoretical framework upon which the intervention was based, with Social Cognitive Theory and the Transtheoretical Model being the most popular. Identifying a stage of readiness to change and then matching an attempt to influence cognitive or behavioural processes (patient beliefs about their ability to increase activity levels or self efficacy) has been the most common approach. The review focused on both behavioural and fitness changes, and highlighted the wide range of measures used, and lengths of study. Only two of the six studies with a greater than six-month follow-up measure of outcome variables showed significantly greater activity or fitness among the intervention group (see Logsdon *et al.*, 1989; ICRF, OXCHECK, 1994). The authors concluded that long-term support and cognitive-behavioural strategies were necessary to ensure sustained change. Finally, Eakin *et al.* (2000) systematically reviewed primary care-based physical activity intervention studies and identified support for short-term effects of counselling and highlighted a need for longer-term interventions.

 Chapter 7 (Inactivity) describes how concepts from the Transtheoretical Model can be developed into practical support.

Unfortunately, some of the more rigorous studies reviewed involved multifactorial health-promotion interventions in PHC, within which exercise advice/counselling was incorporated (Logsdon *et al.*, 1989; Cupples & McKnight, 1994; Family Heart Study Group, 1994; ICRF OXCHECK Study Group, 1994, 1995; Burton *et al.*, 1995; Dowell *et al.*, 1996). While it may be unethical for trial to withhold information on smoking cessation or change in dietary behaviour, the extent of change in physical activity or fitness that is attributable to holistic behaviour change approaches, or to specific physical activity interventions, remains unknown. Multi-factorial health-promotion interventions also make it difficult to determine the cost-effectiveness of the components specifically designed to change physical activity, and this component may become somewhat lost (or time limited) in the complexity of a multiple lifestyle changes for the patient.

These studies are also currently somewhat limited by their dated focus on outcome variables such as the percentage of subjects doing vigorous activity. One final concern is that subjects in such large studies have rarely been selected on the basis of their initial sedentary behaviour, and the sample size in the studies has not usually been determined or powered on the basis of physical activity and expected change. Exclusively selecting patients who are inactive, and targeting an intervention specifically at changing physical activity, may provide more scope for observation of change although such patients may also be more resistant to change.

These large-scale multi-factorial studies will not be reviewed here but their general conclusions point to rather limited long-term change in physical activity at a cost which would not easily be absorbed into general practice. Nevertheless, the large-scale multi-faceted trials provide evidence of reducing CHD risk through health-promotion interventions (Langham *et al.*, 1996; Wonderling *et al.*, 1996a,b; Ashenden *et al.*, 1997; Ebrahim & Davey-Smith, 1997). Further work is needed to determine cost-effectiveness for reducing risk of health outcomes other than CHD, such as mental illness, osteoporosis and hip fracture, and cancer.

Specific physical activity intervention trials

In the past five years there has been a considerable increase in intervention studies that focus on physical activity as the primary outcome. The focus will be on two groups of studies within a PHC setting, one aimed primarily at increasing lifestyle or free-living physical activity, mainly through stage-matched counselling, and the second through a structured exercise programme that is facility based (that is exercise referral schemes), at least initially.

The Activity Counselling Trial (Blair *et al.*, 1998; King *et al.*, 1998; Margitic *et al.*, 1999; Albright *et al.*, 2000; Simons-Morton, 2000; The Writing Group for the ACT Research Group, 2001) is the most rigorous and generalisable study to compare the effects of two physical activity-counselling interventions with normal care in a primary care setting. Subjects included 395 female and 479 male inactive primary care patients aged 35 to 75 years without clinical cardiovascular disease, attending 11 PHC facilities. Participants were randomly assigned to one of three groups: advice (*n*=292) from physician and written educational materials (normal care); assistance (*n*=293), involving 'advice' plus interactive mail and behavioural counselling at physician visits; or counselling (*n*=289), involving 'assistance,' 'advice,' plus regular telephone counselling and behavioural classes. The two patient-counselling interventions were equally effective in women in improving cardio-respiratory fitness over two years compared with recommended care. In men, neither of the two counselling interventions was more effective than normal care.

In an evaluation of the PACE protocol supplemented with a reminder phone call at one month, Norris *et al.* (2000) reported no significant effect of the intervention (compared with a control group) on energy expenditure at the six-month follow-up. Patients receiving the PACE intervention improved their stage of change, particularly those in the pre-contemplation stage, and also pre-disposing factors (that is cognitive and behavioural processes). The implications of the findings were limited by the initially fairly active nature of the participants.

Bull *et al.* (1999a,b) investigated the effects of 'standard' or 'tailored' written information on physical activity on levels of physical activity in 763 sedentary patients recruited through ten family practices. They reported no difference in activity, or stage of change, after 12 months between the two approaches, although short-term differences were observed.

Graham-Clarke & Oldenburg (1994) contrasted the effects of a risk assessment and feedback with the same plus a video, or the same plus video and self-help booklets, and found no difference in energy expenditure after 12 months between the groups.

The findings from these well-funded and rigorous trials paint a rather pessimistic picture of the role of counselling in primary care, without long-term support, and Emmons & Rollnick (2001) warn about the limitations of motivational interviewing in health-care settings. Optimism that exercise counselling would be a cost-effective approach to increasing physical activity have largely not materialised. However, in a study of 883 patients with CHD risk factors (including low-activity levels), Steptoe *et al.* (1999) reported that behavioural counselling, matched to the stage of patient readiness to change, by a trained practice nurse led to significantly greater increases in physical activity than a randomised control group, after 12 months. The size of this effect was greater for those with greater baseline social support, perceived benefits and lower perceived barriers, thereby supporting the need to consider processes (Steptoe *et al.*, 2000).

Recent debate about the effectiveness of GP exercise-referral schemes has followed a review by Riddoch *et al.* (1998), and a report by Harland *et al.* (1999). The latter generated debate regarding the negative conclusions drawn (for example, Craig *et al.*, 2000). The main issue revolved around the conclusions drawn from the Newcastle exercise project (Harland *et al.*, 1999). The study involved 523 patients who were randomised to one of five groups: (1) a control group receiving results from a health screening, an information pack on healthy lifestyles, leaflets on local leisure facilities and activities, and brief advice highlighting individual profiles; (2) a 40-minute motivational interview (Miller & Rollnick, 1991; Rollnick *et al.*, 1999) alone; (3) as (2) plus 30 vouchers entitling free access to leisure facilities; (4) six motivational interviews (over 12 weeks) alone; (5) as (4) plus the 30 free vouchers. The findings revealed no differences in physical activity between the control and intervention groups at one year. However, 23 per cent of the control group had an increased physical activity score at one year, suggesting an effect of the 75-minute physical assessment with brief advice and informational materials. Also, the failure of free leisure-centre vouchers to influence change in behaviour was reported as an indication that exercise-referral schemes are ineffective, and this point has been debated given that all groups reported higher levels of physical activity.

Riddoch *et al.* (1998) reviewed eight trials intended to evaluate a physical activity promotion scheme in PHC, which met the requirements for a systematic review. No study evaluated a scheme that would now match the guidelines on the NQAF although two studies examined GP exercise-referral schemes (Stevens *et al.*, 1998; Taylor *et al.*, 1998).

In one of the studies, Taylor *et al.* (1996, 1998) examined both adherence to a 20-session, ten-week exercise programme at the Hailsham Lagoon leisure centre, East Sussex, and also moderate and vigorous activity, and fitness, at baseline, 8, 16, 26 and 37 weeks. Eighty-seven per cent of referred patients used the prescription and 28 per cent (45 per cent of obese patients) did at least 15 sessions. The mean attendance rate was 9.1 sessions. Referred patients were not significantly different from the control group at 37 weeks on amount of activity. On the basis of the stages of change measure of exercise, the proportion describing themselves as in the active or maintenance stage, increased from 36 per cent at baseline to 97 per cent and 61 per cent at eight per cent and 37 weeks, respectively, compared with 23 per cent, 35 per cent and 23 per cent at the three assessments in the control group. The exercise group was significantly fitter on a sub-maximal cycle test than the control group at 37 weeks (Taylor, 1996). Scope for demonstrating effects within this trial was limited by the fairly high levels of initial activity, limited training of the exercise practitioners in counselling and promoting long-term change, and lower levels of patient support at the leisure centre than now exists. However, patients had significantly enhanced pre-disposing factors (that is, more positive physical self-perceptions and reduced barriers towards exercise) after 37 weeks (Taylor, 1997; Talbot & Taylor, 1998).

Concurrent data (which did not include patients referred through the study) from a previously described large audit with 729 patients, revealed a 22 per cent completion rate (a slightly different criterion measure but one which enables some comparison)(Wealden DC, 1995). In Wealden's second audit (1996) of 627 referred patients, conducted after the study by Taylor (1996), completion rates had increased to 43 per cent.

In Wealden's 1996 audit, a number of factors appeared to be related to programme completion although reporting of statistical analyses were insufficient to enable any conclusions to be drawn. Completion rates varied between referring GPs from less than 30 per cent to more than 50 per cent. Because many patients are referred for more than one reason it was somewhat difficult to interpret differences in completion rates between single referral categories. Nevertheless, those referred for hypertension ($n=73$), asthma ($n=22$), arthritis ($n=61$) had completion rates above 53 per cent, whereas those referred for psychological/stress ($n=90$), general fitness ($n=92$), weight loss ($n=121$) and injury rehabilitation ($n=40$) had completion rates below 39 per cent. Long-term change in activity was not reliably assessed.

The only other rigorous trial to evaluate an exercise-referral scheme that fairly closely matches the guidelines within the NQAF showed some positive effects (Stevens *et al.*, 1998). A net 10 per cent reduction in the proportion of people classified as sedentary in the intervention group compared with the control group, after eight months was reported. Also, the intervention group increased the number of exercise sessions a week by 1.5 more than the control group. Non-response bias was also reported, with the sedentary being the most difficult to attract into the study, through the mailed invitation from the GP. Respondents to the invitation went directly to an exercise-development officer at the local leisure centre for an initial consultation, and then a ten-week exercise programme. The NQAF recommends that a GP is involved in a face-to-face referral which was not the case in this study, nor was it in the study by Taylor.

Clearly, an exercise-referral scheme involves structured exercise, but the NQAF also recommends that resources are directed towards long-term maintenance, through counselling patients about other physical activity options and strategies to remain active. Further research is needed to fully evaluate the effects of a referral scheme that is guided by the NQAF and involves additional long-term support. Evidence from the largest study to compare a structured exercise versus lifestyle intervention (though with no connection to the PHC setting), called Project Active (Dunn *et al.*, 1997, 1998, 1999; Kohl *et al.*, 1998; Sevick *et al.*, 2000) suggested both approaches had an equal impact on changing behaviour after two years. The structured programme had led to greater fitness and energy expenditure at six months. While this rigorous study provides valuable evidence, the generaliseability to less affluent populations and settings must be questioned and further research is needed in settings where high levels of social exclusion and poverty exist. Strategies to recruit such patients through PHC will have to be carefully considered.

The above interventions have focused primarily on intensive interaction with patients either through counselling or referral to a structured exercise programme. However, Kreuter *et al.* (2000) have reported a potential primacy effect in which patients were more likely to be receptive to future information, naturalistic messages and interventions following advice to be more active by a physician. This is in agreement with Taylor (1994) who reported increased intention to increase physical activity following observation of a walking promotion sign, among 300 randomly selected 40–70-year-old adults who had been advised by their GP to exercise more.

Finally, in terms of impact evaluation, it may be that increases in physical activity lead to changes in other health behaviours, such as diet, smoking, alcohol and illegal substance use (Wankel & Sefton, 1994; Ussher *et al.*, 2000). While there is some support for some positive effects, Taylor (1996) reported no effects on smoking status following referral to the exercise programme. Further research is needed to investigate opportunities for multiple-behaviour change.

Phase 9: outcome evaluation

It is beyond the scope of the present chapter to report all changes in health status associated with physical activity interventions in PHC, nor is it necessary. The dose–response relationship between increasing physical activity and health gain has been confirmed for a wide range of health outcomes, and if exercise levels increase in response to an intervention, then assumptions can probably be made about reduced risk or prevalence of such outcomes. Importantly, there are many potential benefits from increasing levels of physical activity. The challenge is to determine how cost-effective interventions are in improving health status once impact evaluations reveal increases in physical activity.

For example, Klaber Moffett *et al.* (1999) provided evidence that a primary care/community-based exercise programme could led to significant health and financial benefits for patients with chronic low-back pain. Eight sessions (two a week for one hour) costing a total of £25.20 per person (with up to 10 people in a class led by a physiotherapist) led to reductions in pain, fewer visits to the GP and physiotherapist services, and fewer days' absence from work, compared with a control group. The fewer visits were estimated to reduce health service costs by £44.55 (in 1996–98). The researchers achieved 75 per cent adherence to the exercise programme. Unfortunately, many other randomised trials involving a physical activity intervention in primary care have not been able to observe effects on outcomes (or physical activity) because of bias in recruitment of subjects (that is, only more active people enter the trial, who have less scope to increase activity levels) and poor retention rates (that is, randomising people into an exercise condition can lead to high withdrawal rates and 'diluted' effects on outcomes). In contrast, prospective evaluations of outcomes among willing participants (who have not been randomised into a condition they wouldn't normally have chosen) are more likely to have an impressive mean group outcome.

Conclusions

The PRECEDE-PROCEED Model has been adapted as a framework for developing ways to promote physical activity though PHC initiatives. It has been used to systematically diagnose current patient behaviour and determinants within the control of PHC, and to review the evidence for the effectiveness of PHC-based interventions aimed at increasing physical activity and health outcomes. The intention was to use this framework to not only structure the chapter, but also provide a model that can be used by students and practitioners for designing and implementing a policy, and evaluating the processes, impact and outcomes of that policy. The chapter identifies a wide range of studies designed to better understand how much physical activity patients are involved in and what factors are associated with the promotion of physical activity in association with PHC. There have also been many interventions designed to increase physical activity promotion, although the quality of these trials has often limited the internal and external validity of the findings. Nevertheless, it is clear that for interventions to be successful a co-ordinated strategy which attempts to address patients' pre-disposing factors, the reinforcing nature of the PHC worker, and which enables patients to change in the most supportive and informative way must be implemented. Without such a whole-system approach, PHC may have little influence on patient levels of physical activity, across a community.

Further research is undoubtedly needed to consider the cost-effectiveness of different strategies, with emerging possibilities using information technology (Prochaska *et al.*, 2000), volunteer support networks (BHF/CA, 2001) and co-ordinated referral processes to structured and lifestyle initiatives. For example, the NQAF (Department of Health, 2001b) provides guidelines for best practice in exercise referral schemes. With only limited evidence to support the role of counselling as a sole strategy, we need to know how effective the optimum GP exercise-referral scheme can be, and whether they can promote long-term change. A combination of structured plus lifestyle promotion of physical activity may well have greatest effects on long-term change in physical activity and health. The psycho-social mechanisms by which people change may be fully understood only through qualitative methods, and there have been few examples of such an approach in the literature (for example, Crone-Grant & Smith, 1999; Hardcastle & Taylor, 2001).

 Chapter 4 (Mental health) provides a justification for using qualitative approaches within exercise and health science.

References

Abenhaim, L., Rossignol, M., Valat, J.-P., Nordin, M., Avouac, B., Blotman, F., Charlot, J., Dreiser, R.L., Legrand, E., Rozenberg, S. & Vautravers, P. for the Paris Task Force (2000) The role of activity in the therapeutic management of back pain: Report of the International Task Force on Back Pain. *Spine*, **25(4)**: 1S–33S.

ACSM (1998) Position stand: Exercise and physical activity for older adults. *Medicine and Science in Sports and Exercise*, **30(6)**: 992–1008.

Albright, C.L., Cohen, S., Gibbons, L., Miller, B., Sallis, J.F., Imai, K. *et al.* (2000) Incorporating physical activity advice into primary care: Physician-delivered advice within the Activity Counselling Trial. *American Journal of Preventive Medicine*, **18**: 225–234.

Ashenden, R., Salagy, C. & Weller, D. (1997) A systematic review of the effectiveness of promoting lifestyle change in general practice. *Family Practice*, **14**: 160–175.

Batty, D. & Thune, I. (2000) Does physical activity prevent cancer? Evidence suggests protection against colon cancer and probably breast cancer. *British Medical Journal*, **321**: 1424–1425.

Biddle, S.J. & Mutrie, N. (2001) *Psychology of Physical Activity: Determinants, Well-being and Interventions*. London: Routledge.

Biddle, S. Fox, K. & Edmunds, L. (1994) *Physical Activity Promotion in Primary Health Care in England*. London: Health Education Authority.

Biddle, S., Fox, K. & Boutcher, S. (eds) (2000) *Physical Activity and Psychological Well-being*. London: Routledge.

Blair, S.N., Applegate, W.B., Dunn, A.L., Ettinger, W.H., Haskall, W.L., King, A.C., Morgan, T.M., Shih, J.A. & Simons-Morton, D.G. (1998) Activity Counselling Trial (ACT): rationale, design and methods. Activity Counselling Trial Research Group. *Medicine and Science in Sports and Exercise*, **30(7)**: 1097–1106.

Blair, S.N. & Jackson, A.S. (2001) Physical fitness and activity as separate heart disease risk factors: a meta-analysis. *Medicine and Science in Sports and Exercise*, **33(5)**: 762–764.

Bouchard, C., Shephard, R.J. & Stephens T. (eds) (1994) *Physical Activity, Fitness and Health: Consensus Statement*, Champaign, Il.: Human Kinetics.

British Heart Foundation/Countryside Agency (2001) *Walking for Health*. website. www.whi.org.uk

Bull, F.C. & Jamrozik, K. (1999a) Advice on exercise from a family physician can help sedentary patients to become active. *American Journal of Preventive Medicine*, **15**: 85–94.

Bull, F.C., Jamrozik, K. & Blanksby, B.A. (1999b) Tailored advice on exercise – does it make a difference? *American Journal of Preventive Medicine*, **16**: 230–239.

Bull, F.C., Schipper, E.C., Jamrozik, K. & Blanksby, B.A. (1995) Beliefs and behaviour of general practitioners regarding promotion of physical activity. *Australian Journal of Public Health*, **19**: 300–304.

Bull, F.C., Schipper, E.C., Jamrozik, K. & Blanksby, B.A. (1997) How can and do Australian doctors promote physical activity? *Preventive Medicine*, **26**: 866–873.

Bull, S. (ed.) (1999) *Adherence Issues in Sport and Exercise*. Chichester: Wiley.

Burton, L.C., Paglia, M.J., German, P.S., Shapiro, S. & Damiano, A.M. (1995) The effect among older persons of a general preventive visit on three health behaviours: smoking, excessive alcohol drinking and sedentary lifestyle. *Preventive Medicine*, **24**: 492–497.

Calnan, M. & Williams, S. (1993) Coronary heart disease prevention in general practice: the practices and views of a national sample of general practitioners. *Health Education Journal*, **52**: 197–203.

Campbell, A.J., Robertson, M.C., Gardner, M.M., Norton, R.N., Tilyard, M.W. & Buchner, D.M. (1998) Randomised controlled trial of a general practice programme of home-based exercise to prevent falls in elderly women. *British Medical Journal*, **313**: 1065–1069.

Chinn, D., White, M., Harland, J., Drinkwater, C. & Raybould, S. (1999) Barriers to physical activity and socio-economic position: implications for health promotion. *Journal of Epidemiology and Community Health*, **53**: 191–192.

Cochrane, T. & Davey, R. (1998) Evaluation of exercise prescription for 25 general practices and a large leisure complex in Sheffield. *Journal of Sport Science*, **16**: 17–18.

Craig, A., Dinan, S., Smith, A., Taylor, A. & Webborn, N. (2000) The Newcastle exercise project. *British Medical Journal*, **320**: 1470.

Crone-Grant, D. & Smith, R.A. (1999) Broadening horizons: A qualitative inquiry into the experiences of patients on an exercise prescription scheme. *Journal of Sport Sciences* (Abstract), **17(1)**: 12.

Cupples, M.E. & McKnight, A. (1994) Randomised controlled trial of health promotion in general practice for patients at high cardiovascular risk. *British Medical Journal*, **309**: 993–996.

Davey, R. & Cochrane, T. (1998) General practice community-based exercise programmes for sedentary adults over 65 years of age. *Journal of Sport Science*, **16**: 18.

Department of Health (2000a) *National Service Framework for Coronary Heart Disease: Modern Standards and Service Models*. London: The Stationery Office.

Department of Health (2000b) *National Service Framework for Mental Health: Modern Standards and Service Models*. London: Department of Health.

Department of Health (2000c) *Health Survey for England 1998: Cardiovascular Disease*. London: The Stationery Office.

Department of Health (2001a) *National Service Framework for Older People*. London: Department of Health.

Department of Health (2001b) *NHS National Quality Assurance Framework: Exercise Referral Systems*. London: Department of Health. www.doh.gov.uk/exercisereferrals.

Dishman, R.K. (ed.) (1994) *Advances in Exercise Adherence*. Champaign, Il: Human Kinetics.

Dowell, A.C., Ochera, J.J., Hilton, S.R., Bland, J.M., Harris, T., Jones, D.R. & Katbamn, S. (1996) Prevention in practice: results of a 2-year follow-up of routine health promotion interventions in general practice. *Family Practitioner*, **13**: 357–362.

Dunn, A.L., Marcus, B.H., Kampert, J.B., Garcia, M.E., Kohl, H.W. & Blair, S.N. (1997) Reduction in cardiovascular disease risk factors: 6-month results from Project Active. *Preventive Medicine*, **26**: 883–892.

Dunn, A.L., Garcia, M.E., Marcus, B.H., Kampert, J.B., Kohl, H.W. & Blair, S.N. (1998) Six-month physical activity and fitness changes in project active, a randomized trial. *Medicine and Science in Sports and Exercise*, **30(7)**: 1076–1083.

Dunn, A.L., Marcus, B.H., Kampert, J.B., Garcia, M.E., Kohl, H.W. & Blair, S.N. (1999) Comparison of lifestyle and structured interventions to increase physical activity and cardiorespiratory fitness: A randomized trial. *Journal of the American Medical Association*, **281(4)**: 327–334.

Dupen, F., Baumen, A.E. & Lin, R. (1999) The sources of risk factor information for General Practitioners: is physical activity under-recognized? *Medical Journal of Australia*, **171(11–12)**: 601–3.

Eakin, E.G., Glasgow, R.E. & Riley, K.M. (2000) Review of primary care-based physical activity intervention studies: effectiveness and implications for practice and future research. *Journal of Family Practice*, **49(2)**: 158–168.

Eaton, C.B. & Menard, L.M. (1998) A systematic review of physical activity promotion in primary care office settings. *British Journal of Sports Medicine*, **32**: 11–16.

Ebrahim, S. & Davey-Smith, G. (1997) A systematic review and meta-analysis of randomised controlled trials of health promotion for prevention of coronary heart disease in adults. *British Medical Journal*, **314**: 1666–1674.

Emmons, K.M. & Rollnick, S. (2001) Motivational interviewing in health care settings: opportunities and limitations. *American Journal of Preventive Medicine*, **20**: 68–74.

Epel, O.B. & Regev, Z. (2000) Quality and correlates of physical activity counseling by health care providers in Israel. *Preventive Medicine*, **31(5)**: 618–626.

Family Heart Study Group (1994) Randomised controlled trial evaluating cardiovascular screening and intervention in general practice: principal results of the British Family Heart Study. *British Medical Journal*, **308**: 313–320.

Fielder, H., Shorney, S. & Wright, D. (1995) Lessons from a pilot study on prescribing exercise. *Health Education Journal*, **54**: 445–452.

Fox, K.R., Biddle, S.J.H., Edmunds, L.E., Bowler, I. & Killoran, A (1997) Physical activity promotion through primary health care in England. *British Journal of General Practice*, **47**: 367–369.

Gould, M.N., Thorogood, M., Iliffe, S. & Morris, J.N. (1995) Promoting exercise in primary care: measuring the knowledge gap. *Health Education Journal*, **54**: 304–311.

Graham-Clarke, P. & Oldenburg, B. (1994) The effectiveness of a general practice-based physical activity intervention on patient physical activity status. *Behavior Change*, **11**: 132–144.

Green, L.W. & Kreuter, M.W. (1991) *Health Promotion Planning: An Educational and Environmental Approach*. London: Mayfield.

Gribben, B., Goodyear-Smith, F., Grobbelaar, M., O'Neill, D. & Walker, S. (2000) The early experience of general practitioners using green prescription. *New Zealand Journal of Medicine*, **113(1117)**: 372–373.

Grzywacz, J.G. & Marks, N.F. (2001) Social inequalities and exercise during adulthood: toward an ecological perspective. *Journal of Health and Social Behavior*, **42(2)**: 202–220.

Hardcastle, S. & Taylor, A.H. (2001) Looking for more than weight loss and fitness gain: Psycho-social dimensions among older women in a primary health care exercise referral scheme. *Journal of Aging and Physical Activity*, **9(3)**: 313–328.

Harland, J., White, M., Drinkwater, C., Chinn, D. & Farr, L. (1997) Does recruitment strategy affect participation and interim outcome in a randomised controlled trial evaluating physical activity promotion in primary health care? *Journal of Epidemiology and Community Health*, **51**: 587–588.

Harland, J., White, M., Drinkwater, C., Chinn, D., Farr, L. & Howel, D. (1999) The Newcastle exercise project: a randomised controlled trial of methods to promote physical activity in primary care. *British Medical Journal*, **319**: 828–832.

Harris, S.S., Caspersen, C.J., DeFries, G.H. & Estes, E.H. (1989) Physical activity counselling for healthy adults as a primary preventive intervention in the clinical setting: Report from the US Preventive Services Task Force, *Journal of the American Medical Association*, **261(24)**: 3590–3598.

Harsha, D.M., Saywell, R.M., Thygerson, S. & Panozzo, J. (1996) Physician factors affecting patient willingness to comply with exercise recommendations. *Clinical Journal of Sports Medicine*, **6**: 112–118.

Health Development Agency (2000) *Coronary Heart Disease: Guidance for Implementing the Preventive Aspects of the National Service Framework*. London: Health Development Agency.

Henry, R.C., Ogle, K.S. & Snellman, L.A. (1987) Preventive medicine: Physician practices, beliefs and perceived barriers for implementation. *Family Medicine*, **19**: 110–113.

Hillsdon, M. & Thorogood, M. (1996) A systematic review of physical activity promotion strategies. *British Journal of Sports Medicine*, **30**: 84–89.

Hillsdon, M., Thorogood, M., Anstiss, T.A. & Morris, J. (1995) Randomised controlled trials of physical activity promotion in free living populations: a review. *Journal of Epidemiology and Community Health*, **49**: 448–453.

Imperial Cancer Research Fund OXCHECK Study Group (1994) Effectiveness of health checks conducted by nurses in primary care: results of the OXCHECK study after one year. *British Medical Journal*, **308**: 308–312.

Imperial Cancer Research Fund OXCHECK Study Group (1995) Effectiveness of health checks conducted by nurses in primary care: final results of the OXCHECK study. *British Medical Journal*, **31**: 1099–1104.

King, A.C., Sallis, J.F., Dunn, A.L., Simons-Morton, D.G., Albright, C.A., Cohen, S., Rejeski, W.J., Marcus, B.H. & Coday, M.C. (1998) Overview of the Activity Counselling trial (ACT) intervention for promoting physical activity in primary care settings. Activity Counselling Trial Research Group. *Medicine and Science in Sports and Exercise*, **30**(7): 1086–1096.

King, A.C., Harris, R.B. & Haskell, W.L. (1994) Effect of recruitment strategy on types of subjects entered into a primary prevention clinical trial. *Annals of Epidemiology*, **4**: 312–320.

Klaber Moffett, J.A., Torgerson, D.J., Bell-Syer, S.E.M., Jackson, D., Llewelyn Phillips, H., Farrin, A. & Barber, J. (1999) A randomised trial of exercise for primary care back pain patients: Clinical outcomes, costs and preferences. *British Medical Journal*, **319**: 279–283.

Kohl, H.W., Dunn, A.L., Marcus, B.H. & Blair, S.N. (1998) A randomised trial of physical activity interventions: design and baseline data from Project Active. *Medicine and Science in Sport and Exercise*, **30**: 275–283.

Kreuter, M.W., Chheda, S.G. & Bull, F.C. (2000) How does physician advice influence patient behaviour? *Archives of Family Medicine*, **9**: 426–433.

Langham, S., Thorogood, M., Normand, C., Muir, J., Jones, L. & Fowler, G. (1996) Costs and cost effectiveness of health checks conducted by nurses in primary care: the OXCHECK study. *British Medical Journal*, **312**: 1265–1268.

Lawlor, D.A., Keen, S. & Neal, D.D. (2000) Can general practitioners influence the nation's health through a population approach to provision of lifestyle advice? *British Journal of General Practice*, **50**: 455–459.

Lewis, B.S. & Lynch, W.D. (1993) The effect of physician advice on exercise behaviour. *Preventive Medicine*, **22**: 110–121.

Logsdon, D.N., Lazaro, C.M. & Meier, R.V. (1989) The feasibility of behavioural risk reduction in primary medical care. *American Journal of Preventive Medicine*, **5**: 249–256.

Long, B.J., Calfas, K.J., Wooten, W., Sallis, J.F., Patrick, K., Goldstein, M., Marcus, B.H., Schwenk, T.L., Chenoweth, J., Carter, R., Torres, T., Palinkas, L.A. & Heath, G. (1996) A multisite field test of the acceptability of physical activity counselling in primary care: project PACE. *American Journal of Preventive Medicine*, **12**(2): 73–81.

Lord, J.C. & Green, F. (1995) Exercise on prescription: does it work? *Health Education Journal*, **54**(4): 453–464.

McDowell, N., McKenna, J. & Naylor, P.J. (1997) Factors that influence practice nurses to promote physical activity. *British Journal of Sports Medicine*, **31**: 308–313.

McKenna, J., Naylor, P.-J. & McDowell, N. (1998) Barriers to physical activity promotion by general practitioners and practice nurses. *British Journal of Sports Medicine*, **32**: 242–247.

McMurdo, M.E., Millar, A.M. & Daly, F. (2000) A randomized controlled trial of fall prevention strategies in old peoples' homes. *Gerontology*, **46**(2): 83–87.

Marcus, B.H., Owen, N., Forsyth, L.H., Cavill, N.A. & Fridinger, F. (1998) Physical activity interventions using mass media, print media and information technology. *American Journal of Preventive Medicine*, **15**(4): 362–378.

Marcus, B.H., Banspach, S.W., Lefebvre, R.C., Rossi, J.S., Carleton, R.A. & Abrams, D.B. (1992) Using the stages of change model to increase the adoption of physical activity among community participants. *American Journal of Health Promotion*, **6**: 424–429.

Marcus, B.H., Goldstein, M.G., Jette, A., Simkin-Silverman, L., Pinto, B.M., Milan, F., Wahburn, R., Smith, K., Radowski, W. & Dube, C.E. (1997) Training physicians to conduct physical activity counselling. *Preventive Medicine*, **26**: 382–388.

Margitic, S., Sevick, M.A., Miller, M., Albright, C., Banton, J., Callahan, K., Garcia, M., Gibbons, L., Levine, B.J. Anderson, R. & Ettinger, W. (1999) Challenges faced in recruiting patients from primary care practices into a physical activity intervention trial. Activity Counselling Trial Research Group. *Preventive Medicine*, **29**(4): 277–286.

Miller, W.R. & Rollnick, S. (1991) *Motivational Interviewing: Preparing People to Change Addictive Behaviour*. New York: Guilford.

Mullen, P. & Tabak, G.R. (1989) Patterns of counselling techniques used by family practice physicians for smoking, weight control, exercise and stress. *Medical Care*, **27**: 694–704.

National Audit Office (2001) *Tackling Obesity in England. Report by Comptroller and Auditor General*. London: The Stationary Office.

Nawaz, H., Adams, M.L. & Katz, D.L. (2000) Physician-patient interactions regarding diet, exercise and smoking. *Preventive Medicine*, **31**: 652–657.

Naylor, P.-J., Simmonds, G., Riddoch, C., Velleman, G. & Turton, P. (1999) Comparison of stage-matched and unmatched interventions to promote exercise behaviour in primary health care. *Health Education Research*, 14: 653–666.

Norris, S.L., Grothaus, L.C., Buchner, D.M. & Pratt, M. (2000) Effectiveness of physician-based assessment and counseling for exercise in a staff model HMO. *Preventive Medicine*, 30(6): 513–523.

Office of Population Censuses and Surveys (1995) *The Health Survey for England 1993*. London: HMSO.

Pate, R.R., Pratt, M., Blair, S.N., Haskell, W.L., Macera, C.A., Bouchard, C. *et al.* (1995) Physical activity and public health: a recommendation from the Centers for Disease Control and Prevention and the American College of Sports Medicine. *Journal of The American Medical Association*, 273: 402–407.

Patrick, K., Sallis, J.F., Long, B.J., Calfas, K.J., Wooten, W.J., Heath, G. & Pratt, M. (1994a) A new tool for encouraging activity: Project PACE. *Physician and Sportsmedicine*, 22(11): 45–55.

Patrick, K., Sallis, J.F., Long, B.J., Calfas, K.J., Wooten, W.J. & Heath, G. (1994b) PACE: physician-based assessment and counseling for exercise, background and development. *Physician and Sportsmedicine*, 22: 245–255.

Patrick, K., Calfas, K.J., Wooten, W.J., Long, B.J. & Sallis, J.F. (1997) The impact of health-care providers on physical activity. In A.S. Leon (ed.) *Physical Activity and Cardiovascular Health*. Champaign, Il: Human Kinetics.

Pender, N.J., Sallis, J.F., Long, B.J. & Calfas, K.J. (1994) Health-care provider counselling to promote physical activity. In: Dishman, R.K. (ed.) *Advances in Exercise Adherence*, Champaign, Il: Human Kinetics, pp. 213–235.

Pinto, B.M., Goldstein, M.G. & Marcus, B.H. (1998a) Activity counselling by primary care physicians. *Preventive Medicine*, 27: 506–513.

Pinto, B.M., Goldstein, M.G., DePue, J.D. & Milan, F.B. (1998b) Acceptability and feasibility of physician-based activity counseling. The PAL project. *American Journal of Preventive Medicine*, 15(2): 95–102.

Pinto, B.M., Lynn, H., Marcus, B.H., DePue, J. & Goldstein, M.G. (2001) Physician-based activity counseling: intervention effects on mediators of motivational readiness for physical activity. *Annals of Behavioral Medicine*, 23(1): 2–10.

Podl, T.R., Goodwin, M.A., Kikano, G.E. & Strange, K.C. (1999) Direct observation of exercise counselling in community family practice. *American Journal of Preventive Medicine*, 17: 207–210.

Prochaska, J.O. & DiClemente, C.C. (1983) Stages and processes of self-change of smoking: toward an integrative model of change. *Journal of Consulting Clinical Psychology*, 51: 390–395.

Prochaska, J.J., Zabinski, M.F., Calfas, K.J., Sallis, J.F. & Patrick, K. (2000) PACE+: interactive communication technology for behavior change in clinical settings. *American Journal of Preventive Medicine*, 19(2): 127–131.

Riddoch, C., Puig-Ribera, A. & Cooper, A. (1998) *Effectiveness of Physical Activity Promotion Schemes in Primary Care: A Review*. London: HEA.

Rollnick, S., Mason, P. & Butler, C. (1999) *Health Behaviour Change: A guide for practitioners*. London: Churchill Livingstone.

Sallis, J.F. & Owen, N. (1999) *Physical Activity and Behavioral Medicine*. London: Sage.

Sevick, M.A., Dunn, A.L., Morrow, M.S., Marcus, B.H., Chen, G.H. & Blair, S. (2000) Cost-effectiveness of lifestyle and structured exercise interventions in sedentary adults; results of project active. *American Journal of Preventive Medicine*, 19: 1–8.

Simons-Morton, D.G., Calfas, K.J., Oldenburg, B. & Burton, N.W. (1998) Effects of interventions in health care settings on physical activity or cardio-respiratory fitness. *American Journal of Preventive Medicine*, 15(4): 413–430.

Simons-Morton, D.G., Hogan, P., Dunn, A.L., Pruitt, L., King, A.C., Levine, B.D. & Miller, S.T. (2000) Characteristics of inactive primary care patients: baseline data from the Activity Counseling Trial. For the Activity Counseling Trial Research Group. *Preventive Medicine*, 31(5): 513–521.

Singh, S. (1997) Why are GP exercise schemes so successful (for those who attend)? *Journal of Management in Medicine*, **11(4)**: 233–237.

Shephard, R.J. (1988) PAR-Q, Canadian Home Fitness Test and exercise screening alternative. *Sports Medicine*, **5(3)**: 282–291.

Smith, R.A. (1998) Health professionals' attitudes towards promoting physical activity. *Journal of Sport Science*, **16**: 104.

Smith, P., Gould, M., See Tai, S. & Iliffe, S. (1996) Exercise as therapy? Results from group interviews with general practice teams involved in an inner-London 'prescription for exercise' scheme. *Health Education Journal*, **55(4)**: 439–446.

Smith, B.J., Bauman, A.E., Bull, F.C., Booth, M.L. & Harris, M.F. (2000) Promoting physical activity in general practice: a controlled trial of written advice and informational materials. *British Journal of Sports Medicine*, **34(4)**: 262–267.

Steptoe, A. & Wardle, J. (1994). What the experts think: A survey of expert opinion in Europe about the influence of lifestyle on health. *European Journal of Epidemiology*, **10(2)**: 195–203.

Steptoe, A., Rink, E. & Kerry, S. (2000) Psychosocial predictors of changes in physical activity in overweight sedentary adults following counseling in primary care. *Preventive Medicine*, **31(2 Pt 1)**: 183–194.

Steptoe, A., Doherty, S., Kendrick, T., Rink, E. & Hilton, S. (1999) Attitudes to cardiovascular health promotion among GPs and practice nurses. *Family Practice*, **16(2)**: 158–163.

Steptoe, A., Doherty, S., Rink, E., Kerry, S., Kendrick, T. & Hilton, S. (1999) Behavioural counselling in general practice for the promotion of healthy behaviour among adults at increased risk of coronary heart disease: a randomised trial. *British Medical Journal*, **319**: 943–948.

Stevens, W., Hillsdon, M., Thorogood, M. & McArdle, D. (1998) The cost of a primary care-based physical activity intervention in 45–74 year old men and women: A randomised controlled trial. *British Journal of Sports Medicine*, **32(3)**: 236–241.

Stott, N.C.H., Kinnersley, P. & Rollnick, S. (1994) The limits to health promotion. *British Medical Journal*, **309**: 971–972.

Swinburn, B.A., Walter, L.G., Arroll, B., Tilyard, M.W. & Russell, D.G. (1997) Green prescriptions: attitudes and perceptions of general practitioners towards prescribing exercise. *British Journal of General Practice*, **47**: 567–569.

Swinburn, B.A., Walter, L.G., Arroll, B., Tilyard, M.W. & Russell, D.G. (1998) The green prescription study: a randomised controlled trial of written exercise advice in general practice. *American Journal of Public Health*, **88**: 288–291.

Talbot, H.-M. & Taylor, A.H. (1998) Changes in physical self-perceptions: findings from a randomised controlled study of a GP exercise referral scheme. *Journal of Sport Sciences*, **16(1)**: 105–106.

Taylor, A.H. (1994) Evaluating the efficacy of exercise promotion signs on Eastbourne seafront: observations and perceptions of over 35-year-olds. *British Journal of Physical Education: Research Supplement*, **14**: 17–22.

Taylor, A.H. (1996) *Evaluating GP Referral Schemes: Findings from a Randomised Controlled Study*. Chelsea School Topic Report No. 6, University of Brighton.

Taylor, A.H. (1997) Changes in perceived barriers towards exercising: findings from a randomised controlled study of a general practitioner exercise referral scheme. *Journal of Sport Sciences*, **15**: 107–108.

Taylor, A.H. (1999) Exercise promotion in primary health care. In: Bull, S.J. (ed.) *Adherence Issues in Exercise and Sport*. Chichester: Wiley Publishers.

Taylor, A.H., Doust, J. & Webborn, A.D.J. (1998) Randomised controlled trial to examine the effects of a GP exercise referral programme in East Sussex, UK, on modifiable coronary heart disease risk factors. *Journal of Epidemiology and Community Health*, **52**: 595–601.

The Writing Group for the Activity Counseling Trial Research Group (2001) Effects of physical activity counseling in primary care: the Activity Counseling Trial: a randomized controlled trial. *Journal of the American Medical Association*, **286(6)**: 677–687.

US Department of Health and Human Services (1996) *Physical Activity and Health: A Report of the Surgeon General*. Atlanta, GA: US Department of Health and Human Services, Centers for Disease Control and Prevention, National Center for Chronic Disease Prevention and Promotion.

Ussher, M.H., West, R., Taylor, A.H. & McEwen, A. (2000) Exercise interventions for smoking cessation (Cochrane Review) In: *The Cochrane Library*, 4. Oxford: Update Software.

Van Tulder, M.W., Koes, B.W. & Bouter, L.M. (1997) Conservative treatment of acute and chronic non-specific low back pain: a systematic review of randomised controlled trials of the most common interventions. *Spine*, **22(18)**: 2128–2156.

Walsh, J.E., Swangard, D.M., Davis, T. & McPhee, S.J. (1999) Exercise counselling by primary care physicians in the era of managed care. *American Journal of Preventive Medicine*, **16**: 307–313.

Wankel, L.M. & Sefton, J.M. (1994) Exercise and other lifestyle behaviours. In: Bouchard, C., Shephard, R.J. & Stephens, T. (eds) *Exercise, Fitness and Health*. Champaign, Il: Human Kinetics.

Wealden District Council (1995) *The Oasis Programme Evaluation Report 1995*. Hailsham, E. Sussex, UK: Wealden District Council Leisure Services.

Wealden District Council (1996) *The Oasis Programme Evaluation Report 1996*. Hailsham, E. Sussex, UK: Wealden District Council Leisure Services.

Williams, S.J., Calnan, M., Cant, S. & Coyle, J. (1993) All change in the NHS? Implications of the NHS reforms for primary care prevention. *Sociology of Health and Illness*, **15**: 107–112.

Williford, H.N., Barfield, B.R., Lazenby, R.B. & Olson, M.S. (1992) A survey of physicians' attitudes and practices related to exercise prescription. *Preventive Medicine*, **21**: 630–636.

Wonderling, D., McDermott, C., Buxton, M., Kinmouth, A.-L., Pyke, S., Thompson, S. *et al.* (1996a) Costs and cost effectiveness of cardiovascular screening and intervention: the British Family Heart Study. *British Medical Journal*, **312**: 1269–1273.

Wonderling, D., Langham, S., Buxton, M., Normand, C. & McDermott, C. (1996b) What can be concluded from the Oxcheck and British Family Heart studies: commentary on cost effectiveness analysis. *British Medical Journal*, **312**: 1274–1278.

CHAPTER 9

Promoting Physical Activity through Schools

KENNETH R. FOX AND JO HARRIS

Chapter Contents

▦ Schools and health promotion

▦ Research base on physical activity promotion in schools

▦ Curricular developments in health-enhancing physical activity

▦ Understanding the nature of physical activity in children

▦ Active school policies

▦ Making physical activity and sport more attractive to youngsters

▦ Influencing young people's activity decision making through schools

▦ The relevance of the physical education curriculum

▦ The importance of quality leadership

▦ Recommendations and needs

Schools and health promotion

One of the primary challenges to public health and health-care delivery is equity across all sectors of the population. This is heavily emphasised in current government health policy (Department of Health, 1997), based on evidence showing that those who are socio-economically disadvantaged are much more likely to engage in clusters of unhealthy behaviours and also experience less healthy living. It is well known to health promoters that these 'health needy' sectors of the population are the most difficult to reach as they are neither easily attracted to health-promotion services nor influenced by health-promotion campaigns.

The school system is therefore very important as a potential site for health promotion because:

- it offers one of the few settings where the full socio-economic spectrum is both represented and in attendance and where sustained exposure to healthy messages and health expertise can be achieved; this is in comparison to health centres, the workplace, or the media where attention is likely to be limited, voluntary, spontaneous and/or selective
- it occupies a good deal of the time of youngsters; in term time, including weekends, the school can influence the behaviour of children for about 40–45 per cent of their waking time; this is second only to the time spent in the home
- it has a primary function to provide a context for learning at a time of development that is characterised by high receptiveness.

Over the decades, governments and schools have taken advantage of these factors to promote several elements of healthy living, such as hygiene, safety, sexual health, nutrition, and physical fitness (sometimes for military preparedness). It is usually the case that the extent of commitment to health promotion is inversely proportional to the degree of pressure at the time to produce high academic standards. Both health education and health promotion are generally seen as curricular activities that compete with more traditional subjects, for example, maths, language, and sciences. The promotion of physical activity in schools has followed a similar track, with the physical education (PE) curriculum and school sport seen as expendable during times of high academic priority. A significant result of this is that the time allocated to physical education in the UK has been consistently among the lowest in Europe at both primary and secondary level. Subsequently, concern regarding the potential health consequences has been frequently expressed in both the UK and the USA (Harris, 1994; Fairclough & Stratton, 1997; Morrow *et al.*, 1999).

This chapter focuses on the need for British schools to be considered as a key site for the promotion of health-enhancing physical activity. In Britain, physical activity levels are noticeably low (Department of Health, 1998), and there are high levels of coronary heart disease, diabetes and obesity. Until recently, in Britain, the role of the school as a vehicle for the promotion of physical activity has not featured overtly in national health policy, although there appears to be a promising wind of change. Successive Ministers of Public Health have announced support for the role of the school in helping to create a healthier nation. This seems to be generating policy such as increased physical education time and improved sports provision that is designed, at least in part, to increase participation in physical activity and sport. As such, Britain appears to be at a point where it is beginning to face up to challenges that may eventually be experienced by other nations as they tackle the problems of sedentary living, largely caused by increasing dependence on high technology. In this chapter, therefore, there is a particular focus on the political context of British schools and their place in the promotion of physical activity for public health.

 Chapter 8 (Primary care) shows another case study of a venue where physical activity can be promoted.

Research base on physical activity promotion in schools

Before discussing the key issues of how health-enhancing physical activity might be most effectively promoted through the school system, it is appropriate to take some time to summarise existing research. Two recent reviews of formally evaluated school-based interventions to promote fitness and physical activity for health have been conducted (Almond & Harris, 1998; Stone *et al.*, 1998). Both reveal that most of the interventions have taken the form of innovative physical education programmes in primary schools in the United States. These have involved additional curricular physical education time allocation and often daily physical education provision. Earlier studies tended to focus primarily or solely on physiological outcomes, such as improvements in aspects of fitness. Studies that are more recent have taken the form of larger-scale interventions incorporating the measurement of multiple behaviours and environmental changes. However, it is difficult to tease out specific effects on physical activity. Almond & Harris (1998) concluded from this limited evidence base that health-related physical education programmes *can* produce improvement in physiological and clinical markers of health. Physical activity and affective measures have been assessed in a smaller number of studies, however most of these showed positive changes. The authors also noted that, even with additional time allocated to PE, there was some evidence that academic performance remained unimpaired.

The review of Stone and colleagues (1998) used stricter study inclusion criteria. Only studies with objective assessment of physical activity and a comparison or control group were considered. They concluded that meaningful improvements in health, knowledge and attitudes, and physical fitness were generally produced. In addition, positive effects on physical activity levels were found in studies that modified the physical education programme. It appeared possible to produce more activity in physical education lessons, but there was little evidence that such programmes influenced out-of-school physical activity. A further review of school-based cardiovascular health-promotion studies (Resnicow & Robinson, 1997) found that physical activity interventions were more effective in achieving their health-behaviour objectives than programmes directly targeting decreases in adiposity and they were equally as effective as dietary-change programmes.

These reviews reveal that curriculum-based intervention studies provide encouraging results. Indeed, Stone and colleagues (1998) consider that school-based physical activity interventions may have a special advantage as they can become institutionalised into the regular curriculum, and influence both staff development and school infrastructures. However, the research base is surprisingly insubstantial with few studies having been conducted outside the USA. The long-term effects remain unknown. There is also insufficient data to determine differential effects by age, gender or ethnicity. There is no conclusive information about the aspects of programme delivery (such as leadership qualities or extra time allocation) that are responsible for the observed positive effects. Furthermore, studies have been primarily limited to curricular change in physical education rather than changes in whole-school policy, which may be equally or more important. Unfortunately, therefore, the existing literature is not sufficiently extensive to provide definitive guidelines for schools about which types of programmes and strategies are most effective in promoting physical activity. Nor do we know the programme factors that determine success. We must therefore focus on existing policy, discuss the grass-roots attempts in schools to promote physical activity, summarise expert opinion, and draw upon the literature on the motivational aspects of children's engagement in physical education, physical activity and sport.

Curricular developments in health-enhancing physical activity

Regardless of the insubstantial research base, there has, since the 1980s, been a well documented and active interest by many UK physical education teachers in promoting health-related physical activity in schools (Williams, 1988). Similarly, interest has been expressed by academics in the USA (Corbin & Laurie, 1978; Corbin *et al.*, 1982) since the 1970s. Grass roots innovation by professionals is not unusual in the health promotion field and has underpinned the tremendous recent growth in 'referral for exercise' schemes, which involve collaboration between primary care and leisure services (Fox *et al.*, 1997; Riddoch *et al.*, 1998). The early approach in schools focused on a re-orientation of the physical education curriculum towards a 'health-related fitness' or 'fitness for life' emphasis, whereby knowledge, attitude and expertise were emphasised. Children were to be 'truly *physically* educated'. They were to be provided with the skills and instilled with the desire to engage in physical activity for the sake of health and well-being. Papers and articles espousing the logic of this approach have featured regularly in teaching journals and specialist texts have been produced (Biddle, 1981, 1987; Almond, 1983; Corbin & Lindsey, 1983; Harris & Elbourn, 1990). However, no rigorous evaluation has taken place and there is little information on its effectiveness in schools in the UK. This perhaps explains why it has struggled to be formally adopted as policy.

The movement was eventually given some consideration in the drafting of the first National Curriculum for Physical Education (NCPE) in 1992. While the NCPE brought with it a formal requirement that health issues should be addressed, its position and mode of expression in the curriculum were vague (Harris, 1997). Health-related physical activity was not afforded the status of a separate programme of study but treated as a theme that should be implicitly embedded in all practical activities and sports on offer in the curriculum. This received some criticism (Fox, 1992; Penney & Evans, 1997) on the basis that without a formal and explicit programme, exercise for health could be easily downgraded or omitted. Harris (1997) noted through her research that the subsequent teaching of health-related aspects of activity in physical education was characterised by confusion among teachers and considerable variation in practice. Health promotion as a key goal of physical education remained neither universally accepted nor well understood (Harris, 1995). Subsequent revisions of the NCPE (Department for Education, and the Welsh Office, 1995; Department for Education and Employment (DfEE) & Qualifications and Curriculum Authority (QCA), 1999) have provided a stronger positioning of health-related issues. This implies a more explicit prompt for health issues to be addressed in curriculum planning and delivery, but there remains only limited guidance on how this can be achieved. There is a belief by many that its effect may be minimal, because many teachers prefer to focus on competitive sport in the curriculum. Furthermore, changes in the terminology towards 'fitness' and 'training' highlight the continued and powerful influence of the focus on sport and performance in physical education in England (Penney & Evans, 1997, 1999; Hargreaves, 2000). Indeed Harris (1997) has noted that many health-related programmes are designed, taught and evaluated with an orientation more towards 'fitness for sports performance' than 'fitness for healthy lifestyles'. Harris & Penney (2000) also found that health-related physical education programmes often reflected, expressed and reinforced gender-specific practices through distinct 'female' and 'male' teacher versions of health-related exercise (HRE). Essentially, the 'female' teacher version of HRE was more holistic in its health-orientation, more lifetime-oriented and individualised in its approach, and more likely to be organised in single-sex groups. In contrast, the 'male' teacher version of HRE was more scientifically and technically oriented, with more emphasis on 'fitness and training', and more likely to be organised in mixed-sex groups. In sociological terms, curricular innovations, it appears, do not escape being shaped by contemporary educational beliefs and discourses.

Recently, there has been a call from the UK government to broaden provision within the physical education curriculum to enhance lifelong learning and healthy lifestyles. This has resulted in the removal of the compulsory requirement to study games (sports) for 14–16-year-olds (DfEE & QCA, 1999). Further, there are now government intentions to arrest the decline and possibly increase curricular physical education time, and to develop HRE guidance material for teachers (Harris, 2000). These are encouraging moves and should help to enhance future provision of education for health enhancing physical activity in schools.

Understanding the nature of physical activity in children

The literature and developments described so far are mainly restricted to how the physical education curriculum has been, or might be, used to influence children's health-related activity. During the past decade, our understanding of issues concerning children's activity and health has improved and we have broadened our perspective on the factors that shape children's physical activity patterns. In particular, the sheer complexity of physical activity as 'lifestyle' behaviour among all populations has become apparent. We now have a better understanding of the variety of activity modes, patterns and settings, together with the way participation in each influences the different aspects of physical functioning, disease risk and mental well-being. This in turn has stimulated a rapid concurrent growth of academic attention within the exercise and sports sciences. Within these developments, the difficulties of measuring and characterising the patterns of children's physical activity in relation to their health has posed a particular set of challenges that has been discussed in detail elsewhere (Fox & Riddoch, 2000; Boreham & Riddoch, 2001) including in this volume (see Cooper, Chapter 5; Boreham & Riddoch, Chapter 2). Clearly, our strategies for the promotion of children's physical activity through the school system should consider these key issues.

 Chapter 2 (Lifespan) details the rationale for promoting physical activity across the lifespan.

Two important consensus conferences have extensively reviewed the relevant research literature on children's physical activity and health. The findings of these reviews have shaped our thinking about children's health-enhancing physical activity. In 1994, a world conference held in San Diego, USA, provided health-related physical activity recommendations aimed specifically at adolescents (Sallis, 1994). A few years later, the English Health Education Authority's 'Young and Active?' conference (Biddle *et al.*, 1998) considered the physical activity needs of 5–18-year-olds. The expert consensus at both conferences was that, although the evidence linking children's physical activity with better health was not strong, it was sufficient to make broad statements about minimal levels of children's physical activity to achieve optimal health benefits. The more recent HEA recommendations were for participation in accumulated activity of at least moderate intensity for an hour a day. In addition, at least twice each week, activities should be included that will enhance muscular strength, flexibility and bone health. More recently, there has been a growing concern about increasing levels of obesity in children and this has resulted in recommendations for greater levels of daily movement and reductions in time spent in sedentary pursuits such as watching TV or playing computer games (National Audit Office, 2001). Therefore, it appears that at least four health-related dimensions of children's physical activity are worthy of consideration:

- accumulated moderate intensity activity for heart and circulatory health
- resistance or weight-bearing exercise for muscular fitness and bone health
- weight-bearing movement for increasing energy expenditure and avoiding obesity
- sedentary time, because of its potential to reduce activity and increase obesity.

Additionally, there are calls for modes of activity that provide mental health benefits for youngsters such as sports and physical activities that can develop a sense of achievement and satisfaction (Calfas & Taylor, 1995; Biddle *et al.*, 2000).

 Chapter 4 (Mental health) discusses the role of physical activity in promoting mental health.

Of critical importance to school policy for the promotion of physical activity is: (a) the *types* of activity that can produce these health benefits; (b) the free living and formalised *settings* in which they might take place; and (c) how each of these may vary among age, gender and ethnic groups. In this respect, greater attention is now being paid by researchers to the daily physical activity *patterns* of youngsters. Using diaries that section the day, and accelerometers that quantify minute-by-minute movements, comprehensive objective data from both school and weekend days can now be collected (see Cooper, Chapter 5). From this work, and evidence from the recent National Dietary and Nutrition Survey for 4–18-year-olds (Gregory *et al.*, 2000), it has become clear that youngsters' physical activity occurs in a range of settings, in a variety of modes and at particular times in the day:

- active transport to and from school, mainly through walking
- informal play during school breaks and lunchtimes, mainly for younger children
- informal play after school, mainly for younger children
- formal sports, PE and exercise training, particularly for older children
- active jobs for older children.

It is important to realise that the balance between these ways of being active varies considerably between individual children. For example, young children's activity is characterised by short, brisk bursts of 'kiss-and-chase' or 'kick-and-run' activities. The engagement of teenagers is more akin to adult activity and is likely to involve sustained moderate-intensity activity produced through sports or exercise, for example, jogging or aerobic dance. At all ages, but particularly from 12–13 years onwards, girls are consistently less active than boys, with many teenage girls achieving little or no moderate-to-vigorous activity at all. Weekend activity patterns are much more varied and inconsistent, compared to weekdays, probably due to a greater free choice of activities. However, on-going research at Bristol University using accelerometers suggests that weekends and holidays are no more active than schooldays and can even be less active, at least for boys. Additionally, children of all ages watch on average between two and three hours of television a day, with longer periods of viewing occurring at weekends.

Innovative research of this type is beginning to show how schools can contribute towards the achievement of optimal levels and patterns of physical activity in children. One message that emerges is that the focus on physical education provides only one part of the solution. Even with the proposed minimum of two hours a week of physical activity in schools, this represents at most only 1–2 per cent of the child's waking time. It is clear that whereas physical education time may be very important with respect to its ability to influence children's decisions about activity, physical activity shortfalls cannot be compensated in that time alone. Therefore, the design of health-related aspects of the physical education curriculum needs to be very carefully thought out (see later section). What does become evident is that other factors within the school system are also very important in determining children's physical activity patterns. Examples might include accessibility of the school from children's homes, the school routine, play facilities, and the extent of organised extra-curricular sport and exercise provision. All of these considerations suggest that it may be useful for schools to consider the physical activity *profiles* of children, because individuals or sub-groups of children might accrue their total amount of exercise in very different ways. Profiles would incorporate activity through transport, informal play, sports practice and games, work, and sedentary time (Fox, 1996). Recent work by Biddle and Wang has indicated that such profiles exist and that various clusters of activity profiles can be identified. Profiles are likely to vary according to the socio-economic and demographic characteristics of the neighbourhoods that constitute the school's catchment area.

The activity profiles of two children are shown in Figure 9.1. It can be seen that the activity patterns of Francis and Bobby contrast starkly, even though both are obviously quite active youngsters. In reality, Francis derives activity from formal sport at school, weekends and during the evenings but engages in little spontaneous play. Bobby, who lives on a council estate, is active through playing sport on the local recreation ground, walking to school, and

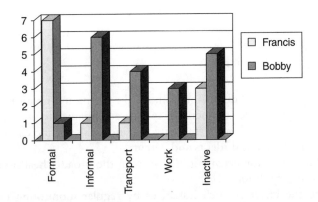

Figure 9.1 Contrasting activity profiles in hours per week

a half-hour paper round each morning. Greater use of this profile approach may help policy makers look beyond the confines of sport provision and physical education to a more comprehensive range of initiatives. It may also help to draw out important gender, age, ethnic and social group differences in activity needs.

Active school policies

It is now possible to achieve formal recognition as an 'active school'. The concept of the 'active school' implies that a broad and comprehensive approach is required for optimal effectiveness in the promotion of children's physical activity. In much the same way that schools might be considered 'healthy', they might be judged as 'active' by their environment, ethos, procedures and the curriculum they offer. The active school will be aware of the need to promote healthy physical activity in *all* children and will constantly be developing strategies that will (a) provide children with activity opportunities, and (b) increase their desire and knowledge base to sustain active lifestyles. Elements of the 'active school' concept have resonance with the environmental approach to activity promotion described and endorsed by Kerr, Eves & Carroll (Chapter 10).

 Chapter 10 (Environment) describes how changing enviromental factors help to encourage physical activity in public places.

There are many ways to achieve active school status, and each school will have unique characteristics that reflect the nature of the locality and the ethnic, gender, socio-economic mix of staff and pupils. In a climate of increasing prioritisation of human and physical resources and time, it is essential to have well-established policy-making machinery to ensure that physical activity promotion remains on the school agenda. A champion of the cause, capable of strong argument and with abilities to motivate staff and governors, will facilitate the process. This person might be supported by an 'active-school committee' whose function is to:

- act as a gateway and discussion point for incoming information on central or regional policy and commercially sponsored initiatives to promote activity
- develop short- and long-term strategies and goals for increasing physical activity among staff, students and parents
- co-ordinate physical activity initiatives with the broader health-promotion policies of the school
- evaluate the effect of such initiatives by regular monitoring of physical activity patterns among staff and students.

Strategies to promote physical activity can be achieved through changes in the environment, procedures or the curriculum, so that the influence of the school may extend far beyond its gates. Examples of strategies, many of which are already in operation in schools, some of them in collaboration with other organisations, are listed in Table 9.1. For more examples, see the recent *Young@heart* campaign documents (National Heart Forum, 2002).

Increasingly, government policy, commercial organisations and charitable trusts are supporting the development of sports and activity participation in

Table 9.1 Strategies for promoting activity through schools

Environmental change

- Developing a 'safe routes to school' initiative to encourage walking and cycling
- Installing secure cycle storage
- Working with local councils to develop safe play areas
- Producing a traffic free zone outside the school at critical hours
- Marking out the playground to encourage games playing

Procedural change

- Allowing access to sports facilities and playgrounds after school hours
- Developing a fitness and health appraisal scheme for staff
- Forging stronger links with local leisure facilities and sports clubs
- Involving year-11 and -12 pupils in the organisation and officiating of intra-mural sports competitions
- Producing a booklet for parents to help them work with children to reduce TV watching
- Developing a scheme to monitor playground bullying
- Developing a public-relations policy that helps build the reputation of the school as being healthy and active

Curricular change

- Offering cycle safety and maintenance courses
- Promoting active lessons in other subjects – for example mapping (geography), nature walks (biology) and measurement (mathematics)
- Exposing children through class projects to environmental issues around traffic, pollution, town planning for activity and safety

the school setting and schools will need to be well organised to take advantage of this. Indeed, the government's National Healthy School Standard (Department of Health & Department for Education and Employment, 2000) is already in place to promote physical activity as one of its three health themes. It is possible for schools to join award schemes to encourage activity and sport involvement such as Activemark, Sportsmark and the Youth Sport Trust's TOP programmes. The most recent government initiatives (DfCMS, 2001) explicitly aim to address issues relating to 'increasing participation by young people' and 'lifelong participation'. The implementation policy has a particular focus on social inclusion (reaching out to sections of the community who participate in less activity). Strategies include investment in school sports facilities, prevention of the sale of school playing fields, creation of 200 specialist Sports Colleges, extending out-of-school-hours learning opportunities to include physical education and sport for all pupils, and establishing 1000 school sports co-ordinators in communities of greatest need. It is interesting to note that access to finances for these developments is dependent on collaboration with local health-service providers. This may offer schools an excellent opportunity to add a stronger health focus to what are currently seen as developments in sport provision.

Other organisations will collaborate with schools to promote safe and healthy physical activity. These include the 'Safe Kids Campaign' launched by the Child Accident Prevention Trust in 1999, the School Travel Advisory Group (STAG), and Sustrans, who create 'Safe Routes to School' schemes. Active-schools resource packs and curricular materials for the teaching of health-enhancing physical activity have been produced by the British Heart Foundation and YMCA, respectively. Exercise-education schemes for teachers have been developed by the YMCA and the Keep Fit Association, and for sport leaders by the Central Council for Physical Recreation and most governing bodies of sport. The National Children's Bureau has developed computer materials for school children to map their travel to school routes, identify danger spots and plan for improvements. The Children's Play Council is developing traffic-restricted residential areas (home zones) to encourage safe play. Furthermore, several commercial organisations such as Glaxo-Wellcome, Nike, the Food and Drink Federation, and Mars have produced health, activity and sport schemes or materials for schools.

Therefore, a wide variety of resources is available to assist schools to develop their activity-promotion policy. However, the initial commitment by the school to establish policy-making machinery seems critical. The diverse range of agencies associated with children's sport and physical activity promotion suggests that lack of co-ordination at the school level may prove to be the critical barrier. An expectation that physical education teachers will increase their workloads at a time of staffing shortages is probably unrealistic. It may be that failing to provide the most important link – an active schools co-ordinator – could prove to be a serious omission and lead to wasted activity opportunities.

Making physical activity and sport more attractive to youngsters

Active-school policies could have a significant effect on several aspects of children's physical activity, simply by providing a greater number of opportunities. Many children report that they would prefer to walk or cycle to school (Balding, 1998), probably because it offers opportunities to talk to friends or possibly because it can be quicker and cheaper. Successful 'safe routes to school' policies might therefore have substantial impact on daily physical activity for large numbers of children. Road traffic and associated air pollution might also be reduced. Similarly, young children will become more active if the school playground is well designed and conducive to physical activity. There is also evidence that lack of sports facilities and sport opportunities are prohibitive where formal sport engagement is concerned (Coakley & White, 1992). Additional provision of physical resources should therefore have an impact.

Clearly, education is concerned both with influencing children's decision-making for the present, and their behaviour beyond the curriculum and the school years. The latter can be achieved only if the child's experiences of physical activity at school are delivered in a way that makes them seem attractive, worthwhile, and important. This may seem an obvious statement, but there is disturbing evidence that this is may not be the case. There is a gradual decline in physical activity, particularly engagement in sport or exercise participation, throughout the secondary-school years (Gregory *et al.*, 2000). Girls in particular, but also a large percentage of boys, exhibit very low rates of participation and most are clearly opting out when they have a choice to do so. This is at a time when the government is planning to dramatically increase access to sport and increase physical activity time in schools. In this regard, there may be a lesson to be learned from the experiences of many large corporations in America who, in the 1980s, invested heavily in expensive on-site exercise facilities for their workers, only to be disappointed that they were not widely used. The challenge here is to make sure that these extra opportunities are designed and offered in such a way that more of our youngsters are attracted to regular exercise and sport and that they become convinced of the value and importance of daily and lifelong physical activity. This applies to youngsters of all shapes, size, and ability.

 Chapter 2 (Lifespan) details the rationale for promoting physical activity across the lifespan, including childhood and adolescence.

The reasons why children do, and do not, engage in sport and exercise has been the subject of scientific investigation. Although speculative models of psychosocial determinants of physical activity participation have been around for some time (Sonstroem, 1976), sport and exercise psychologists have now produced a body of evidence that has identified critical factors in the sport and exercise motivation of children. These factors are closely tied to the components of human need identified by psychologists such as Epstein (1973), Rogers (1951), and Deci & Ryan (1996). It seems that sport and exercise are judged by individuals according to their capacity to provide personal fulfilment and affirmation. Briefly put, these are as follows:

The need to feel competent and capable　By the time youngsters leave school, there is a strong association between their perceptions of competence in sport and fitness activities and their levels of engagement. As children progress through early adolescence, they become increasingly able to accurately assess their level of ability in the range of pursuits on offer and there is naturally a strong tendency to opt out of those where a sense of inevitable failure, fear or embarrassment is perceived. Avoidance or disengagement is an obvious solution, as it preserves self-worth. Recent evidence suggests that development of a sense of mastery may be the key to experiencing feelings of competence in children throughout the range of ability. A mastery approach to teaching which encourages children to focus on self-improvement and task-completion and to avoid reliance on comparisons with others has been shown to produce higher levels of motivation in sport and exercise (Lloyd & Fox, 1992; Ntoumanis & Biddle, 1999; Papaioannou & Goudas, 1999). A focus on effort and progress makes sense when, by definition, excellence in performance can be achieved only by a small minority of children. An acknowledged problem of both physical education and coaching is that they are often designed to produce positive experiences for a limited range of children, generally of higher ability.

 Chapter 7 (Inactivity) describes how other theoretical concepts can be developed into practical support.

The need to feel autonomous and self-determined　Closely tied to mastery is the notion that individuals are better motivated when they experience responsibility for their own achievements. Such a sense of ownership develops through the belief that personal efforts and wise decisions, rather than innate ability, have produced the successful results. Allowing young people to experience responsibility and personal control and to take their place in the decision-making process regarding exercise and sport seem an important aspect of good teaching (Biddle, 1999).

The need to belong and feel valued　Although less well researched than might be expected, feeling a part of a group has a powerful effect on adolescents. They are busy striving to develop an individual identity but they also feel insecure and vulnerable and need the reassurance of affiliation to groups. Sports teams and exercise groups offer an opportunity to nurture such a sense of belonging. Additionally, young people will join groups because their friends already take part. In this sense, a crowd often forms a crowd. Unfortunately, adolescent girl cultures do not appear to value membership of sports groups as it is currently offered and this poses a serious challenge to the success of planned increases in provision of sports facilities. Increasing children's access to sport needs to consider psychosocial as well as physical availability. An essential precursor to joining a sports group is that individuals or peer groups see personal value in being associated with sports settings. Surprisingly, although peer-group membership has been studied extensively, this has not been extended to its impact on sport and exercise participation. An ongoing school-based intervention study in the UK, the Nike Girls in Sport Partnership, which focuses on helping to make physical education and sport more inclusive and attractive to girls (Kirk *et al.*, 2000), is currently addressing this issue.

Influencing young people's activity decision making through schools

The deep-seated self-enhancement motives discussed above will feed into young people's decisions about participation in sport and exercise, through their influence on beliefs, attitudes and values. Activities presented in a way which allows youngsters to experience competence and achievement, self-expression, responsibility for and ownership of success, and a sense of affiliation, will be fundamentally attractive to more youngsters. Activities also need to be seen to be enjoyable for their own sake, particularly by younger children who, unlike adolescents and adults, are unable to delay gratification – which is needed when fitness and skill improvements, and perhaps social benefits are sought. Additionally, if schools are to influence children's broader activity patterns such as increasing levels of walking and cycling, or reducing the amount of sedentary time, then children will need convincing of the benefits. They might also need to be shown specific strategies that can effect change.

For young children, the decision-making formula is relatively simple. If activity is fun, then it is worthwhile. As youngsters enter adolescence, they become much more body conscious and sensitive, and are able to make judgements that are more accurate and attributions[1] about their performances. Their behavioural choices are based on the relative risks, rewards and costs of sport or exercise participation within the range of options that the adolescent world has to offer. Early adolescence is a particularly difficult time as children's bodies are changing rapidly and they know little about what the future holds regarding the development of physiques and physical abilities. Ironically, this is a time when decisions are made, which can affect the individual for the rest of their life. Indirect evidence for this comes from the Allied Dunbar National Fitness Survey (Sports Council/HEA, 1992) indicating that one of the main reasons that adults report lack of regular exercise is 'because I am not the sporty type'. Presumably, for many, this identity statement and confusion between sport and physical activity was established early in life. To prevent this becoming a common perception that prohibits physical activity participation in adult life, positive childhood experiences of sport and exercise are needed. In this way, these behaviours can become central to the identities of young people.

The relevance of the physical education curriculum

Time allocated to physical education is meagre and cannot alone satisfy the physical activity needs of children. This means that the content of the programme has to be efficient and effective. It is clear that the traditional programme, dominated by team games, currently has limited appeal to a large proportion of children. Although there is little robust evidence to support the effectiveness of alternative programmes, the psychosocial factors discussed above would suggest that certain key features might, if incorporated, produce successful programmes. For example:

- Facilitating the early development of a range of motor and sports skills in children of all abilities. Remedial help may be offered to small, weak, poorly co-ordinated or obese youngsters, or to children who miss activity opportunities through chronic or episodic illness.
- Introducing more individual sports such as racket sports, orienteering or golf, and individualised fitness activities such as aerobics, fitness circuits, weight-training, and swimming for fitness. This would allow more opportunity for the measurement and experience of personal improvement.
- Providing activities acceptable to a range of adolescent subcultures. Girls are more likely to engage in activities seen as relevant to the values of their peer group. Aerobic dance, step aerobics or aquafit may be more acceptable than field hockey or netball.
- Teaching the 'why' of physical activity within the formal curriculum, so that youngsters understand and accept the importance of physical activity for health and well-being.
- Teaching the 'how' of physical activity, so that youngsters gain the expertise and confidence to exercise effectively and safely.
- Helping youngsters to develop self-management skills that equip them to make lifestyle changes perceived to be important.
- Creating a teaching or coaching climate where children can develop a sense of responsibility for their personal improvement in fitness and sport skills.
- Helping youngsters to understand the environmental impact of over-reliance on motorised transport. Additionally, encouraging a critical perspective on local planning and how the design of localities can be improved to make them 'activity friendly'.
- Helping youngsters to see how activity can resonate with the particular characteristics of their own, and other ethnic groups.

The importance of quality leadership

A common finding in health-service research is that the quality of leadership or professional contact is critical to programme success. For young people, physical educators, fitness leaders and sport coaches have a crucial role to play in developing both short- and long-term motivation to be physically active. Taking the perspective that activity itself is a neutral experience, then the way it is presented can have a positive or negative impact. Teachers who embrace a philosophy that the central feature of education and schooling is the welfare, development and health of the child are more likely to make child-centred decisions and produce positive experiences regardless of the nature of the activity. Additionally, understanding and applying developmental and motivational psychology in children would appear critical to the stimulation of physical activity involvement. Unfortunately, few physical educators have been adequately trained to address the health-enhancing aspects of physical activity promotion in children (Harris, 1997; Pate *et al.*, 1999), although broadening competitive sport participation is a recurrent theme.

School-based intervention studies in the USA have shown that specific training for physical education teachers can make a difference to the amount of physical activity achieved during lessons (Sallis & Owen, 1999). Sallis and colleagues (1999) have also demonstrated that physical-education specialists can improve children's physical activity much more than classroom teachers, and the latter provided better results than untrained teachers. A few studies have also indicated the long-term effects of teacher training (McKenzie *et al.*, 1997), especially where the physical education programme is delivered by specialists or trained classroom teachers receiving on-site support. For example, the Child and Adolescent Trial for Cardiovascular Health (CATCH) study in the USA demonstrated that after three academic years of training and assistance in using the health-related curriculum, intervention students were active for 51 per cent of physical education class time, compared with 42 per cent for control students (McKenzie *et al.*, 1996). Although these studies do not show the kinds of impact we might look for in children's physical activity decision-making and overall levels of activity, they do show that intensive input to teacher education can make a difference to the experiences of children in physical education.

Preparation of physical educators in the UK continues to face several challenges. Nearly all three- or four-year undergraduate specialist courses in physical education have disappeared. The common route to qualified physical education teacher status is through a three-year undergraduate programme in sports studies or sports science, followed by a one year post-graduate teaching certificate in physical education. Due to increasingly large student intakes and cost-cutting measures, few undergraduate programmes offer adequate practical sports or exercise-teaching experience. Only one-third of the post-graduate certificate year is available for study of health-related concepts, child develop-ment and motivational principles – all of which are necessary to fully appreci-ate patterns of physical activity engagement and how they vary between different types of children. Usually the time is spent developing technical coaching skills in a range of sports. Secondary-level trainee teachers then enter schools where curricular values are set by teachers who have had minimal exposure to, and have limited acceptance of, a health-related physical activity perspective. Many are unaware of the health-related physical activity recom-mendations for children or indeed of the 'paradigm shift' from fitness to life-style activity that has been the main theme of adult physical activity promotion over the past 20 years (Cale & Harris, 2001). The situation in pri-mary schools, where children should be learning important physical skills, is even worse, as physical education is normally taught by non-specialist teach-ers. With the progressively greater involvement of volunteer sports coaches in the system, these inadequacies are likely to worsen. Certainly, with the current organisation of teacher education, there is little opportunity for the required positive change and innovation.

Recommendations and needs

Over recent years, several recommendations for physical activity promotion through schools have been published in the UK (Health Education Authority, 1998; Harris, 2000; National Audit Office, 2001; National Heart Forum, 2002) and in the USA (Centers for Disease Control and Prevention, 1997, 2000; Morrow *et al.*, 1999). These share many common themes.

Firstly, there is a need for a whole-school approach that incorporates:

- The development of school policies that promote lifelong physical activity.
- The provision of social and physical environments at school and in the local community that encourage and enable safe and enjoyable physical activity.
- Frequent access to high-quality, adequately-resourced physical education designed to promote physical activity and delivered by appropriately trained and supported staff.
- The promotion of classroom health education that complements physical education.
- The expansion of inclusive extra-curricular programmes that feature a selection of competitive and non-competitive, structured and unstructured, team and individual activities that meet the needs and interests of young people with a wide range of abilities.
- Access to community physical activity programmes that meet the needs and interests of all young people.

- Training for individuals who can play a role in promoting physical activity among young people to help them provide developmentally appropriate, safe and enjoyable activity experiences.
- Parental education and involvement in school and community programmes that directly support their children's physical activity.

Secondly, there is a need to target particularly needy populations. The President's Council on Physical Fitness and Sports (Morrow *et al.*, 1999) has called for interventions differentiated on the grounds of gender, age/life-stage and socio-economic status – separate strategies for different age groups formulated around recognised age-specific determinants such as opportunities for play, support of friends and competence in physical activities. Such a proposal will emphasise that, for all life-stages, enjoyment of physical activity, success and peer and family support are key features. Priority groups for further investigation have included young people from black and minority ethnic groups, individuals with physical and mental disabilities, and those with clinical conditions such as obesity, clinical depression or diabetes. The Health Education Authority (Biddle *et al.*, 1998) proposed interventions specifically targeted at girls aged 12–18 years, young people of low socio-economic status, and older adolescents.

Thirdly, investment in research is needed to determine the effectiveness of different school-based approaches to the promotion of young people's physical activity. Given the potential impact of the school on the lifestyles of young people, it is worrying that so little systematic and sequential research has been undertaken, particularly in UK and mainland Europe. Many environmental and curricular interventions have been attempted at grass-roots level. However, because rigorous research and evaluation requires skills and funding that are rarely available, there has been little opportunity to build an evidence base regarding programme effectiveness and mechanisms of change. Most of the important questions remain unanswered. For example, little is known about the effectiveness of safe routes to schools, or elements such as 'walking buses', new cycle routes, cycle storage, improved access, traffic-reduction schemes or the ways in which each of these changes the lifestyles of children and their families. Within the school, neither the effectiveness of formal programmes of teaching health-enhancing activity concepts, nor the effects of extra-curricular sport and exercise programmes have been investigated. Although the positive impact of a mastery-oriented teaching climate has been indicated in several studies, the most effective way of facilitating the adoption of such an approach by teachers and coaches has not been established. The importance of active school co-ordinators has been suggested, but this has yet to be researched. The answers to critical questions such as these can be achieved only through serious commitment to long-term research funding by the research councils, trusts and charities. Until such an evidence base is constructed then the design and delivery of effective activity-promotion initiatives will remain uninformed, undirected and sporadic. Hopefully, this chapter has made the case that the contribution of the school as vehicle for physical activity and public-health promotion is too great to be left to chance.

Note

1 Attributions are reasons individuals provide for their successes and failures. For example a child may think they won a tennis match because they tried really hard or because their opponent did not play well.

References

Almond, L. (1983) A rationale for health related fitness in schools. *Bulletin of Physical Education*, **19(2)**: 5–10.

Almond, L. & Harris, J. (1998) Interventions to promote health-related physical education. In: Biddle, S., Sallis, J. & Cavill, N. (eds) *Young and Active? Young People and Health-enhancing Physical Activity – Evidence and Implications*, London: Health Education Authority, pp. 133–149.

Balding, J. (1998) *Young People in 1997*. Exeter: Schools Health Education Unit.

Biddle, S. (1981) The why of health-related fitness. *Bulletin of Physical Education*, **17(3)**: 28–31.

Biddle, S.J.H. (1999) Motivation and perceptions of control: Tracing its development and plotting its future in exercise and sport psychology. *Journal of Sport and Exercise Psychology*, **21**: 1–23.

Biddle, S.J.H., Fox, K.R. & Boutcher, S.H. (2000) *Physical Activity and Psychological Well-being*. London & New York: Routledge.

Biddle, S., Sallis, J. & Cavill, N. (1998) *Young and Active? Young People and Health-enhancing Physical Activity – Evidence and Implications*. London: Health Education Authority.

Cale, L. & Harris, J. (2001) Exercise recommendations for young people: An update. *Health Education*, **101(3)**: 126–138.

Calfas, K.J. & Taylor, W.C. (1994) Effects of physical activity on psychological variables in adolescents. *Pediatric Exercise Science*, **6**: 406–423.

Centers for Disease Control and Prevention (1997) Guidelines for school and community programs to promote lifelong physical activity among young people. *Morbidity and Mortality Weekly Report*, **46**: RR–6.

Centers for Disease Control and Prevention (2000) *Promoting Better Health for Young People through Physical Activity and Sports*. A report to the President from the Secretary of Health and Human Services and the Secretary of Education.

Coakley, J. & White, A. (1992) Making decisions: gender and sports participation among British adolescents. *Sociology of Sport Journal*, **9**: 20–35.

Corbin, C. & Laurie, D. (1978) Exercise for a lifetime: An educational effort. *Physician and Sportsmedicine*, **6**: 50–55.

Corbin, C. & Lindsey, R. (1983) *Fitness for Life. (2nd ed.)* Glenview, IL: Scott, Foresman and Company.

Deci, E.L. & Ryan, R.M. (1996) Human autonomy: The basis for true self-esteem. In: Kernis, M. (ed.) *Agency, Efficacy, and Self-esteem*, New York: Plenum, pp. 31–49.

Department for Culture, Media and Sport (DfCMS) (2001) *A Sporting Future for All. The Government's Plan for Sport*. London: DfCMS.

Department for Education, and the Welsh Office (DfE and WO) (1995) *Physical Education in the National Curriculum*. London: HMSO.

Department for Education and Employment (DfEE) & Qualifications and Curriculum Authority (QCA) (1999) *Physical Education. The National Curriculum for England*. London: HMSO.

Department of Health (1997) *Our Healthier Nation*. London: HMSO.

Department of Health (1998) *Health Survey for England: Cardiovascular Disease*. London: The Stationery Office.

Epstein, S. (1973) The self-concept revisited or a theory of a theory. *American Psychologist*, **28**: 405–416.

Fairclough, S. & Stratton, G. (1997) Physical education curriculum and extra curriculum time: A survey of secondary schools in the North West of England. *British Journal of Physical Education*, **28**: 21–24.

Fox, K.R. (1992) Education for exercise and the National Curriculum proposals: A step forwards or backwards? *British Journal of Physical Education*, **23**: 8–11.

Fox, K.R. (1996). Physical activity promotion and the active school. In N. Armstrong (ed.) *New Directions in Physical Education – Volume III* (pp. 94–109), London: Farmer.

Fox, K.R. & Riddoch, C.J. (2000) Charting physical activity patterns in contemporary young people. *Proceedings of the Nutrition Society*, **59**: 1–8.

Fox, K.R., Biddle, S.J.H., Edmunds, L.E., Bowler, I. & Killoran, A. (1997) Physical activity promotion through primary health care in England. *British Journal of General Practice*, **47**: 367–379.

Gregory, J., Lowe, S., Bates, C.J., Prentice, A., Jackson, L., Smithers, G., Wenlock, R. & Farron, M. (2000) *National Diet and Nutrition Survey: Young People Aged 4–18 years.* London: The Stationery Office.

Hargreaves, J. (2000) Gender, morality and the national physical education curriculum. In: Hansen, J. & Nielsen, N. (eds) *Sports, Body and Health*, Odense University Press.

Harris, J. (1994) Physical education in the National Curriculum: Is there enough time to be effective? *British Journal of Physical Education*, **25**: 4.

Harris, J. (1995) Physical education: a picture of health? *British Journal of Physical Education*, **26**: 25–32.

Harris, J. (1997) *Physical Education: A Picture of Health? The Implementation of Health-Related Exercise in the National Curriculum in Secondary Schools in England.* Unpublished doctoral thesis, Loughborough University.

Harris, J. (2000) *Health-related Exercise in the National Curriculum. Key Stages 1 to 4.* Champaign, IL: Human Kinetics.

Harris, J. & Elbourn, J. (1990) *Action for Heart Health. A Practical Health Related Exercise Programme for Physical Education.* Loughborough University: Exercise and Health Group.

Harris, J. & Penney, D. (2000) Gender issues in health-related exercise. *European Physical Education Review*, **6**: 249–273.

Kirk, D., Fitzgerald, H., Wang, J. & Biddle, S. (2000) *Towards Girl-friendly Physical Education: The Nike/YST Girls in Sport Partnership Project. Final Report.* Institute of Youth Sport, Loughborough University.

Lloyd, J. & Fox, K.R. (1992) The effect of contrasting interventions on the achievement orientation and motivation of adolescent girls to exercise. *British Journal of Physical Education Research Supplement*, **11**: 12–16.

McKenzie, T.L., Nader, P.R., Strikmiller, P.K., Yang, M., Stone, E., Perry, C.L. *et al.* (1996) School physical education: Effect of the child and adolescent trial for cardiovascular health. *Preventive Medicine*, **25**: 423–431.

McKenzie, T.L., Sallis, J.F., Kolody, B. & Faucett, F.N. (1997) Long-term effects of a physical education curriculum and staff development work: SPARK. *Research Quarterly in Exercise and Sport*, **68**: 280–291.

Morrow, J.R., Jackson, A.W. & Payne, V.G. (1999) Physical activity promotion and school physical education. *President's Council on Physical Fitness and Sports Research Digest*, **3**: 1–7.

National Audit Office (2001) *Tackling Obesity in England.* London: The Stationery Office.

National Heart Forum (2002) *Young@Heart: A Healthy Start for a New Generation.* London: National Heart Forum.

Ntoumanis, N. & Biddle, S.J.H. (1999) A review of motivational climate in physical activity. *Journal of Sports Sciences*, **17**: 643–665.

Papaioannou, A. & Goudas, M. (1999) Motivational climate of the physical education class. In: Vanden Auweele, Y., Bakker, F., Biddle, S., Durand, M. & Seiler, R. (eds) *Psychology for Physical Educators*, Champaign, IL: Human Kinetics, pp. 51–68.

Pate, R.R., Small, M.L., Ross, J.G., Young, J.C., Flint, K.H. & Warren, C.W. (1999) School physical education. *NASPE Speak II Advocacy Kit*, pp. 19–26.

Penney, D. & Evans, J. (1997) Naming the Game. Discourse and domination in Physical Education and sport in England and Wales. *European Physical Education Review*, **3**: 21–32.

Penney, D. & Evans, J. (1999) *Politics, Policy and Practice in Physical Education*. London: EdFN Spon.

Resnicow, K. & Robinson, T.N. (1997) School-based cardiovascular disease prevention studies: Review and synthesis. *Annual of Epidemiology*, 7: S14–S31.

Riddoch, C.J., Puig-Ribera, A. & Cooper A. (1998) *The Effectiveness of Physical Activity Promotion Schemes in Primary Care: A Systematic Review*. London: Health Education Authority.

Rogers, C.R. (1951) *Client-centered Therapy*. Boston: Houghton Mifflin.

Sallis, J.F. (1994) Physical activity guidelines for adolescents. *Pediatric Exercise Science (Special issue)*, 6: 299–463.

Sonstroem, R.J. (1976) The validity of self-perceptions regarding physical and athletic ability. *Medicine and Science in Sports*, 8: 126–132.

Sports Council/Health Education Authority (1992) *Allied Dunbar National Fitness Survey: Main findings*. London: Author.

Stone, E.J., McKenzie, T.L., Welk, G.J. & Booth, M.L. (1998) Effects of physical activity interventions in youth: Review and synthesis. *American Journal of Preventive Medicine*, 15: 298–315.

Wang, J.C.K. & Biddle, S.J.H. (2001) Young people's motivational profiles in physical activity: A cluster analysis. *Journal of Sport and Exercise Psychology*, 23: 1–22.

Williams, A. (1988) The historiography of health and fitness in physical education. *British Journal of Physical Education Research Supplement*, 3: 1–4.

CHAPTER 10

The Environment: the Greatest Barrier?

JACQUELINE KERR, FRANK EVES AND DOUGLAS CARROLL

Chapter Contents

Introduction

The physical activity crisis

In population terms, the visible fitness boom of the 20th century has failed to compensate for the loss of more traditional sources of energy expenditure (King *et al.*, 1999). Changing patterns of transport and work, electronic communication, internet shopping, energy-saving devices such as escalators, motorised lawn mowers, washing machines, and remote controls, as well as sedentary entertainment such as television and computer games, make it possible to be virtually inactive but occupied. While the loss of any one traditional activity is likely to have only a marginal impact on energy expenditure, the composite effect of such lifestyle changes is now appreciated to be substantial

(Hill *et al.*, 2000). It is estimated that over 80 per cent of the population in industrialised nations is insufficiently active (ADNFS, 1992). Further, the Healthy People 2000 target for physical activity, that no more than 15 per cent of the population be completely sedentary, is unlikely to be met until 2024, if at all (King *et al.*, 1999). To date, cognitive behavioural exercise interventions have been largely unsuccessful (Sallis, 1998) and educational efforts have been ineffective in reversing a seemingly inexorable population trend toward inactivity (King *et al.*, 1999).

 Chapter 12 (Anthropology) illustrates how populations can change their activity levels.

Ideologically, behavioural and educational interventions tend to hold individuals liable for their inactive behaviour, and respond by intervening at an individual level. Behavioural choices, however, are not made in a vacuum (Breslow, 1996) and it may be unreasonable to expect individuals to become more active when inactivity is so strongly reinforced by their environment and prevailing social norms (Schmid *et al.*, 1995). Thus, not only have current behavioural and educational approaches proved insufficient to change population exercise behaviour, only perverse optimism could continue to sustain the belief that they should. In addition, the behavioural approach may not only be unrealistic, it may also be counter-productive in contemporary social and physical infrastructures (Schmid *et al.*, 1995; Sallis *et al.*, 1998; Minkler *et al.*, 2000). Encouraging activity, *per se*, could actually increase exposure to health hazards – for example, in the absence of safe cycle lanes, active transport initiatives may increase the incidence of cycling accidents. Encouraging jogging in low income neighbourhoods, where pavements are poorly maintained and frequented by drug users, might increase exposure to a range of risks. Children playing without adequate sun protection may also be at greater risk for skin cancer. In this context, it is important to appreciate that pressuring drivers to abandon their cars for more active commuting options, however well intentioned, amounts to little more than empty rhetoric in the absence of an integrated and reliable public transport system. It is also worth pointing out that the facilities required for some activities, such as watersports, can damage fragile ecosystems (House of Commons, 1995).

Behavioural and educational interventions have focused principally on leisure-time activity. Most people, however, spend more of their time at work, in transit, and performing household chores (King *et al.*, 1999). Encouraging activity at these times and in these environments may be the most profitable focus for addressing low levels of physical activity. Lifestyle activities or task-oriented physical activities that are sufficiently intense to result in the recommended health benefits (Pate *et al.*, 1995), may be more likely to respond to intervention (Hillsdon, 1995; Dunn *et al.*, 1998). Such activities are also more susceptible to environmental change (King *et al.*, 1999). Walking and stair-climbing, for example, could be undertaken easily by large segments of the population throughout the week, and may be particularly amenable to environmental reinforcement (King *et al.*, 1999).

In general terms, it has been argued that the modification of social, economic, and environmental factors can yield greater population-health dividends than individual lifestyle approaches (Nutbeam, 1997). Environmental interventions can reach larger and broader constituencies (Bauman *et al.*, 1999), including low-income groups where environmental barriers may be particularly constraining (Sallis *et al.*, 1998). Environmental approaches may also result in longer-lasting effects as environmental change is assimilated into structures, systems, policies, and sociocultural norms (Swinburn *et al.*, 1999). It is perhaps hardly surprising, then, that a number of researchers have begun to advocate environmental solutions to physical inactivity (King *et al.*, 1995; Schmid *et al.*, 1995; Sallis *et al.*, 1998; Sallis & Owen, 1999).

In the context of physical activity, various environmental manipulations, likely to sponsor increased activity, have been proposed. At the outset, though, it is worth pointing out that the environmental approach is not only intuitively appealing, it also has strong theoretical foundations. Nevertheless, a number of questions remain. For example, are perceived environmental barriers to physical activity merely proxies for poor individual motivation (Sallis *et al.*, 1998)? If actual physical and social environmental barriers do exist, will removing them result in increased physical activity? In addition, environmental change can be difficult to implement; it requires, *ipso facto*, a multi-disciplinary approach and the collaboration of a range of expertises: commercial, political, academic, and health-related. Further, proposed environmental interventions may be working against prevailing economic, social, and technical trends, as well as those who supply and support the efficiency of the new technologies, such as employers and manufacturers (Sallis *et al.*, 1998; Hill *et al.*, 2000; Sparling *et al.*, 2000).

Theoretical foundations for environmental change

The idea of an environmental approach to public health is not new. Many successful public-health initiatives have involved environmental and/or policy change: sanitation, water purification, road safety, for example (Schmid *et al.*, 1995; King *et al.*, 1999). Health promotion has long been regarded as best served by a combination of educational and environmental approaches (Sallis *et al.*, 1998). Education, however, has proved a far more popular tool of late than environmental manipulation, despite persuasive arguments that environmental interventions ought to take precedence over educational ones (Sallis *et al.*, 1998; King *et al.*, 1999). For example, a review of 44 health-promotion programmes concluded that programmes targeting intra- and inter-personal change substantially outnumbered ecological interventions (Richard *et al.*, 1996). Ease of implementation is undoubtedly a factor here (Green *et al.*,

1996). So too, though, is the ideology of personal responsibility and the construction of behaviour, including healthy behaviour, as volitional, an expression of free will and choice. Such an ideology regards education as the simple dissemination of information to help inform personal choice whereas environmental-level intervention is regarded as transcending or even subverting free will and choice (Schmid *et al.*, 1995). These sorts of considerations have been used to explain, why, in contrast to behavioural interventions, the environmental approach has been little used in, for example, cardiovascular disease prevention (Sallis *et al.*, 1998).

A theoretical foundation is essential for any health-promotion intervention and an environmental approach can be supported from many theoretical perspectives. Dwyer (1997) regards Organisational Development Theory as offering the means for moving from isolated physical activity promotion initiatives to a systematic and co-ordinated national approach. Reciprocal Determinism from Bandura's Social Cognitive Theory describes how individuals' behaviour and the environment continuously interact and influence each other (Sallis *et al.*, 1993). A Human Ecological approach maintains that the environment largely controls or sets limits on the behaviour that occurs in it and that environmental modification results in changes to behaviour (Green *et al.*, 1996). The Social Ecological approach goes beyond behavioural and environmental change strategies by offering a theoretical framework for understanding the dynamic interplay among persons, groups, and their social and physical *milieus* (Stokols, 1992). Stokols (1996) argued that a Social Ecological approach evolved from and incorporates other theoretical models, such as the Biopsychosocial Model of Health, the Person-Environment Fit Theory, the Ecology of Human Development, and Community Health Promotion. The Theory of Diffusion of Innovations can also be regarded as relevant here (Schmid *et al.*, 1995), as it postulates that only early adopters of a new behaviour make positive choices based on new information. Late adopters, the majority, require a supportive environment to instigate change (Schmid *et al.*, 1995). Behavioural Choice Theory also describes how we make decisions in the context of external stimuli and reinforcements (Epstein, 1998).

Considered together, these theoretical frameworks provide an eclectic and multi-layered conceptualisation of the environment. Duhl (1996) describes the environment as a web of relationships: biologic, spatial, physical, social, political, and cultural. Stokols (1992) defines the physical environment as geographic, architectural, and technical, and the social environment as cultural, economical, and political. Environmental manipulations can also operate at individual, corporate, community, regional, national or global levels. It is this complex representation of the environment that demands a multi-disciplinary approach, and, by extension, the implementation of environmental change necessitates extensive, structured, and systematic collaborative endeavour (Wandersman *et al.*, 1996; Harris & Wills, 1997; Kickbusch, 1997; Cohen *et al.*, 2000). No ecological model makes the claim that environmental variables are

the only influences on behaviour (Sallis *et al.*, 1998); rather they stress the reciprocal and dynamic interaction of people and the environment. As a consequence,
environmental change has to be regarded from a similarly interactive perspective
(Sparling *et al.*, 2000). A good example of the benefits of the synergy between
passive and active public-health strategies is the 50 per cent reduction in
motor-vehicle fatality rates per mile driven over the past 25 years (Schmid
et al., 1995). The structure of roads and cars has improved, legislation, which
is enforced, for seat belts, speed limits and drink-driving is in place, and there
has been a sea change in the attitudes and behaviours of individual drivers
with regard to the risk (Schmid *et al.*, 1995). Thus, health-promotion strategies should match environmental and policy-intervention strategies to the
behavioural needs of the population groups targeted. At the same time,
though, it is important to recognise that different groups in different settings
will react differently to environmental contingencies (King *et al.*, 1999).
Clearly, a range of considerations should inform an environmental approach
to health promotion, such that the broadest possible audience is reached by
an intervention.

The potential of environmental change in physical activity promotion

It is difficult to escape the conclusion that this sort of complex conceptualisation of the environment, with its radical implications for intervention, has
yet to be fully accommodated by many of those engaged in the promotion
of physical activity. However, a number of suggestions for environmental
change have been made and these are presented in Table 10.1. In some
instances, proposals were made to stimulate further research (Sallis *et al.*, 1998).
Few, if any of them, have attracted anything approaching proper empirical
investigation. The contents of Table 10.1 are derived from several sources.
(Environmental working groups in the USA; the Department for the Environment, Transport and the Regions, UK: National Cycling Strategy; Blair
et al., 1996; Corti *et al.*, 1996; Booth & Samdal, 1997; Holman, 1997; Sallis
et al., 1998; King *et al.*, 1999; Sallis & Owen, 1999; Swinburn *et al.*, 1999;
Brownson *et al.*, 2000; Price *et al.*, 2000; Richter *et al.*, 2000; Wechsler *et al.*,
2000).

The example of a cyclist commuting to work can be elaborated to demonstrate how barriers to physical activity arise and how environmental changes
might be deployed to counter them. First, since our cycling commuter needs
a reliable bicycle, cost might be the first barrier. A company-subsidised bicycle
could help reduce costs, as could reduced sales tax. Payment per mile of
cycling by the company or a tax break might act as a further incentive. After
all, companies throughout the world provide free or heavily subsided motor
cars to some of their employees. If the ability to cycle is a problem, safe cycle
training could be provided through local government or local charities. Scouts

Table 10.1   Environmental proposals for physical activity promotion

In the community

City centres   pedestrian zones; green zones; displaced parking so people walk further; exclude cars from town centres; increase parking charges; continuous paths around town.

Facilities   availability of low-cost facilities; activities appropriate to environment, for example, cross-country skiing or indoor facilities when cold, outdoor swimming pools when hot; liability legislation; subsidise exercise-equipment manufacturers and leisure-facility providers; accessible stairways; out-of-hours shopping-centre walking; longer opening hours.

Parks   availability of toilets, drinking water, lighting, shaded areas; use spaces around institutions for example hospitals; safety features; well-used so no crime; parks with trees and walking paths, not just open space for organised team sports.

Residential areas   neighbourhood clean-ups in parks, roads and beaches; neighbourhood-watch walking groups.

In transport

Separate walkways for pedestrians, pedestrian-friendly sidewalks, handrails, bricked crosswalks, change patterns of lines.

Increase accessibility to facilities by short trips; link cycle and walking paths to public transport, businesses and shops; link urban routes to countryside.

Enable combinations of cycling and public transport, cycle carriers on buses and trains

Improve cycle safety, reduce traffic speeds, restrict heavy goods vehicles (HGVs), improve road-user courtesy, education and enforcement of driving laws.

'Think cycling' in all highway management and public transport schemes; reallocate road space; secure and ample cycle parking; reduce cycle theft; cycle-loan schemes

Raise public awareness of physical activity options with transport providers, cyclists, other road users, retailers and so on.

At work

Businesses adjacent to residential areas with connecting paths.

Showers, changing facilities, cycle racks, activity areas, team 'stroll, strut, stride' schemes, sponsored team sports.

Management support, exercise breaks, compensatory time, point of choice information, recognition, human-resources involvement, screen-saver reminders, exercise personnel.

Subsidised health clubs; guest memberships; pay mileage costs for active transport; home postcodes determine parking permits.

Commuting policies, federal/government worksites should set example, economic incentives from government, commercial sponsorship of local facilities.

Building construction legislation, building codes requiring centrally located and inviting stairways, with escalators and lifts available only to those unable to climb stairs.

In schools

Active field trips and homework; safe, active playground areas; non-competitive sports programmes; children design exercise schemes, longer recess periods, structured activities, greater choice of activities, shock-absorbing surfaces; sunscreen and hats available, walk-to-school groups, road and cycle safety tests.

Child-parent aerobic classes, parental support and involvement, facilities available to community, longer opening hours.

Example set by staff, provide support and cues, not using exercise as a punishment, teacher training.

State educational legislation, physical activity curriculum, school policies.

In the home

VAT on labour-saving devices, tax rebates on energy-making goods which are also energy saving in terms of electricity, reduced household insurance for exercise equipment.

Build homes with stairs.

Free TV ads for exercise promotion, physically active computer games.

and other youth groups could offer inexpensive bicycle-maintenance services, for example. Having to wear a cycle helmet or other cycling paraphernalia might also be an obstacle; inexpensive but fashionably designed gear might help to overcome this hurdle. Before actually beginning the journey, the cyclist has to resist taking the car; not only a powerful status symbol but fun to drive, comfortable, acclimatised, radio-entertained and fast. The car would be less enticing if the government made running costs higher and employers provided less and/or more expensive worksite parking. The revenues generated here could be used to support cycling. Communication campaigns, sponsored by environmental groups, could change the image of driving as well as demonstrate that local journeys that take half an hour by car can be undertaken just as, if not more, quickly by bicycle given traffic congestion and parking time. Government-sponsored designers could work to make bicycle seats more comfortable and equip cycle helmets with stereos, fans, and mobile phones. Advertising space could be sold on cycle helmets to reduce the costs. Special rucksack computer bags could also be provided by all employers or computer manufacturers as part of 'equality for cyclists' initiatives.

We now have a well-equipped, state-of-the-art, highly subsidised cyclist, but no suitable cycle path and a fear of traffic. Cycle trails adjacent to all main roads should be provided by transport departments, and made a condition of contracts for all new road construction projects. Cycle paths would have to be properly maintained and, if possible, form part of the pavement rather than the road, achieved through pavement expansion and road reduction. If slots for car parking were removed from roadsides more space would be available for cycle paths. Even if our commuter could cycle all the way to work without hindrance from other road users, he/she might not start the journey if it were raining. Ventilated but covered cycle paths would make cycling possible in all weathers. Finally, the cyclist arrives at work, in record time, but sweating profusely. Without showers and changing facilities, he/she may be hesitant to continue to cycle on a daily basis. The provision of such facilities could be made mandatory as part of health-and-safety requirements, and/or tax breaks introduced for companies that install them. In addition to suitable changing facilities, secure parking for cycles is essential. With fewer car-parking duties, traffic wardens could help patrol street-based cycle stands. Workplace water dispensers and later start times for cyclists would also provide encouragement. Although this example may seem extravagant, it does demonstrate that most obstacles to physical activity can be surmounted by environmental solutions that do not depend on individual effort. The practicality, effectiveness, and cost of such changes have yet to be determined. It is worth noting, however, that many of the fiscal and structural workplace initiatives described here find parallels in the provisions and facilities already available to those who commute by car. In addition, many of the conditions necessary to foster commuting by bicycle are already being addressed by the UK National Cycling Strategy (www.local-transport. detr.gov.uk).

Environmental barriers to physical activity

In the main, the proposals summarised in Table 10.1, like the ones elaborated above for cycling, have yet to receive the scrutiny necessary to assess the extent to which environmental barriers exist and whether they would yield to the solutions proposed. Nevertheless, a few surveys of environmental barriers to physical activity have been conducted. It should be noted, however, that these are generally cross-sectional studies of self-reported behaviour. Poor weather, for example, is often reported as a barrier to physical activity (Sallis & Owen, 1999). Individuals living in coastal (Bauman *et al.*, 1999), or rural rather than suburban or inner city areas (Potvin *et al.*, 1997), are more likely to engage in physical activity. In rural communities, physically demanding occupations and easier access to energetic leisure activities undoubtedly contribute to higher levels of activity (Potvin *et al.*, 1997). In a study of rural activity levels, farmers were found to have higher levels of 'sweat' activities (Eaton *et al.*, 1995). Among older Australians, access to footpaths and local parks were associated with increased levels of walking (Booth *et al.*, 2000). In a cross-sectional study, 38.8 per cent of those who had access to walking trails reported using them (Brownson *et al.*, 2000). Scenery might also be an issue here; in one study, physically active women were found to be more likely to live in neighbourhoods with enjoyable scenery and hills (King *et al.*, 2000). It has also been reported that older women do more activity indoors while older men are more active outdoors (Bennett, 1998). In this context, safety appears to be an important environmental barrier for women (Pinto *et al.*, 1996), as well as for ethnic-minority youths (Garcia *et al.*, 1995). However, safety did not emerge as a significant obstacle to physical activity in one multivariate study of barriers to exercise (King *et al.*, 2000). Women have also been reported to have experienced reduced self-efficacy when exercising in front of a full-length mirror (Katula *et al.*, 1998). This has obvious implications for the design of exercise environments.

In a community care home, residents, regardless of functional ability, made use of the supportive services provided, such as lifts and motorised vehicles. Thus, the usual instrumental activities of living, like walking and stair-climbing, disappeared from the daily routines of even those with reasonable functional capacity (Shipp & Branch, 1999). A study of non-institutionalised older Dutch persons also found that those who lived in housing without stairs were 2.0–2.7 times more likely to have lower overall levels of physical activity compared to those living in housing with stairs (Van Den Hombergh *et al.*, 1995). However, studies of the effects of access to exercise facilities and exercise equipment have produced mixed results (Sallis *et al.*, 1998; King *et al.*, 1999). Sallis *et al.* (1998) found that although perceived access to facilities was unrelated to exercise levels, actual access plotted on a map showed a significant effect (Sallis *et al.*, 1998). Similarly, awareness of facilities was not associated with physical activity levels in Australian college students (Leslie *et al.*, 1999). In contrast, the availability of facilities has been found to contribute to active, but not inactive, adolescents' activity levels (Gordon-Larson *et al.*, 2000). In general, children have been found to be more active outdoors than indoors, particularly when play spaces are available (Baronowski *et al.*, 1993; Sallis *et al.*, 1993). Finally, positive associations have been reported between physical inactivity and television watching (Robinson *et al.*, 1993; Andersen *et al.*, 1998; Sallis *et al.*, 1998; Owen *et al.*, 2000). Most recently, computer use has been associated with reduced activity levels (Fotheringham *et al.*, 2000; Owen *et al.*, 2000).

 Chapter 3 (Epidemiology) describes the relationships between physical activity and health indices.

Environmental interventions for physical activity

The environment can clearly throw up barriers to activity. This strongly suggests that the environment could be exploited to promote exercise. However, intervention studies testing environmental manipulations have yielded mixed results. School physical education programmes reliably increased physical activity at least during class (Sallis *et al.*, 1998). Similarly, painting fluorescent markings in a school playground led to an increase of 11 per cent in play time at a moderate-to-vigorous heart rate in the experimental site compared with no increase in the control site (Stratton, 2000). In contrast, several studies have found that introducing fitness facilities at the workplace did not increase activity levels (Sallis *et al.*, 1998). However, adding showers and changing rooms and using lotteries to enhance motivation for active commuting yielded a 7 per cent increase in activity levels, although lotteries and prizes did not lead to greater attendance at university aerobics classes (Sallis *et al.*, 1998). Environmental improvements on a military base, including introducing a cycle path, extending gymnasium hours, purchasing new equipment, opening a women's centre, running courses and clubs, allowing time off duties was associated with an improvement in the fitness of personnel relative to those at a control site (Linenger, 1991).

A case study – stair climbing

Work places, retail outlets, public buildings, and the domestic environment provide ample opportunities for stair-climbing and regular stair-climbing has well-documented health benefits, such as increased fitness and strength, weight loss, improved lipid profiles, and reduced risk of osteoporosis (Olson *et al.*, 1991; Loy *et al.*, 1994; Coupland *et al.*, 1999; Boreham *et al.*, 2000). Indeed, all-cause mortality has been found to be lower in individuals reporting regular stair use (Paffenbarger *et al.*, 1993) and higher in those who reported difficulties in climbing stairs (Haapanen-Niemi *et al.*, 1996). In a UK national fitness survey, however, only 18 per cent reported climbing 300 or more stairs a week (ADNFS, 1992). Similarly, in the US, only 24 per cent of older adults surveyed claimed to climb three or more flights of stairs a day (Clark, 1999). Observational studies of stair use at escalator/stair choice points paint an even bleaker picture. Only 5.6 per cent opted for the stairs in a train station, 7.2 per cent in a shopping mall, and 5.9 per cent at a bus terminal in an early study in Philadelphia (Brownell *et al.*, 1980). In a more recent study in Baltimore, baseline stair use in a shopping mall was a meagre 4.8 per cent (Andersen *et al.*, 1998). Similarly, only 8 per cent chose stairs over escalators in a Glasgow train station (Blamey *et al.*, 1996). Clearly, regular stair-climbing, although positively related to health, remains a minority activity, and, given a choice, people will select mechanical rather than energetic means of ascent.

Several studies, however, have shown that cues in the environment can increase stair use by as much as 9 per cent (Brownell *et al.*, 1980; Blamey *et al.*, 1996; Andersen *et al.*, 1998). The cues appear to alter the decision-making context and promote stair use. Further investigation into stair-climbing interventions was recommended at a recent physical activity conference (Epstein, 1998; Sallis *et al.*, 1998), which concluded that the most successful exercise interventions in the past 20 years were stair-climbing initiatives. Our research group, therefore, accepted this challenge and attempted to find the optimal stair-promoting environment. Some of the results of these investigations are presented below. Observations were made at escalator/stair choice-points. In some instances, baseline observations acted as the control condition. In all the studies, participants' gender was noted and overall pedestrian traffic volume was recorded. Logistic regression analyses were employed with escalator/stair use as the dichotomous (0–1) dependent variable. Logistic regression analyses provide odds ratios (ORs) for the independent variables. For the variable 'intervention', for example, an odds ratio of 1.15 can be interpreted as 15 per cent more people on the stairs during the intervention. An odds ratio of 0.70 would mean 30 per cent fewer. The figures here present the results as percentage stair use; a baseline stair use of 10 per cent would increase to 11.5 per cent with an odds ratio of 1.15, for example. All results reported here were significant (p < .01), thus specific confidence intervals, normally found with odds ratios, are not given.

Study 1   Escalator and stair users (N = 14 760) were observed in a city-centre shopping centre. Within the same shopping centre, three stairwells, with adjacent escalators, were monitored. The three sites had different staircase heights. The lowest staircase had nine steps (144 cm climbed), the middle staircase had 18 steps (306 cm), and the longest staircase had 24 steps (408 cm). Observations were made once a week over four weeks between 11.00 and 13.00 hours. The results are presented in Figure 10.1 as percentage stair use. There was a significantly increased likelihood of using the 18-step staircase (OR: 2.15, that is, 115 per cent) and the 9-step staircase (OR: 5.06, that is, 406 per cent)

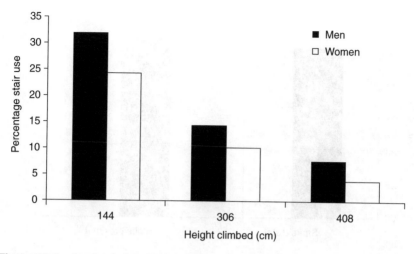

Figure 10.1 As stair height increased, stair use decreased, especially in women

than the 24-step staircase. There was also an interaction between staircase height and gender. The odds ratios for gender at each height indicate that as staircase height increased, the gender gap in stair climbing widened: nine step (OR: 1.52), 18 step (OR: 1.84), 24 step (OR: 2.17). These odds ratios indicate that on the nine-step staircase men were 52 per cent more likely to be on the stairs than women, at the 18-step staircase 84 per cent more likely and on the 24-step staircase 117 per cent more likely than women to be using the stairs. The findings for stair height were also reflected in a workplace study, where the floor on which employees worked affected their stair use; those on higher floors reported less stair use (Kerr *et al.*, 2001a).

Study 2 Escalator and stair users (N = 17 644) were observed exiting from two different train platforms in a city-centre train station. On one platform the stairs were the nearer option, on the other the escalators were closer. Observations were made twice a week over four weeks between 8.00 and 10.00 hours. The results for percentage stair use are presented in Figure 10.2. Commuters were more likely to use the stairs when they were the closer option (OR: 1.37). There was also a platform by gender interaction with women using the stairs less than men when the stairs were distal to the platform (OR: 1.23, that is, men were 23 per cent more likely to be on the stairs) compared with the proximal platform (OR: 1.08, that is, men only 8 per cent more likely to be on the stairs).

Study 3 (Kerr *et al.*, 2001b) Shoppers' (N = 12 588) and commuters' (N = 25 319) choice of escalators or stairs was observed over a six-week period. The first two observation weeks acted as the baseline period. In the second two weeks, an A1-size poster reading 'Stay healthy, use the stairs' (designed by Greater Glasgow Health Board) was placed between the escalators and stairs in both the shopping centre and train station. During the last two weeks

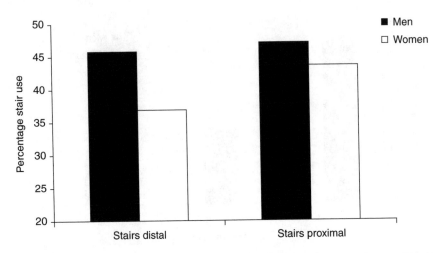

Figure 10.2 When stairs were the closest option stair use increased, especially in women

the poster was altered to read 'Stay healthy, save time, use the stairs', previously tested in Glasgow (Blamey *et al.*, 1996). Poster size had already been established as an important factor in stair use (Kerr *et al.*, 2001b). In the train station, stair use increased with both the first (OR: 1.12, that is, 12 per cent) and the second (OR: 1.22, that is, 22 per cent) posters. There was also a significant gender by poster interaction (p<.01) with female commuters responding more to the second poster. In the shopping centre, stair use also increased with both posters (OR: 1.49) and (OR: 1.39) respectively. There was also a gender by poster interaction (p<.01) with female shoppers responding less to the second poster. The results for percentage stair use are presented in Figure 10.3.

   Study 4 (Kerr *et al.*, 2001c) Escalator and stair users (N=23979) were observed in two city-centre shopping centres twice a week between 11.00 and 13.00 hours over a six-week period. In both sites, a two-week baseline period was followed by a two-week A1-size poster intervention, with the message 'Stay healthy, use the stairs'. In the last two weeks, the poster remained in the control shopping centre. In the experimental shopping centre, however, multiple messages were placed as colourful banners on the stair-risers. Shoppers in street interviews had selected the messages on the stair-riser banners and their effectiveness had been examined in an earlier study (Kerr *et al.*, 2001d – see illustration 10.1). In both shopping centres, the poster was associated with increased stair use (OR: 2.18). In the second intervention period there was an interaction between sites (OR: 2.06) such that stair use was higher in the experimental site with the stair-riser banners.

   These studies clearly demonstrate the active interaction of individuals with their environment. The design of the environment affected stair use with

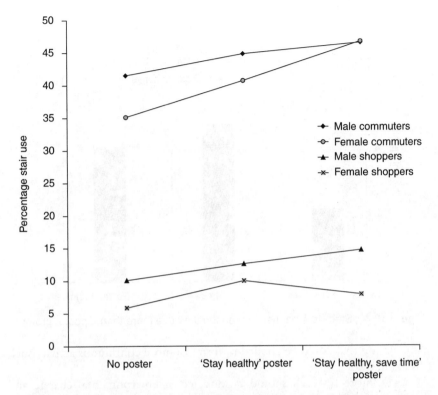

Figure 10.3 Female shoppers and commuters responded differently to the second poster

more women using the stairs when they were easily accessible and lower in height. The context in which the cue was received was also important with female shoppers and commuters reacting differently. Finally, transforming the environment with bright stair-riser banners suggested that, by making stairs more noticeable and attractive, stair use can be increased dramatically. It is important to note, however, that the gender differences revealed by the observational studies were not apparent in self-reported stair use from a sub-sample of interview respondents. As Sallis and associates (1998) emphasise, where possible, objective data collection methods are preferable, especially when assessing environmental influences on behaviour.

The potential health benefits of stair-climbing, outlined earlier, result from regular, continuous use. The studies summarised constitute rather time-limited examples of increased stair use. However, we have recently found that messages can maintain stair use over a three-month period (Kerr *et al.*, 2001e). Thus, our results hold out the possibility that strategies of the sort employed here could effect long-term shifts in stair-climbing behaviour that would achieve concerted improvements in overall energy expenditure levels. Moreover, our studies might also afford a model of environmental

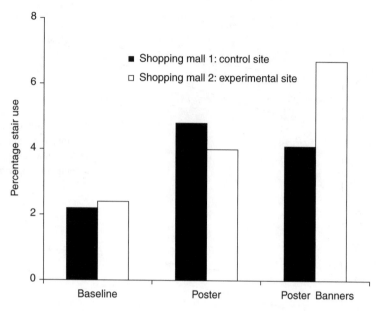

Figure 10.4 Stair-riser banners increased stair use more than a poster prompt

manipulation that could be applied to forms of more continuous activity such as walking.

Clearly, more research should be directed at environmental change and physical activity. Even in the relatively simple example of stair climbing, further work is needed. The research, to date, indicates that cue formats and messages work. Recently, music and art has been used to encourage stair use (Boutelle *et al.*, 2001). There is further scope, though, for examining alternatives to determine the optimum message characteristics as well as the lifetime of the effect of such messages. Restricting escalator use is another untested strategy. Stair climbing preferences have been monitored for other purposes; for example, in a transport engineering study of the Hong Kong Mass Transit Railway, pedestrians were observed to choose the stairs more quickly when faced with congestion on the descending rather than the ascending escalator (Cheung & Lam, 1998). The observation methods and findings of town planners, architects and engineers should be heeded more frequently. Objective observation tools, such as SOPLAY (system for observing play and leisure activity in youths), should also be considered (McKenzie *et al.*, 2000). At present, reliable, valid instruments for measuring the effects of environmental change are scarce (Booth & Samdal, 1997; Richter *et al.*, 2000).

The commitment of management is essential for stair-banners to become permanent features of, for example, shopping centres. Since this would entail further cleaning and maintenance expense, management would have to be convinced of added value to the shopping centre. However, our research

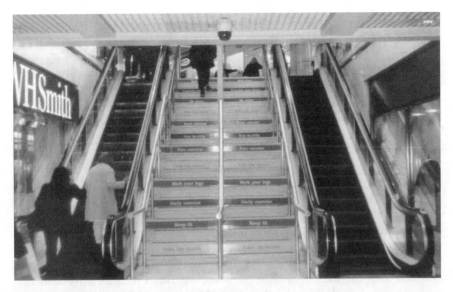

Illustration 10.1 Stair-riser banners with multiple messages in a city-centre shopping centre

received the full support of management who attested that the stair banners 'cheered up' the shopping centre. Securing co-operation, as well as additional resources for the production of further stair banners, however, will involve expertise in negotiation and sales tactics that are not necessarily part of the usual skills portfolio of research workers. It is important to recognise that additional skills are required to implement an environmental programme, and that the deployment of the appropriate personnel can be critical to its success (St Leger, 1997).

To implement even the simplest environmental initiative, such as banners on stair risers, at a national level would involve a different level of organisation. It would be necessary to recruit the support of those national retailers with outlets in most towns. Retailers, however, would have to be convinced that the intervention would not inhibit customers' spending. In addition, retailers need to be persuaded against exploiting this relatively new advertising medium for their own promotions. Again, tax breaks for stores participating in initiatives involving exercise, but not commercial messages, would help. Our research on stair-climbing also revealed that the physical design of the environment was associated with variations in stair use. However, architectural initiatives would require changes to building-code legislation, and the necessary co-operation of town planners, architects, and construction firms. Before design changes are implemented, research using photo manipulation may indicate whether changing staircase designs would lead to behaviour change.

Guidelines for researching and implementing environmental change

Several authors provide models and frameworks for understanding the process of environmental change (Stokols, 1996; Wandersman *et al.*, 1996; Dwyer, 1997; Sallis *et al.*, 1998; Sallis & Owen, 1999; Swinburn *et al.*, 1999). Some coalitions for promoting physical activity already exist, for example, the National Coalition to Promote Physical Activity, Partnership for Walkable America, and the New South Wales Physical Activity Task Force (Sallis *et al.*, 1998; Sparling *et al.*, 2000). It is important to learn from the experiences of these groups. Lessons learned from the Healthy Cities project have also been reported (Duhl, 1996) and the World Health Organisation guidelines, 'Twenty steps for developing a healthy cities project', are available on the internet (Kickbusch, 1997: www.who.int). All too frequently, however, environmental approaches, because of their complexity, have not been worked out in great detail (Green *et al.*, 1996). Administrative conflicts and difficulties coupled with the inexact science of measuring often relegate environmental programmes into the 'too-hard basket' (Nutbeam, 1997). Certainly, implementing initiatives that require complex networks and multiple-level strategies is a daunting task.

In Table 10.2, we have tried to outline the different stages involved in developing environmental change and to identify possible courses of action. Our experience as behavioural scientists encompasses some but far from all the expertise needed to implement complex environmental programmes. The main message of this chapter, however, is that successful environmental change requires skills unavailable to any one discipline and necessitates the pooling of expertise from a range of disciplines. The competencies of most behavioural scientists run out after the first three levels of tasks identified in Table 10.2 and orthodox cause and effect epidemiology would appear to be similarly limited (Ewan, 1997).

Conclusions

Self-report data suggests that the environment is a barrier to physical activity. Importantly, studies involving direct observation of behaviour also indicate that the environment can be a major limiting factor. For example, stair location and structure were consistently associated with variations in stair climbing. Further, environmental change, by, for example, introducing cues in the form of stair barriers, can increase stair use. In general, it would appear that redesigning the environment, whether by introducing cycle lanes or making car-driving less attractive economically, offers the most likely means of affecting sustained changes in physical activity levels. Given the number of environmental barriers to physical activity, comprehensive environmental solutions are required.

Table 10.2 Environmental change research framework

	Tasks	Examples
1	Validate research tools, conduct needs assessments and feasibility appraisals	Questionnaires, interviews and observations for physical-activity prevalence, other health risks, readiness for change, potential environments where change would be easy to implement and so on
2	Research environmental barriers to physical activity in target communities and locations: perceived or actual?	Questionnaires and interviews of active and inactive people Use objective measures where possible and collect observations at exercise choice points, for example, escalators, bus stops, car parks, cycle paths Cross reference observations with self-report, for example, safety with crime
3	Check whether changing the environment would lead to behaviour change	Enhance environment with cues and test what signs work, size, message, creative formats; test environment changes using photo manipulation Remove environmental barriers, for example, free access to facilities Create alternative barriers, for example, increased parking costs
4	Through brain-storming, identify a potential physical activity coalition, key leaders, and find existing programmes into which physical activity could fit	*Beneficiaries:* individuals, residents, consumers, employees *Potential collaborators:* environmental conservation groups, recreation groups, park managers, medical and health providers, employers, transport services, energy conservationists, educators, sports organisations, religious organisations, civic leaders, tourist agencies, senior-citizen groups, retailers *Existing schemes:* smoking cessation, weight watchers, ramblers' association *Funding bodies:* local government, insurance companies, corporations *Facilitators:* lobbyists, lawyers, advocates, media gate-keepers *Decision-makers:* politicians, local councillors, managers, head teachers, and so on *Implementers:* architects, town planners, police, local councils, constructors *Communicators:* health promoters, teachers, advertisers, PR, journalists
5	Identify problem areas and potential opponents and try to engage support	For example, technology industry, automobile manufacturers, computer manufacturers, software developers, computer-service industries, employers, transport unions, transport planners, construction industry Sell sponsorship of activity initiatives as positive PR opportunity
6	Development	Motivate and secure co-operation of members of all the above subgroups Find common goals, define roles, delegate, develop systems, identify opportunities and high-impact leverage points, set targets Provide training where necessary

Table 10.2 (*Cont'd*)

	Tasks	Examples
7	Decision-making	Work together, test network, get sponsorship, initiate political lobbying, convince decision-makers, infiltrate committees
8	Implementation	Amend current facilities, paths, parks; build new facilities, paths, parks Provide subsidies, rebates, funding Policy and legislation implementation and enforcement
9	Communication and education	News reports, mass media communication, point of choice cues Supportive help-lines, telephone reminders, skills-development courses
10	Evaluate	Short- and long-term outcomes; continuous feedback into programmes Cost effectiveness
11	Maintain	Co-operation of police for enforcement of legislation, protection from vandalism; neighbourhood-watch groups, conservationists to ensure facilities are used appropriately Local council support for cleaning, pavement maintenance Continuous re-launches of facilities, dedicated action weeks, new deals

If environmental change is to be successfully implemented, a flexible multi-disciplinary approach that entails interaction with key individuals and communities is required. The greatest barrier to environmental change appears to be its sheer complexity. Further research could identify systems and procedures that could simplify the process of environmental change. It should be noted, however, that persuading corporations and communities to engage in environmental initiatives may be just as difficult as convincing individuals to take up exercise. There is now a general consensus that behavioural and educational approaches to exercise promotion have had, at best, very limited impact. We need to heed the lessons from the shortcomings of such approaches and not apply the same blunt instruments, and do so at a higher level. Environmental tactics would also have to be applied at this level, in, for example, the form of tax and other incentives from governing bodies. Many of the difficulties of engaging different groups could be mitigated if the political process rewarded environmental initiatives directed at increasing physical activity.

Ultimately, the aim of environmental change should be to facilitate increased activity in all sections of society (Richter *et al.*, 2000). The potential benefits of environmental change in this context are clear. Unlike behavioural and educational approaches, environmental initiatives do not hold individuals responsible for change. Given that the contemporary environment increasingly limits the opportunities for physical activity, environmental initiatives are the only ones likely to yield substantial population dividends. In addition, environmental initiatives should produce longer effects, since such initiatives become embedded and affect social norms. The environment approach is also more likely to encompass those social groups limited by time and/or income from conforming to educational initiatives. Judging from their rhetoric, most Western governments are eager to improve health, transport, and the environment. By helping to establish environments that foster increased physical activity, they would be able to contribute substantially to improvements in all three areas of life.

References

Allied Dunbar National Fitness Survey (1992) London, Sports Council and Health Education Authority.

Andersen, R.E., Franckowiak, S.C., Snyder, J., Bartlett, S.J. & Fontaine, K.R. (1998) Can inexpensive signs encourage the use of stairs? Results from a community intervention. *Annals of Internal Medicine*, **129**: 363–369.

Andersen, R.E., Crespo, C.J., Bartlett, S.J., Cheskin, L.J. & Pratt, M. (1998) Relationship of physical activity and television watching with body weight and level of fatness among children. *Journal of the American Medical Association*, **279**: 938–942.

Baronowski, T., Thompson, W.O., DuRant, R.H., Baranowski, J. & Puhl, J. (1993) Observations on physical activity in physical locations: Age, gender, ethnicity and month effects. *Research Quarterly for Exercise and Sport*, **64**: 127–133.

Bauman, A., Smith, B., Stoker, L., Bellew, B. & Booth, M. (1999) Geographical influences upon physical activity participation, evidence of a 'coastal effect'. *Australian and New Zealand Journal of Public Health*, **23**: 322–324.

Bennett, K.M. (1998) Gender and longitudinal changes in physical activities in later life. *Age and Ageing*, **27**: 24–28.

Blair S.N., Booth, M., Gyarfar, I., Iwane, H., Mart, B., Matsudo, V., Morrow, M.S., Noaker, T. & Shephard, R. (1996) Development of public policy and physical activity initiatives internationally. *Sportsmedicine*, **21**(3): 157–163.

Blamey, A., Mutrie, N. & Aitchison, T. (1996) Promoting active living: A step in the right direction. *Journal of the Institute of Health Education*, **34**: 5–9.

Booth, M.L. & Samdal, O. (1997) Health-promoting schools in Australia: models and measurement. *Australian and New Zealand Journal of Public Health*, **21**: 365–370.

Booth, M.L., Owen, N., Bauman, A., Clavisi, O. & Leslie, E. (2000) Social-cognitive and perceived environment influences associated with physical activity in older Australians. *Preventive Medicine*, **31**: 15–22.

Boreham, C.A.G., Wallace, W.F.M. & Nevill, A. (2000) Training effects of accumulating daily stair climbing exercise in previously sedentary young women. *Preventive Medicine*, **30**: 277–281.

Boutelle, K., Jeffery, R.W., Murray, D.M. & Schmitz, K.H. (2001) The use of signs, artwork, and music to promote daily lifestyle activity in a public building. *American Journal of Public Health*, **91**: 2004–2006.

Breslow, L. (1996) Social ecological strategies for promoting healthy lifestyles. *American Journal of Health Promotion*, **10**: 253–257.

Brownell, K.D., Stunkard, A.J. & Albaum, J.M. (1980) Evaluation and modification of exercise patterns in the natural environment. *American Journal of Psychiatry*, **137**: 1540–1545.

Brownson, R.C., Housemann, R.A., Brown, D.R., Jackson-Thompson, J., King, A.C., Malone, B.R. & Sallis, J.F. (2000) Promoting physical activity in rural communities. *American Journal of Preventive Medicine*, **18**: 235–241.

Cheung, C.Y. & Lam, W.H.K. (1998) Pedestrian route choices between escalator and stairway in MTR stations. *Journal of Transportatio n Engineering*, **124**: 277–285.

Clark, D.O. (1999) Physical activity and its correlates among urban primary care patients aged 55 years or older. *Journal of Gerontology*, **54B**: S41–S48.

Cohen, D.A., Scribner, R.A. & Farley, T.A. (2000) A structural model of health behaviour: A pragmatic approach to explain and influence health behaviours at the population level. *Preventive Medicine*, **30**: 146–154.

Corti, B., Donovan, R.J. & Holman, C.D.J. (1996) Factors influencing the use of physical activity facilities: Results from qualitative research. *Health Promotion Journal of Australia*, **6**: 16–21.

Coupland, C.A.C., Cliffe, S.J., Bassey, E.J., Grainge, M.J., Hosking, D.J. & Clivers, C.E.D. (1999) Habitual activity and bone mineral density in postmenopausal women in England. *International Journal of Epidemiology*, **28**: 241–246.

Duhl, L.J. (1996) An ecohistory of health: The role of 'Healthy Cities'. *American Journal of Health Promotion*, **10**: 258–261.

Dunn, A.L., Andersen, R.E. & Jakicic, J.M. (1998) Lifestyle physical activity interventions: History, short- and long-term effects, and recommendations. *American Journal of Preventive Medicine*, **15**: 398–412.

Dwyer, S. (1997) Improving delivery of a health-promoting-environments program: experiences from Queensland Health. *Australian and New Zealand Journal of Public Health*, **21**: 398–402.

Eaton, C.B, Nafziger, A.N., Strogatz D.S. & Pearson, T.A. (1995) Self-reported physical activity in a rural county: A New York county health census. *American Journal of Public Health*, **84**: 29–32.

Environmental Working Group. www.ewg.org/pub/home/Reports/meanstreets/meanrecs.html

Epstein, L.H. (1998) Integrating theoretical approaches to promote physical activity. *American Journal of Preventive Medicine*, **15**: 257–265.

Ewan, C. (1997) Can the environment promote health? And how will we answer that question? *Australian and New Zealand Journal of Public Health*, **21**: 417–419.

Fotheringham, M.J., Wonnacott, R.L. & Owen, N. (2000) Computer use and physical activity in young adults: Public health perils and potentials of new information technologies. *Annals of Behavioral Medicine*, **22**: 269–275.

Garcia, A.W., Broda, M.A.N., Covial, C., Pender, N.J. & Ronis, D.L. (1995) Gender and developmental differences in exercise beliefs among youth and prediction of their exercise behaviour. *Journal of School Health*, **65**: 213–219.

Gordon-Larson, P., McMurray, R.G. & Popkin, B. (2000) Determinants of adolescent physical activity and inactivity patterns. *Pediatrics*, **105**: 1327–1328.

Green, L.W., Richards, R. & Potvin, L. (1996) Ecological foundations of health promotion. *American Journal of Health Promotion*, **10**: 270–281.

Haapanen-Niemi, N., Miilunpalo, S., Vuori, I., Oja, P. & Pasanen, M. (1996) Characteristics of leisure time physical activity associated with decreased risk of premature all-cause and cardiovascular disease mortality in middle-aged men. *American Journal of Epidemiology*, **143**: 870–880.

Harris, E. & Wills, J. (1997) Developing healthy local communities at local government level: lessons from the past decade. *Australian and New Zealand Journal of Public Health*, **21**: 403–412.

Hill, J.O., Wyatt, H.R. & Melanson, E.L. (2000) Genetic and environmental contributions to obesity. *Medical Clinics of North America*, **84**: 333–347.

Hillsdon, M., Thorogood, M., Anstiss, T. & Morris, J. (1995) Randomised controlled trials of physical activity promotion in free-living populations – A review. *Journal of Epidemiology and Community Health*, **49**: 448–453.

Holman, C.D. (1997) Measuring the occurrence of health-promoting interactions with the environment. *Australian and New Zealand Journal of Public Health*, 21: 360–364.

House of Commons (1995) Environment Committee. *Fourth Report: The Environmental Impact of Leisure Activities*. Volume 1. London, HMSO.

Katula, J., McAuley, E., Mihalko, S.L. & Bane, S.M. (1998) Mirror, mirror on the wall . . . exercise environment influences in self-efficacy. *Journal of Social Behavior and Personality*, 13: 319–332.

Kerr, J., Eves, F.F. & Carroll, D. (2001a) Can posters prompt stair use in a worksite environment? *Journal of Occupational Health*, in press.

Kerr, J., Eves, F.F. & Carroll, D. (2001b) The influence of poster prompts on stair use: The effects of setting, poster size and content. *British Journal of Health Psychology*, 6(4): 397–405.

Kerr, J., Eves, F.F. & Carroll, D. (2001c) Encouraging stair use: stair-riser banners are better than poster prompts. *American Journal of Public Health*, 91(8): 1192–1193.

Kerr, J., Eves, F.F. & Carroll, D. (2001d) Getting people on the stairs: The impact of a new message format. *Journal of Health Psychology*, in press.

Kerr, J., Eves, F.F. & Carroll, D. (2001e) Six-month observational study of prompted stair climbing. *Preventive Medicine*, 33(5): 422–427.

Kickbusch, I. (1997) Health-promoting environments: the next steps. *Australian and New Zealand Journal of Public Health*, 21: 431–434.

King, A.C. (1999) Environmental and policy approaches to the promotion of physical activity. In: Rippe, J. (ed.) *Lifestyle Medicine*. Norwalk, CT Blackwell Science.

King, A.C., Castro, C., Wilcox, S., Eyler, A.A., Sallis, J.F. & Brownson, R.C. (2000) Personal and environmental factors associated with physical inactivity among different racial-ethnic groups of US middle-aged and older-aged women. *Health Psychology*, 19: 354–364.

King, A.C., Jeffery, R.W., Fridinger, F., Dusenbury, L., Provence, S., Hedlund, S.A. & Spangler, K. (1995) Environmental and policy approaches to cardiovascular disease prevention through physical activity: Issues and opportunities. *Health Education Quarterly*, 22: 499–511.

Leslie, E., Owen, N., Salmon, J., Bauman, A., Sallis, J.F. & Lo, S.K. (1999) Insufficiently active Australian college students: Perceived personal, social and environmental influences. *Preventive Medicine*, 28: 20–27.

Linenger, J.M., Chesson, C.V. & Nice, D.S. (1991) Physical fitness gains following simple environmental change. *American Journal of Preventive Medicine*, 7: 298–310.

Loy, S.F., Conley, L.M., Sacco, E.R., Vincent, W.J., Holland, G.J., Sletten, E.G. & Trueblood, P.R. (1994) Effects of stair climbing on $\dot{V}O_{2max}$ and quadriceps strength in middle-aged females. *Medicine and Science in Sports and Exercise*, 26: 241–247.

McKenzie, T.L., Marshall, S.J., Sallis, J.F. & Conway, T.L. (2000) Leisure-time physical activity in school environments: An observational study using SOPLAY. *Preventive Medicine*, 30: 70–77.

Minkler, M., Schauffer, H. & Clements-Nolle, K. (2000) Health promotion for older Americans in the 21st century. *American Journal of Health Promotion*, 14: 371–379.

Nutbeam, D. (1997) Creating health-promoting environments: overcoming barriers to action. *Australian and New Zealand Journal of Public Health*, 21: 355–359.

Olson, M.S., Williford, H.N., Blessing, D.L. & Greathouse, R. (1991) The cardiovascular and metabolic effects of bench stepping exercise in females. *Medicine and Science in Sports and Exercise*, 23: 1311–1318.

Owen, N., Leslie, E., Salmon, J. & Fotheringham, M.J. (2000) Environmental determinants of physical activity and sedentary behaviour. *Exercise and Sport Science Reviews*, 28: 153–158.

Paffenbarger, R.S., Hyde, R.T., Wing, A.L., Lee, I.M., Jung, D.L. & Kampert, J.B. (1993) The association of changes in physical activity level and other lifestyle characteristics with mortality among men. *New England Journal of Medicine*, 328: 538–545.

Pate, R.R., Pratt, M., Blair, S.N., Haskell, W.L., Macera, C.A., Bouchard, C., Buchner, D., Ettinger, W., Heath, G.W., King, A.C., Kriska, A., Leon, A.S., Marcus, B.H., Morris, J., Paffenbarger, R., Patrick, K., Pollock, M.L., Rippe, J.M., Sallis, J. & Wilmore, J.H. (1995)

Physical activity and public health: A recommendation from the Centers for Disease Control and Prevention and the American College of Sportsmedicine. *Journal of the American Medical Association*, 273: 402–407.

Pinto, B.M., Marcus, B.H. & Clark, M.M. (1996) Promoting physical activity in women: The new challenges. *American Journal of Preventive Medicine*, 12: 395–400.

Potvin, L., Gauvin, L. & Nguyen, N.M. (1997) Prevalence of stages of change for physical activity in rural, suburban and inner-city communities. *Journal of Community Health*, 22: 1–13.

Price, G., Mackay, S. & Swinburn, B. (2000) The Heartbeat Challenge program: promoting healthy changes in New Zealand workplaces. *Health Promotion International*, 15: 49–55.

Richard, L., Potvin, L., Kishchuk, N., Prlic, H. & Green, L.W. (1996) Assessment of the integration of the ecological approach in health promotion programs. *American Journal of Health Promotion*, 10: 318–328.

Richter, K.P., Harris, K.J., Paine-Andrews, A., Fawcett, S.B., Schmid, T.L., Lankenau, B.H. & Johnston, J. (2000) Measuring the health environment for physical activity and nutrition among youth: A review of the literature and applications for community initiatives. *Preventive Medicine*, 31: S98–S111.

Robinson, T.N., Hammer, L.D., Killen, J.D., Kraemer, H.C., Wilson, D.M., Hayward, C. & Taylor, C.B. (1993) Does television viewing increase obesity and reduce physical activity? Cross-sectional and longitudinal analyses among adolescent girls. *Pediatrics*, 91: 273–280.

Sallis, J.F., Nader, P.R., Broyles, S.L., Berry, C.C., Elder, J.P., McKenzie, T.L. & Nelson, J.A. (1993) Correlates of physical activity at home in Mexican-American and Anglo-American preschool children. *Health Psychology*, 12: 390–398.

Sallis, J.F. (1998) Reflections on the Physical Activity Interventions Conference. *American Journal of Preventive Medicine*, 15: 431–432.

Sallis, J.F., Bauman, A. & Pratt, M. (1998) Environmental and policy interventions to promote physical activity. *American Journal of Preventive Medicine*, 15: 379–397.

Sallis, J.F. & Owen, N. (1999) *Physical Activity and Behavioural Medicine*. Newbury, CA Sage Publications.

Sallis, J.F., Zakarian, J.M., Hovell, M.F. & Hofstetter, C.R. (1998) Ethnic, socioeconomic, and sex differences in physical activity among adolescents. *Journal of Clinical Epidemiology*, 49: 125–134.

Schmid, T.L., Pratt, M. & Howze, E. (1995) Policy as intervention: Environmental and policy approaches to the prevention of cardiovascular diseases. *American Journal of Public Health*, 85: 1207–1211.

Shipp, K.M. & Branch, L.G. (1999) The physical environment as a determinant of the health status of older populations. *Canadian Journal on Ageing*, 18: 313–327.

Sparling, P., Owen, O., Lambert, E. & Haskell, W. (2000) Promoting physical activity: The new imperative for public health. *Health Education Research*, 15: 367–376.

St Leger, L. (1997) The education and training framework for health-promoting environments. *Australian and New Zealand Journal of Public Health*, 21: 420–424.

Stokols, D. (1992) Establishing and maintaining healthy environments: Toward a social ecology of health promotion. *American Psychologist*, 47: 6–22.

Stokols, D. (1996) Translating social ecological theory into guidelines for community health promotion. *American Journal of Health Promotion*, 10: 282–298.

Stratton, G. (2000) Promoting children's physical activity in primary school: An intervention study using playground markings. *Ergonomics*, 43: 1538–1546.

Swinburn, B., Egger, G. & Raza, F. (1999) Dissecting obesogenic environments: The development and application of a framework for identifying and prioritizing environmental interventions for obesity. *Preventive Medicine*, 29: 563–570.

The Department for the Environment, Transport and the Regions: National Cycling Strategy. www.local-transport.detr.gov.uk.

Van Den Hombergh, C.E.J., Schouten, E.G., Van Staveren, W.A., Van Amelsvoort, L.G. & Kok, F.J. (1995) Physical activities of noninstitutionalised Dutch elderly and characteristics of inactive elderly. *Medicine and Science in Sports and Exercise*, 27: 334–339.

Wandersman, A., Valois, R., Ochs, L., de la Cruz, D., Adkins, E. & Goodman, R. (1996) Toward a social ecology of community coalitions. *American Journal of Health Promotion*, **10**: 299–307.

Wechsler, H., Devereaux, R.S., Davis, M. & Collins, J. (2000) Using the school environment to promote physical activity and healthy eating. *Preventive Medicine*, **31**: S121–S137.

SECTION IV

THE BIOLOGY AND ANTHROPOLOGY OF PHYSICAL ACTIVITY

In this final section, two important themes are addressed, each of which can be easily overlooked. The oversight is unfortunate, because each makes extremely important contributions to a full understanding of physical activity. Firstly, Viru and Harro address a range of potential biological mechanisms – or aetiological pathways – by which physical activity leads to structural and functional changes in the human body that result in improved health status. Biological plausibility is a key factor in the acceptance of observational evidence, and in the field of physical activity and health this type of evidence predominates. It is therefore important to address the issue of 'how' physical activity confers health benefits, as well as 'whether' and 'how strongly' it does this. We already know a great deal about the acute and chronic physiological responses of the human body to physical activity. This evidence has been obtained largely from well-designed and controlled laboratory studies, often relating to sports science, and has a history of over half a century. Observational studies relating Physical activity levels to health outcomes have followed a similar time course. In order to establish cause-and-effect – that is, that increased physical activity *causes* improved health – it is essential to establish plausible biological pathways that are known to be modifiable via physical activity and have definite influences on health. In effect, we need to 'marry' the evidence from exercise physiology and epidemiology in order to establish causal links.

In Chapter 12, the final contribution to this book, Panter Brick takes an anthropological perspective regarding how physically active we, as human beings, are 'supposed' to be. In other words – what level of physical activity

227

have humans evolved to do? There is a logical train of thought that if we have evolved to do a certain amount and type of physical activity then we really ought to do it. Evolution rarely (in fact never) gets it wrong – it is the critical connection between how man survives in his environment. This discussion of our 'natural' level and type of physical activity supports – and may even explain – some of the observational evidence relating types and levels of physical activity to health. Taken together, the combined evidence may eventually be the cornerstone of public-health Physical activity recommendations.

CHAPTER 11

Biological Aspects of Physical Activity and Health

ATKO VIRU AND MAARIKE HARRO

Chapter Contents

In contemporary society physical activity is no longer a major feature of human everyday life. Nevertheless, physical activity influences the development and maturation of the human body and has a major influence on health status throughout life. There is no doubt that an active body develops in a healthy manner and maintains a higher level of health and well-being. These relationships between physical activity and health constitute the background for studying the influence of physical activity on the healthy formation and maintenance of the body and its organs. Conversely, a lack of physical activity promotes a range of degradation processes and causes a concomitant deterioration in body function. This chapter discusses the biological mechanisms involved in the promotion of good health through physical activity.

Chapter 2 (Lifespan) describes the rationale for a lifecourse approach for promoting physical activity.

How physical activity affects body systems and structures

It has been suggested that an intracellular mechanism exists which relates the function of cellular structures to the genome in cells (Meerson, 1965). Through this mechanism, the variability in intensity with which the cellular structures function determines the level of activity of the cell's genetic apparatus and, thereby, causes a specific stimulation of protein synthesis (adaptive protein synthesis). It has been hypothesised (Viru, 1994) that physical activity and exercise cause an accumulation of metabolites which specifically induce adaptive synthesis of structural and enzyme proteins of the most active cellular structures. Hormonal changes induced by activity further amplify the inductor effect of the metabolites and ensure that protein synthesis is maintained by a constant supply of 'building materials'. In this way there is an effective constant renewal and enlargement of protein structures and an increase in the number of molecules within the most important enzymes (Figure 11.1).

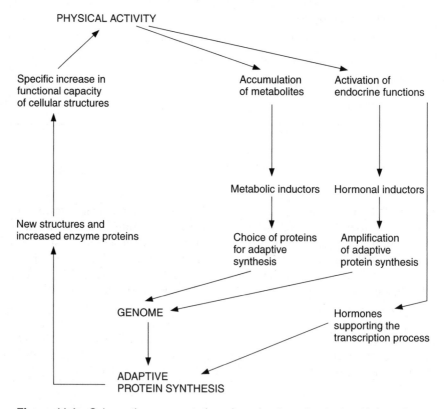

Figure 11.1 Schematic representation of mechanisms for the health benefits of physical activity

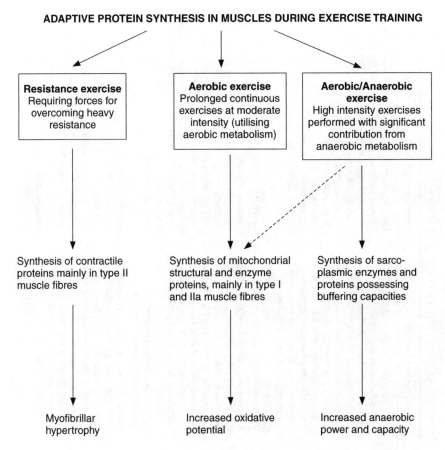

ADAPTIVE PROTEIN SYNTHESIS IN MUSCLES DURING EXERCISE TRAINING

Resistance exercise	Aerobic exercise	Aerobic/Anaerobic exercise
Requiring forces for overcoming heavy resistance	Prolonged continuous exercises at moderate intensity (utilising aerobic metabolism)	High intensity exercises performed with significant contribution from anaerobic metabolism

Synthesis of contractile proteins mainly in type II muscle fibres

Synthesis of mitochondrial structural and enzyme proteins, mainly in type I and IIa muscle fibres

Synthesis of sarcoplasmic enzymes and proteins possessing buffering capacities

Myofibrillar hypertrophy

Increased oxidative potential

Increased anaerobic power and capacity

Figure 11.2 Contribution of different types of physical activity to the health effect

In skeletal muscular activity, adaptive protein synthesis takes place to augment a range of structural and enzymatic proteins in the muscles, depending on the degree of muscle force applied and the intensity and duration of the activity (Figure 11.2, for references see Booth & Thomason, 1991; Viru, 1995). Through mechanisms such as these, physical activity and exercise improve the function of cardiovascular and respiratory systems, refine nervous and hormonal regulation, augment energy stores and induce changes in connective tissue (Table 11.1).

It has been suggested (Reindell *et al.*, 1957) that heart enlargement takes place when Physical activity intensity is sufficient to raise the stroke volume of the heart to its maximum. This suggestion arose through observation of the pattern of stroke volume during incremental exercise testing. At low-exercise intensities, increases in heart rate are directly related to increases in stroke volume. At moderate intensities of exercise – eliciting heart rates of 120–140 beats a minute – stroke volume reaches its highest level and remains stable despite

Table 11.1 Effects of physical activity on various organs and tissues

Organs or tissues	Types of physical activity	Effects of physical activity	Effects on health	Key references
Bone	Strong muscular contractions and weight-bearing exercise Vigorous, prolonged, repetitive exercise, callisthenics, sports, games	Stimulates bone formation and growth. Tensile and compressive forces associated with muscular contractions cause intermittent compression of growth plates Activation of osteocytes alters the delicate balance between bone resorption and formation, increases bone mineral density and bone mineral content and/or reduces the rate of bone loss	Primary prevention of osteoporosis due to increased peak bone mass during adolescence/ young adulthood Primary and secondary prevention of osteoporosis in adults Prevention of fractures	(Sorock et al., 1988; Suominen, 1993; Vuori, 1995)
	Note: High volume endurance training	Demineralization of bones	Contributes to osteoporosis	
Joints, ligaments, tendons, endomyoseal connective tissue	Gymnastics, weight bearing, prolonged high-intensity exercise	Increases and maintains range of movement and flexibility Increases tendon strength and joint stability by (a) increasing the strength of insertion sites between ligaments, tendons, and bones and (b) increasing cross-sectional area of ligaments and tendons Increases supportive function of endomyoseal connective tissue	Minimises physical limitation of reduced flexibility Limits the effects of degenerative arthritis Reduces injury risk, especially at older ages Reduces the risk of muscular disease	(Tipton et al., 1967; Booth & Gould, 1975; Kovanen & Suominen, 1989; Kannus et al., 1992; Brown & Holloszy, 1993)
Skeletal muscle	Resistance exercises for improved strength Aerobic exercises Anaerobic and aerobic–anaerobic exercises	Increases muscular strength by myofibril-lar hypertrophy and neural adaptation Increases oxidation potential by increasing quantity of mitochondria and enhancing activity of oxidative enzymes Increases density of capillaries Augments stores of glycogen and phosphocreatine	Improves coping ability in various habitual and job activities Reduces effects of age and chronic disease on the reserve capacity for exercise Increases ability to be physically active	(Saltin & Gollnick, 1983; Marks, 1992; Bailey & Martin, 1994; Viru, 1995; Vuori, 1995)

		Increases density of Na$^+$, K$^+$ pumps in the sarcolemma and improves function of the sarcoplasmic reticulum	
		Improves lipid utilization and spares glycogen stores during prolonged exercise of moderate intensity	
		Improves endurance capacity for prolonged exercise	
		Increases potential for anaerobic synthesis of ATP and increases buffering capacity	
		Increases oxidation potential (aerobic–anaerobic exercise)	
		Improves function of ionic pumps	
		Improves performance in anaerobic or aerobic–anaerobic exercises	
Cardiovascular system	Aerobic exercise Aerobic–anaerobic exercises [Note: Exercise intensity has to be sufficient to elicit maximal stroke volume (heart rate > 130 bpm) and duration must be greater than 15–20 minutes]	Heart enlargement as result of (a) pronounced eccentric hypertrophy (increases capacity of heart ventricles) and (b) modest concentric hypertrophy (increases cross-sectional diameter of myocytes) and (c) augmented number of capillaries per myocardial fiber	Increases coronary blood flow
		Better coronary blood supply by (a) increased capillary diffusion capacity, (b) increased pre-capillary vascularity, (c) increased size of coronary tree, and (d) development of additional coronary collateral capillaries	Improves myocardial blood supply
		Increases contractility of myocytes	Improved potential for collateral vascularisation
		Improves capacity of myocardial sarcoplasmic reticulum	Decreases cardiac function at rest and at submaximal exercise
		Increases maximal stroke volume, cardiac output, and blood flow rate in working muscles and maximal oxygen uptake	Reduces the ratio between sympathetic/ parasympathetic drives at rest and during submaximal exercise
			Decreases regional ischaemia of myocardium
			Increases ventricular fibrillation threshold

(Teppermann & Pearlman, 1961; Komadel et al., 1968; Mole et al., 1978; Malhorta et al., 1981; Keul et al., 1982; Koerner & Terjung, 1982; Ho et al., 1983; Åstrand & Rodahl, 1986; Lauglin & Tomanek, 1987; Rost, 1989; Haskell et al., 1992)

Table 11.1 *(Cont'd)*

Organs or tissues	Types of physical activity	Effects of physical activity	Effects on health	Key references
		Reduces heart rate and cardiac output at rest and at submaximal exercise in connection with increased economy of energy metabolism	Reduces risk of spasm in proximal coronary arteries and arterioles Reduces blood pressure in mild hypertension Ameliorates the effects of age and chronic disease (including coronary heart disease)	(Moor & Gollnick, 1982; Åstrand & Rodahl, 1986; Dempsey, 1986)
Respiratory system	Aerobic exercise Aerobic–anaerobic exercises	Increases maximal rate of pulmonary ventilation Improves efficiency of alveolar ventilation and pulmonary gas diffusion Improves abilities of respiratory muscles Increases capillarisation of lung alveoli Improved respiratory control	Maintain efficient respiration Prevention of chronic obstructive pulmonary disease	
Blood	Aerobic exercise Aerobic–anaerobic exercise	Increased blood and plasma volume Modest increase of erythrocyte and hemoglobin quantity Reduction in concentration of total and LDL-cholesterol, increase in HDL-cholesterol Decreases platelet aggregation and increases fibrinolysis	Improves blood supply to tissues Decreases progression of coronary atherosclerosis by increased ratio of HDL-cholesterol/LDL-cholesterol Decreases potential for blood clots	(Åstrand & Rodahl, 1986; Rauramaa et al., 1986; Szygula, 1990; Berg et al., 1994; Sawka et al., 2000)
Endocrine functions	Aerobic exercise Aerobic–anaerobic exercises	Decreases hormonal response in submaximal exercises Increases responses of catecholamines, corticotropin, cortisol, growth hormone and β-endorphin during maximal and supramaximal exercise	Enhanced homeostatic regulation Enhanced adaptivity Avoids hyperinsulinaemia and glucose intolerance	(Galbo, 1983; Holloszy et al., 1987; Viru, 1995)

		Effects	Benefits	References
		Increased secretion of hormones related to hypertrophy of endocrine glands and structural changes in cells producing hormones	Increases insulin sensitivity	
		Increases sensitivity of tissues to hormones due to (a) changes in the density of intracellular and membrane hormone receptors, (b) their affinity, and (c) efficiency of events that occur beyond the receptors	Reduces risk of NIDDM (Type II diabetes)	
Central nervous system	Callisthenic exercises Sports and games	Neural adaptation manifested by improved coordination of muscles	Improved nervous regulation of body functions	(Keul *et al.*, 1982; Dunn & Dishman, 1991; Petruzzello *et al.*, 1991; Sale, 1992; Biddle, 1995)
		Rapid and effective triggering of motor functions	Reduced anxiety and depression	
		Increases activation of prime mover muscles	Improved ability to cope with activities of daily living – especially in the elderly	
		Improved co-ordination of activity of agonistic motor units	Possibility of amelioration of stress-related conditions	
		More labile regulatory influences of autonomic nerves	Improved mood and memory	
		Increased parasympathetic and decreased sympathetic drive at rest	Increased self-esteem	
		Rapid activation of sympathetic drive during exercise		
		Structural changes in neurons		

further increases in exercise intensity. At near maximal intensities – heart rates of 180–190 bpm – maximal values of cardiac output occur with maximal stroke volume being maintained (Musshoff *et al.*, 1959; Åstrand *et al.*, 1964). It has been postulated that certain types of exercise training can improve diastolic function, which has the effect of enabling stroke volume to increase to near maximal levels of activity (Gledhill *et al.*, 1994). However, it seems also to be the case that at very high heart rates (over 180 bpm) stroke volume actually *reduces* due to incomplete filling of ventricles – caused by a short duration of diastole. In terms of effective exercise training, it should be noted that maximal oxygen uptake (an integral index of the power of the oxygen transport system) increases when the intensity of exercise is in the heart rate range 130–180 bpm (Åstrand & Rodahl, 1986).

The benefits of training are also related to neural adaptations (Sale, 1992). Training effects are directly related to the formation of new co-ordination mechanisms at various levels of the central nervous system. For example, appropriate training can develop the ability to recruit a *larger* number of motor units when a strong muscular contraction is required. Alternatively, appropriate training can result in an *optimal* number of motor units being recruited – in order to achieve *economical* muscular contractions. In effect, neural mechanisms ensure optimal activation of agonist motor units and optimal inhibition or co-contraction of antagonist muscles. Neural adaptation can also be general as well as specific, as evidenced by the identification of 'cross-training' effects. In studies where the muscles of one limb have been trained for strength, increases in the strength of the muscles of the contralateral (untrained) limb are also observed. Animal experiments have shown that training-induced neural adaptation occurs via morphological and metabolic changes in nervous structures (see Viru, 1995).

Similar effects can be seen in cardio-respiratory physiology. Fitness training improves neural control of both cardiovascular and respiratory systems. This is evidenced by changes in autonomic balance, more labile regulatory influences, more rapid reaction to activity by autonomic responses, and increased general sensitivity to regulatory influences (see Scheuer & Tipton, 1977; Rowell, 1986).

Blood levels of most hormones change both during and after physical activity providing the intensity reaches a critical threshold or alternatively that the duration of activity reaches a critical 'duration threshold' (Viru, 1992). Typically, exercise training reduces – and can even eliminate – the hormonal response to submaximal exercise because the training raises both the intensity and duration thresholds (Galbo, 1983; Viru, 1992). However, supramaximal exercise performed by elite endurance athletes can elicit very pronounced responses by the catecholamines, corticotrophin, cortisol, growth hormone, and β-endorphin. Thus, high level exercise training can increase secretion of hormones (Kjaer, 1992; Viru, 1995) and this is related to structural changes in endocrine cells (Viru & Seene, 1985).

The concentration of hormones in the blood depends on both rate of hormone release and rate of clearance. Acute exercise bouts have been shown to decrease the rate of sex-hormone elimination from blood (Keiser *et al.*, 1980) and also the metabolism of endorphins (Viru & Tendzegolskis, 1995). The effects of training on blood-hormone clearance are mainly observed in regard to adrenaline. Kjaer *et al.* (1985) demonstrated that a moderate decline in hormone clearance (by 15–22 per cent) occurred in trained subjects at higher intensities of exercise and were more pronounced than in untrained subjects.

The training effects described above – on metabolism, the functional capacities of organs, and on neural and hormonal regulation – have the combined effect of increasing both metabolic efficiency and functional efficiency. These changes also favour functional stability – this is, the ability to maintain metabolic, muscular and mechanical efficiency during prolonged periods of activity.

During endurance exercise in untrained individuals a 'cardiovascular drift' appears, which is characterised by a progressive decline in stroke volume after about 20 minutes of exercise (Coyle & Conzalez-Alonso, 2001). For example, 16 weeks of endurance training resulted in an enhanced ability to maintain higher levels of stroke volume and mean arterial pressure during a 60-minute steady exercise compared to pre-training values (Ekblom, 1970). However, in elite triathletes, echocardiography recordings have indicated impaired relaxation characteristics and reduced contractility of the left ventricle immediately after competition (Whyte *et al.*, 2000).

Health benefits of physical activity

Population studies have shown unequivocally that a strong relationship exists between health and physical activity (for reviews see Blair *et al.*, 1989, 1992; Bouchard *et al.*, 1994; US Department of Health and Human Services, 1996; Wareham & Jakes – this volume). Consistently, physically active people display lower morbidity and mortality rates in regard to a number of diseases, compared to physically inactive people. A problem arises as to whether the positive health effects of activity are related to the physical activity *per se* or to the improved physical fitness that can result from physical activity. A meta-analysis of 23 sex-specific cohorts (representing 1 325 004 person-years of follow-up) revealed that the risk of both CHD and CVD decreased linearly in association with increasing physical activity. In contrast, fitness improvement was reflected in health improvement only when its level was greater than the 25th percentile of the fitness distribution. Above this threshold the reduction in risk was precipitous, with a more gradual gradient towards the higher centiles. Nevertheless, the level of risk reduction was more strongly associated with fitness than with physical activity at all centiles (Williams, 2001). Actually, this outcome indicates that (1) a threshold amount of physical activity is necessary to improve fitness, and (2) increases of physical activity may be most effective when it evokes a training effect – expressed as a fitness improvement. In this meta-analysis fitness was assessed by either direct or indirect measures of maximal oxygen uptake ($\dot{V}O_2$max).

Chapter 3 (Epidemiology) describes the relationships between physical activity and health indices. Chapter 5 (Measurement) shows the importance of accurate and specific measurement of physical activity.

However, there may well be training effects essential for reduction in CVD risk which are not reflected by the level of $\dot{V}O_2$max. All in all, it is difficult to believe that health improvement (reduction of risk of disease) is possible without any structural or functional change in the body. The question is whether the critical changes that promote health are measurable, by what means they are best measured, and whether improved fitness is a mediator of reduced risk or a parallel outcome. This final point is difficult to assess, because physical activity and cardio-respiratory fitness are related in a dose-response fashion. For example, in a study of 619 healthy men and 497 healthy women (age range 18–95 years), it was found that leisure-time physical activity accounted for 12.9 per cent of peak $\dot{V}O_2$ variance for men and 10.6 per cent for women. Peak $\dot{V}O_2$ correlated most strongly with the high-intensity physical activity ($r=0.33$ in men and $r=0.27$ in women). Correlations with moderate-intensity activity were $r=0.12$ for men and $r=0.17$ for women. With low-intensity activity, correlations were $r=0.08$ and $r=0.06$ respectively (Brill *et al.*, 2000). Whereas these correlations are not strong, they do indicate that different types of physical activity have differential effects on cardio-respiratory fitness.

Three theoretical concepts exist to assist our understanding of the relationship between health status and physical activity/physical fitness: (1) counteraction of the effects of hypokinaesia, (2) specific preventive effects on body systems, and (3) increased 'adaptivity'. These concepts will provide the framework for our understanding of the health-promoting physiological effects of physical activity. Each concept is discussed in detail below.

Counteraction of the effects of hypokinaesia

In this case, the beneficial effects of physical activity mediate the degenerative – and therefore harmful – consequences of sedentary living. Experiments have been performed to assess the effects of hypokinaesia, most commonly utilising enforced periods of bed-rest (up to three weeks) in the supine position. These studies have shown decrements in cardiovascular function (decreases in $\dot{V}O_2$max, maximal cardiac output, maximal stroke volume and myocardial contractility; slight increase in resting heart rate) which are proportional to the duration of the bed-rest (Saltin *et al.*, 1968; Bloomfield & Coyle, 1993). Simultaneously, glucose intolerance and hyperinsulinaemia (Lipman *et al.*, 1972) are increased, nitrogen and calcium balances (evidencing loss of protein and of bone mass, respectively) increased, and plasma volume substantially decreased (Bloomfield & Coyle, 1993). Decrements in skeletal-muscle mass (disuse atrophy) are also observed and are associated with reduced cross-sectional area for both slow-twitch and fast-twitch muscle fibres and loss of muscle strength. In muscle tissue there is a loss of capillary density, a decline in aerobic enzyme activity and reduced stores of phosphocreatine and glycogen (see Saltin & Gollnick, 1983; Bloomfield & Coyle, 1993). It is clear, therefore, that there are definite degenerative and potentially harmful consequences of extreme physical inactivity (bed-rest). However, such extremes of physical inactivity are not typical of ordinary people, even if their physical activity is minimal. Therefore, what we are really concerned with is 'relative hypokinaesia', which might be defined as a lack of sufficient physical activity to avoid disuse atrophy. The actual amount of physical activity that corresponds to a critical level of hypokinaesia is discussd later.

A specific preventive effect

According to this concept, the biological changes caused by physical activity reduce the risk of development of various pathogenic processes (Table 11.1). These biological changes include: (1) improved functional status, (2) an anti-atherosclerotic effect, (3) improved metabolic control, (4) avoidance of excess deposition of adipose tissue, and (5) an anti-carcinogenic effect.

Improved functional status

Regular physical activity induces functional and morphological adaptations that are specifically related to the activities performed and improves our capacity to perform these activities (increases fitness). Increased functional capacity of the cardiovascular system results in more effective oxygen transport to contracting muscles and is generally accepted as a mechanism of prevention of coronary and other cardiovascular diseases. Maximal oxygen uptake is an integral measure of the capacities of the cardiovascular and respiratory systems and demonstrates a strong, inverse correlation with cardiovascular morbidity and mortality (Ekelund *et al.*, 1988; Williams, 2001; Arraiz *et al.*, 1992).

Increased functional *reserve* (the difference between maximal functional capacity and basal capacity) may actually be more essential for health than the maximal level *per se*. This functional reserve can be enhanced 'at both ends', as endurance training results in higher maximal cardiac output or stroke volume during maximal exercise as well as a decreased basal level of heart rate and cardiac output (see Åstrand & Rodahl, 1986). This increased functional reserve enables the body to more easily cope with physical stresses on the cardiovascular system using a portion of the reserve rather than the maximum capacity. In this case, the necessary functional adjustments are within the person's capacity and are not over-stressful.

At the 'other end' of the reserve, low basal values are an indication of high functional economy – the ease with which life requirements are met with minimal functional activity. Mellerowicz introduced this principle of 'functional economy' to exercise physiology in 1956. He was probably the first person to emphasise the significance of 'economy' in reducing risk of cardiovascular disease (Mellerowicz, 1956). In endurance-trained persons, functional economy is also reflected in less pronounced functional adaptation, and more rapid recovery from submaximal exercise, compared to untrained persons.

Whereas the expression of functional economy in heart rate changes is clear, this is not reflected in regard to basal levels of stroke volume and how this changes with exercise. For example, after endurance training heart rate has been shown to decrease and stroke volume to increase, both at rest and during exercise at 60 per cent $\dot{V}O_2$max. Cardiac output (a function of heart rate and stroke volume) was decreased at rest but slightly increased during submaximal exercise (Wilmore *et al.*, 2001). Barnard (1975) did not find any changes in post-training cardiac output at the same exercise intensity. However, Andrew *et al.* (1966) and Ekblom *et al.* (1968) have shown that training causes a reduced oxygen uptake during a standard workload (increased work efficiency), and that cardiac output declines in a similar fashion (−3.5%). Obviously, these contradictory results might be related to other training effects on the economy of metabolic processes (for example, increased mechanical efficiency), or it may be due to increases in blood volume and/or decreased neural influences.

It has been shown that endurance training increases plasma volume and resting stroke volume by about the same amount (Green *et al.*, 1990). An increased volume of circulating blood favours the venous return of blood to heart and, thereby, the filling of the ventricles during diastole (Seals *et al.*, 1994). There is also a compensatory increase in erythrocytes. However, plasma volume expansion occurs immediately at the onset of training, whereas the increase of erythrocyte volume takes several weeks (Sawka *et al.*, 2000). This can give rise to a relative dilutional affect and can give rise to conditions such as 'athletic anaemia'.

It is known that the heart hypertrophies as a result of regular exercise and one possible adjustment for this may be decreased myocardial contractility in resting conditions. This possibility is supported by the fact that the residual (post-systolic) amount of blood in the heart is increased in people with cardiac hypertrophy (Reindell *et al.*, 1957). The increased residual volume appears to exist only at rest and this suggests that it has a neural origin.

Endurance training induces pronounced changes in coronary vessels, and this may be critically important for health. In particular, these changes prevent regional ischaemia of the heart. The following adaptations may all be highly significant:

- increased number of capillaries per myocardial fibre (Komadell *et al.*, 1968; Tharp & Wagner, 1982)
- increased capillary diffusion capacity (Laughlin & Tomanek, 1987)
- improved pre-capillary vascularity (Ho *et al.*, 1983)
- increased total size of the coronary tree (Tepperman & Pearlman, 1961)
- development of extra collateral coronary capillaries (Koerner & Terjung, 1982).

The preventive significance of these various changes in the heart may relate to increased contractility of the myocytes (Scheuer & Tipton, 1977; Mole, 1978) and to an improved capacity of the myocardial sarcoplasmic reticulum (Penpargkul *et al.*, 1977; Tibbits *et al.*, 1978). Raab (1970) has suggested that improved balance of sympathetic/parasympathetic drives may be important for prevention of diffuse ischaemic changes. Keul *et al.* (1982) pointed out the plausible significance of increased β-adrenergic receptors in combination with decreased sympathetic drive for increased heart efficiency in a trained organism. Haskell *et al.* (1992) emphasised that exercise training decreases the risk of regional ischaemia of myocardium. They also cite experimental studies on rats performed by Noakes *et al.* (1983), where exercise training increased the ventricular fibrillation threshold of isolated rat heart during conditions of both hypoxia and regional ischaemia. Laughlin (1994) has also indicated the potential of training to induce a reduction of spasm risk in proximal coronary arteries and arterioles. Finally, a meta-analysis has shown that endurance exercise for coronary rehabilitation decreased the risk of sudden cardiac death even among people with advanced coronary atherosclerosis (O'Connor *et al.*, 1989).

Training improves the control of blood coagulation by decreased platelet adhesion and aggregation (prevents clot formation) and enhanced enzymatic fibrinolysis (breakdown of clots). It may be that this is mediated by prostanoid prostacyclin (Rauramaa, 1986) and tissue plasminogen activator (Stratton *et al.*, 1991).

Physical activity is effective for reducing arterial pressure in mild hypertension (Paffenbarger *et al.*, 1991) and, thereby, preventing the development of advanced hypertension. In physically inactive and/or unfit persons, the risk of development of hypertension is 30–50 per cent greater than in more fit and active persons (Blair *et al.*, 1984).

The effects of physical activity and exercise on the respiratory system probably have preventive significance for certain lung diseases and for maintaining effective respiration in other diseases. However, in this field the data is rather sparse. The following effects may contribute to such benefits: increased maximal rate of respiration, improved efficiency of alveolar ventilation and pulmonary diffusion (Åstrand & Rodahl, 1986; Dempsey, 1986) and improved function of respiratory muscles and their energy stores (Moor & Gollnick, 1982).

With respect to nearly all of the above effects, it is apparent that performing a wide variety of habitual physical activities promotes a wide range of physical benefits that are related to health. It should be noted that for improved health it is important to develop strength, agility, flexibility and aerobic and muscular endurance (Brown & Holloszy, 1993). Most importantly, it is not the *maximal* performance that is necessary, but rather some optimal level – which probably varies between the different dimensions of both physical activity and health.

Studies have shown that regular moderate physical activity has a potential role as a protective factor for mechanical low-back pain, as well as a role in treatment and rehabilitation (Biering-Sörenson *et al.*, 1994). In this respect, it is often postulated that developing muscular fitness in the lower back and abdominal muscles is important. Development of these muscles maintains the position of individual vertebrae and, thereby, optimises posture. However, it should be noted that in susceptible individuals the muscular effort involved in such exercises may provoke low-back pain if not performed correctly.

The above principles can in reality be applied to just about any joint. That is, development of the skeletal muscles around the joint regulates the degree of freedom of movements within the joint. The co-ordination between these muscles determines the actual direction of movement of the limb or its parts. This interplay between the relative actions of the agonist and antagonist muscles in effect works to prevent excessive and injurious amplitude of movement by the joint.

There are a range of other considerations whereby the effects of physical activity improve health. Being habitually active can help prevent traumatic injuries. For example, in elderly people improvement of balance and gait significantly decreases the risk of falls (Tinetti *et al.*, 1994). Further, should a fall occur the effects may be less serious if the strength and elasticity of ligaments, tendons and bones is higher. It has been shown that physical activity reduces fracture risk by improving the density – and hence the strength – of bone tissue (Tipton *et al.*, 1967; Booth & Gould, 1975; Sorock *et al.*, 1988; Kovanen & Suominen, 1989). In this respect, the mechanical load on bones during muscular activity stimulates bone formation. There are increases in bone-mineral density and a more optimal balance between bone formation and resorption. Conversely, inactivity results in a decline in bone mass (Layon, 1996).

Physical activity during adolescence may be particularly important in order that a high peak bone mass is achieved. In this case, the deleterious effects of the age-related decline in bone mass may be minimised (Grington *et al.*, 1993; Kirchner *et al.*, 1996). Physical activity during adulthood also helps to maintain bone mass and bone-mineral density as we age (Talmage *et al.*, 1986). Even osteoporotic women can minimise bone loss or even achieve a modest gain in bone-mineral density with appropriate physical activity (Krølner *et al.*, 1983). Physical activity contributes to the primary (due to increased peak bone mass during adolescence) and secondary (due to reduced rate of bone loss in elderly) prevention of osteoporosis (Suominen, 1993; Vuori, 1995). When we consider the extreme case of physical activity we consistently see that athletes, especially those who are strength-trained, have greater bone-mineral density than non-athletes (Chilibeck *et al.*, 1995).

 Chapter 2 (Lifespan) details the rationale for a lifecourse approach for promoting physical activity to optimise bone development.

An antisclerotic effect

Two types of antisclerotic effects are evoked by physical activity and exercise (Viru & Smirnova, 1995).

The *metabolic* antisclerotic effect is seen largely in changes in the lipoprotein profile and total concentration of cholesterol in blood. Regular physical activity has the following metabolic actions:

1. Increases the content of high-density lipoprotein cholesterol (HDL-cholesterol), encouraging the return of cholesterol into the liver, where it is oxidised and removed from the body.
2. Decreases the content of low-density lipoprotein cholesterol (LDL-cholesterol) – mainly LDL2 cholesterol. This lipoprotein contributes to the fixation of cholesterol in sites of formation of atherosclerotic plaque on the internal wall of blood vessels
3. Increases levels of apolipoprotein-A and decrease levels of apolipoprotein B (see Berg *et al.*, 1994). Both of these changes are in the 'healthy' direction.

In addition to the above measures that take place in the blood, there are also observable effects on body organs. For example, a training-induced increase in cholesterol degradation has been found in the liver (Hebbelnick & Casier, 1966).

Taken overall, the metabolic antisclerotic effect of improving the blood-lipoprotein profile provides benefits by (a) preventing cardiac ischaemia, (b) reducing the risk of hypertension, and (c) decreasing the risk of stroke. It is sometimes argued that an association between activity or fitness and reduced risk of stroke or peripheral vascular diseases is not convincingly established (Blair *et al.*, 1992). Several but not all population-based studies do report an inverse association between physical activity and the risk of stroke (US Department of Health and Human Services, 1996). Inactive men have also been shown to be more likely to have a hemorrhagic stroke than active men. However, ischaemic stroke seems not to be related to levels of physical activity (Abbott *et al.*, 1994).

The *mechanical* antisclerotic effect of physical activity is related to the protection of tissues from sclerotic changes that are induced by inactivity. In this respect, the protection – by regular activity – of muscles, tendons and ligaments from sclerotic changes can promote higher levels of flexibility in older people. A second form of mechanical effect is from exercises that involve frequent and dynamic changes in body position or movements in a range of directions. In activities such as these, rapid changes in vascular tone are necessary in order to ensure sufficient blood supply to various parts of body. In effect, the blood vessels themselves are physically 'trained'.

Improved metabolic control

Physical activity influences metabolic control at three important levels: (1) cellular auto-regulation, (2) hormonal control, and (3) neural control. Improvement of cellular auto-regulation is based on the effects of activity on enzyme systems. Usually, training simultaneously increases both the concentration and activity levels of enzymes. This makes control easier to achieve. Physical activity also influences the susceptibility of enzymes to both stimulating and inhibiting factors, and this promotes a minimal rate of biochemical reaction related to energy production at rest. Also, exercised-induced increases in the rate can be more efficiently achieved.

The endocrine system reacts in two ways – firstly by enhancing hormone production and, secondly, by improving the sensitivity of hormone receptors. Improvements in neural control are related to the rapid activation of hormone responses during activity, and this possibly helps to achieve optimum balance between the regulatory activities of the endocrine system and sympathetic/parasympathetic nervous drive. Other aspects of improved metabolic control include enhanced stores of energy substrates, augmented number of mitochondria (improving control of oxidative processes) and an increase in number of a range of transporter proteins (see Jakovlev, 1977; Keul *et al.*, 1982; Saltin & Gollnick, 1983; Hargreaves, 1995; Viru, 1995).

A major factor in regard to the prevention of health disorders through activity is the prevention of hyperinsulinaemia and improvement of glucose tolerance. These appear to be central actions in many aspects of the health benefits of physical activity. Blood glucose is homeostatically controlled in that the ratio between blood levels of insulin and glucagon needs to be optimised (Wolfe *et al.*, 1986). Insulin inhibits glucose output by liver and stimulates glucose transport into muscle cells and other tissues, where it is stored as glycogen. Conversely, glucagon (a 'counter-regulatory' hormone, that is, it has an action opposite to that of insulin) enhances hepatic glucose output. So, elevations in blood-glucose concentrations stimulate increased insulin levels and inhibit glucagon secretion. Conversely, a fall in blood-glucose level suppresses insulin release and enhances glucagon secretion. In this way, an optimal balance is achieved between hepatic glucose output and glucose deposition in cells.

Maintaining a constant blood-glucose level is highly significant in that it ensures that carbohydrates are available as a fuel for tissues. There are two potential problems that this avoids – hypoglycaemia and hyperglycaemia. In hypoglycaemia, virtually all muscular and neural function is impaired. Hyperglycaemia has a strong action on various metabolic processes. For example, it suppresses hepatic glucose output and lipolysis in adipose tissue. In this way, the availability of both, carbohydrates and lipids decreases and a situation of 'tissue starving' will develop. Hyperglycaemia also suppresses secretion of adrenaline, noradrenaline, cortisol and growth hormone, thus impairing the adaptive responses controlled by these hormones. Sustained hyperglycaemia is a plausible condition for destruction or damage to cellular insulin receptors in tissues, resulting in a condition of glucose intolerance. In this condition, glucose administration or a meal provoke pronounced and prolonged hyperglycaemia, and there is increased 'insulin resistance' (decreased sensitivity to insulin). Both hyperinsulinaemia and glucose intolerance are known to enhance risk of several pathological processes, including coronary artery disease (Ducimetiere *et al.*, 1980).

Sustained hyperglycaemia is caused by either (1) deficiency of circulating insulin due to pathological destruction of pancreatic beta islet cells (insulin-dependent diabetes mellitus – IDDM), or (2) insulin resistance (non-insulin dependent diabetes mellitus – NIDDM). Physical activity improves glucose intolerance when the abnormality is primarily caused by NIDDM. In cases of IDDM, the effects of physical activity are minimal (Holloszy *et al.*, 1987). Physical activity appears to be most beneficial in preventing the progression of NIDDM during the earlier stages of the pathological process, in combination with appropriate diet manipulations (Barnard *et al.*, 1994).

Evidence for a preventive role of physical activity against NIDDM has been provided by a prospective study of the University of Pennsylvania alumni. In this study, physical activity was inversely related to the incidence of NIDDM. Each 500 kcal increment of weekly leisure-time physical activity was associated with a 6 per cent decrease in risk (adjusted for age, basal metabolic rate, history of high blood pressure, and parental history of diabetes) of developing NIDDM (Helmrich *et al.*, 1991).

 Chapter 3 (Epidemiology) describes the science supporting the determination of the relationships between physical activity and health.

Physical activity in the form of endurance training reduces the activity of pancreatic β-cells, which produce insulin (King *et al.*, 1990). This is one of the main means of improving the effectiveness of homeostatic control of blood glucose levels (euglycaemia) (Vranic & Wasserman, 1990). Improved blood-glucose control is manifested in a less pronounced increase in blood glucose and insulin concentrations after a meal or after the administration of glucose into the bloodstream (Lindgårde & Saltin, 1981). A further important adaptive effect occurs at the level of cellular reception of insulin. In this case the sensitivity of tissue to insulin is markedly enhanced (Craig *et al.*, 1981; Rönnemaa *et al.*, 1986; Dohm *et al.*, 1987).

A prolonged bout of exercise of submaximal intensity suppresses the release of insulin and this is seen in reduced blood-insulin levels during the exercise. As a result, hepatic-glucose output can increase, and the lipolytic action of the catecholamines and other lipolytic hormones (for example, growth hormone, glucagon, thyroid hormones, and corticotrophin) are freed from the blockade that insulin exerts. As a consequence, blood levels of free fatty acids increase and lipid oxidation is enhanced. In this way there is a 'sparing' of muscle glycogen usage and enlarged supply of blood glucose for the nerve cells during prolonged exercise. Despite the decreased level of circulating insulin during exercise, glucose transport into contracting muscle fibres is actually increased (Plough *et al.*, 1987). This enhancement persists for 24 hours or more after the end of exercise and this enables muscle glycogen to be replenished more effectively and efficiently. Accordingly, it has been suggested that the positive influence of regular physical activity on glucose metabolism may be, in part, related to the overlapping effects of repeated Physical activity sessions (Harris *et al.*, 1987). In terms of health, therefore, the beneficial effects of physical activity on the body may be particularly enhanced by a lifestyle that involves a large number of short activity bouts, rather than a fewer number of longer sessions.

An interesting and more recent area of research has focused on the role of Glucose Transporter 4 (GLUT4), which is a transporter protein. GLUT4 is the predominant transporter in skeletal muscle and adipose tissue and essentially acts to allow glucose to enter the cell where it can be processed by the body into more usable forms of energy. Interestingly, physical activity is known to be beneficial in the prevention and treatment of diabetes mellitus as it increases the rate of glucose uptake into the contracting skeletal muscles, which is the same action as insulin. The process is regulated by the translocation of GLUT4 glucose transporters to the plasma membrane and transverse tubules. However, physical activity and insulin appear to achieve this effect through different signalling pathways. Namely, physical activity seems to increase GLUT4 expression, which in turn contributes to an increase in the responsiveness of muscle-glucose uptake to insulin. Therefore, physical activity appears to promote glucose uptake by muscle independent of the actions of insulin. For a more detailed discussion of these processes, see Goodyear & Kahn (1998).

Reduced body fat

Obesity is possibly the major overt health problem facing 21st-century industrialised nations. Obesity is associated with reduced longevity and increased incidence of cardiovascular disease, non-insulin dependent diabetes mellitus (NIDDM), osteoarthritis, and certain types of cancer (Blair *et al.*, 1996). A simplistic approach to obesity is that the mass of adipose tissue reduces as a result of systematic physical activity when the total energy expenditure is higher than the energy intake by eating food. This is essentially true, but in order to *sustain* this reduction of body fat there is a need to improve metabolic *control* – most particularly the insulin-related control mechanisms. As discussed above, such improvements can be evoked by regular physical activity that can initiate beneficial adaptations to an individual's energy metabolism. In recent years, there has been considerable interest in the role of the hormone leptin. Whereas the importance of leptin has yet to be ascertained, it is worth noting that plasma levels of leptin are proportional to body-fat levels. As far as we know, leptin acts as a messenger to the brain and it is responsive to disruptions in energy balance caused by changes in energy stores (Caro *et al.*, 1996).

A further important effect of physical activity on adiposity is the potential for redistribution of regional fat stores. The development of related disorders such as insulin resistance, hyperinsulinaemia, and glucose intolerance are related to an accumulation of fat around the waist, abdomen, upper body, and within the abdominal cavity (Harris *et al.*, 1987). Increased low-density lipoprotein (LDL) cholesterol is common in people having this type of fat distribution (Kanaley *et al.*, 1993). However, abdominal fat is more responsive than gluteal or lower-body fat to adrenaline stimulation (Wahrenberg *et al.*, 1991). Accordingly, physical activity such as systematic endurance exercise preferentially decreases subcutaneous fat stores of the trunk (Després *et al.*, 1988).

Influence on carcinogenesis

Several epidemiological studies indicate a limited preventive influence of physical activity with regard to some cancers, most notably cancer of the colon (Blair *et al.*, 1989; Lee, 1995). Conversely, it has been argued that physical inactivity increases the risk of cancer (Lee, 1995). The risk of cancer among sedentary people in comparison with physically active people is between 1.4- and 3.7-fold (Lee, 1995). An association between either physical activity or physical fitness and the risk of other cancers (for example, rectal cancer, female and male reproductive cancers) has yet to be proven (Lee, 1995; US Department of Health and Human Services, 1996). However, there are interesting results from a longitudinal study performed at the Cooper Institute for Aerobics Research in Dallas. This study included 10224 men and 3120 women who were observed for an average of eight years. In this study the age-adjusted total death rates per 10000 persons-years of observation for individuals of low, moderate and high aerobic fitness were 20, 7 and 5 for men, and 16, 10 and 1 for women, respectively (Blair *et al.*, 1989).

The foundation for an anti-carcinogenic effect may lie in the enhancement of the number and activity of natural killer cells as a result of physical activity (Lee, 1995; Nieman, 2000). It has been observed that regular exercise training significantly enhances resting blood levels of natural killer cell activity in previously sedentary people (Nieman *et al.*, 1990) and increased activity has been established in elite athletes (Petersen & Ullum, 1994). In high-intensity physical activity, natural killer cell cytotoxic activity increases 40–100 per cent. However, between one and two hours post-exercise there is a decrease of 25–35 per cent *below* the pre-activity level (Nieman, 1994). With physical activity of moderate intensity there is also enhanced cytotoxic activity of natural killer cells. This response is usually less pronounced than with vigorous activity, but the post-activity immunosuppression does *not* seem to occur (Pedersen & Ullum, 1994). It has been suggested that physical activity effect on natural killer cells activity is mediated by adrenaline, as well as by interleukin-1, interleukin-6, and tumour necrosis factor-α (Nieman, 1994; Pedersen & Ullum, 1994).

In addition to changes in immune activity, the acute bouts of physical activity may inhibit carcinogenesis through other mechanisms. For instance, decreased colon-cancer risk may be related to shortening the transit time of food within the intestinal system. This results in a decreased contact time of potential carcinogens and co-carcinogens in the faecal stream. Since the rectum is filled with faecal material only just before evacuation, the protective effect on the rectum is negligible. This may explain the marked difference in the protective effect of physical activity on the colon, compared with the lack of effect on the rectum (Lee, 1995).

Increased 'adaptivity'

Figure 11.3 shows how the human body strives for a state of well-being or health by adapting to events that disturb it. It does this by mobilising its resources to 'fight' the disturbances. This fight for maintaining and/or restoring the state of well-being uses an array of physiological adaptation processes as weapons. This ability to fight for a state of well-being can be generalised into the term 'adaptivity'. Adaptivity can be defined as the ability of an organism to mobilise adaptation processes in two ways. Firstly, it facilitates normal life activities despite changes within the body or in the external environment. Secondly, it makes adaptive alterations in both cellular structures and in the quantities of enzymes which can aid restoration of normality. In this way, the body achieves a form of resistance to the influence of a broad range of chronic influences that might act to disturb the body's function.

A broad range of factors can adversely affect the body's adaptivity. These include an unhealthy lifestyle, for example, poor nutrition, lack of physical activity, and, in particular, alcohol, nicotine and illicit-drug use. Diseases and the pollution of air, water and food also decrease adaptivity. It is interesting to note that only one non-pharmacological strategy has been found to increase the body's adaptivity to adverse influences – physical activity. In animal studies it has been found that exercise-trained rats are more resistant to the influences of hypoxia, irritation, high or low ambient temperatures and the actions of

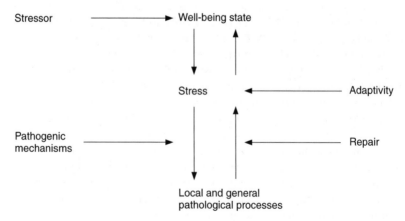

Figure 11.3 Schematic representation of how the body attempts to maintain a 'normal' state of well-being

various toxins, compared to sedentary rats. However, in rats that had been forced to exercise at very high levels, the resistance to various stressors was *lower* than levels found in sedentary rats (Zhimkin, 1961). Thus, the exercise training induced an increase in adaptivity that disappeared when the training regime was too hard. Such an 'exhausted' adaptivity can be termed the 'over-training syndrome', which is often seen in athletes. Overtraining syndrome is characterised by persistent fatigue, reduced performance, neuroendocrine changes, alterations in mood states, and frequent illness, especially upper-respiratory-tract infection (Mackinnon & Hooper, 2000). The overtraining appears to be a result of too much exercise and too little time for the body to recover. A range of factors can exacerbate the condition, including nutritional factors, travel, psychological strain, a stressful job or studies, and a genetic predisposition (Lehmann *et al.*, 1999). The overtraining syndrome can require medical treat-ment, but sufficient rest is normally all that may be necessary. However, persuading athletes to rest is a problem to which no one has yet discovered an answer.

The positive effect of physical activity on adaptivity may reside in improved mechanisms for general body adaptation (Viru, 1992). The optimal level of physical activity for achieving such an effect seems to be that point where physical working capacity is seen to improve. In other words, a visible training effect – that is, improved physical fitness – seems to be required (Viru & Smirnova, 1995). However, as seen above, it seems unnecessary to strive for very high levels of fitness gain. At this optimum level, the main categories of physical adaptations are listed in Table 11.2, together with examples of physical activities thought to optimally improve them.

One of the main effects of physical activity and exercise is improved oxida-tive capacity. This takes place as a result of increased numbers of mitochondria in the muscle cell, and an improved ratio between production of free radicals

Table 11.2 The benefits of exercise training that increase the adaptivity of the body

The benefits of exercise training	Effective activities
Improvement of nervous regulation and functions of the central nervous system	Gymnastics and callisthenics
Increased capacity of endocrine system and altered sensitivity of hormones	Aerobic exercise
Increased energy stores of muscles and liver	Aerobic exercise
Improved capacity of oxygen transport system	Aerobic exercise
Efficiency of oxidation processes	Aerobic exercise
Increased metabolic and functional economy	Aerobic exercise
Increased functional stability	Aerobic exercise
Increased number of Na^+ and K^+ pumps	Callisthenics and repetitive exercise
Positive influence on immunoreactivity	Most exercises
Antisclerotic effect of training	
Metabolic	Aerobic exercise
Mechanical	Callisthenics

Source: for references see Viru & Smirnova, 1995.

and the activity of antioxidant enzymes. The former of these is well described in exercise physiology textbooks, but the second effect is worthy of discussion. Increased free-radical activity occurs in certain conditions where oxygen molecules convert into an active form of oxygen. In this way, the so-called free radicals are produced. Free radicals may have destructive and even lethal effects on cells. Their main effect is to oxidise polyunsaturated fatty acids that are the essential components of cellular membranes. They are able to oxidise some of these cellular enzymes, thus damaging cellular metabolic systems. Free radicals can also modify nucleic acids, proteins and lipids in cells (Yu, 1994). These harmful effects of free radicals are opposed by an antioxidant system, consisting principally of multiple enzymes that actually remove free radicals. The harmful consequences of the production of free radicals is experienced only when an imbalance, called oxidative stress, occurs between the production of free radicals and the activity of the antioxidant system (Buettinger, 1993).

Vigorous physical activity may actually induce oxidative stress as it causes an accumulation of free radicals and subsequent oxidative damage to lipids, protein and DNA in skeletal muscles (Powers *et al.*, 1999; Sen, 2001). Systematic exercise training that results in increased activity of antioxidant enzymes (Powers *et al.*, 1999) can reduce the level of exercise-induced oxidative stress. In a study of swimmers it was shown that both long-distance and short-distance exercise training increases the activity levels of antioxidant enzymes (Inal *et al.*, 2001).

There are important relationships between the observed 'training effect' of physical activity on the body's adaptivity and changes in immune activity. Exercise training may enhance the body's capacity for specific antibody formation in response to immunogenic challenge (Eskola *et al.*, 1978). For example, exercise-trained elderly people show an enhanced lymphocyte proliferative response and T-cell function compared to sedentary people (Nieman, 1997). We have already discussed the way in which physical activity enhances the actions of natural killer cells in the acute phase. However, it should be mentioned that moderate amounts of physical activity (3–5 sessions a week, 15–60 minutes a session = at 40–60 per cent $\dot{V}O_2$max) have little if any *chronic* effect on immune function (Nieman, 1997). In athletes, a pronounced drop in immunoreactivity may follow exhaustive exercise-training sessions and competitions which include a decrease in both natural killer cell and cytotoxic activity (Nieman, 1997). Studies on high-level athletes showed similar decreases in the indices of secretory immunity during preparation for international competition – specifically, low levels of immunoglobulins IgA, IgG and IgM in both blood and saliva. This may be associated with (a) a low antiviral immune defence, (b) inefficiency of anti-influenza vaccination (Levando *et al.*, 1988), and (c) suppressed production of interferon α and interleukin 2 (Gotovtseva *et al.*, 1998). These changes are transitory when sufficient time for recovery is allowed after such hard training or competition (Pershin *et al.*, 1988).

In the above discussion it has been noted that moderate and vigorous physical activity seem to have differential effects. This is also reflected in the fact that regular moderate-intensity exercise training reduces the risk of upper-respiratory-tract infection (URTI), whereas vigorous-intensity-exercise training increases the risk (Nieman, 1994, 2000). Usually, suppressed immunoreactivity and increased risk of URTI appear in athletes as, or just after, their performance level has reached an individual peak. Therefore, the specific cause appears not to be a manifestation of overtraining itself but rather a chronic development of an exhausted adaptive capability – resulting from the physical efforts required to reach such a peak of performance. Nevertheless, the true mechanism of exhausted adaptivity in athletes during the time of their peak performance is still relatively unclear. One possibility is that there exists a certain level of fatigue of the cellular genetic apparatus that prohibits further adaptive responses such as adaptive synthesis of proteins. Another possibility is that exhausted adaptivity is related to changes in regulatory function, particularly hormonal metabolic control (Viru, 1995). Athletes are not clinically immune deficient (Mackinnon, 2000) and the condition is not serious. Accordingly, the combined effects of moderate changes in several immune parameters appear only to compromise resistance to minor illnesses such as URTI (Mackinnon, 2000). However, such illnesses do impair and interrupt training programmes and are a serious problem for some athletes.

The effects of exhausted adaptivity on immunoreactivity may, therefore, appear as suppressed natural killer cell activity, nitrogen-induced lymphocyte proliferation, upper airway neutrophil phagocytosis, and reduced salivary IgA concentration several hours into recovery from acute prolonged or intensive exercise. During this 'window of decreased immunoreactivity', viruses and bacteria may gain a foothold, thus increasing the risk of infection (Pederson & Bruumsgaard, 1995, 1997). This is a plausible explanation as to why athletes going through repeated cycles of heavy training loads appear to be at increased risk of infection (Payne, 1994).

Quantitative aspects of health enhancement exercises

The above concepts exploring the health-promoting effect of physical activity should not be thought of as alternatives. Their relative significance and contribution depends on both the volume and intensity of the physical activity performed. From the mechanisms discussed so far, it seems that in terms of health, five levels of human physical activity can be identified:

- very low activity (hypokinaesia)
- modest activity, enough to be distinguishable from hypokinaesia
- moderate activity that can produce specific preventive effects that reduce the risk of a range of pathological processes

- moderate-to-vigorous (optimal) activity that produces training effects and increases the body's adaptivity
- excessive activity, causing overstrain phenomena.

It should be noted that it is difficult, if not impossible, to identify specific (absolute) amounts and intensities of activity with the above categories, as each depends on an individual's level of fitness, age and gender. For each category, the absolute level of activity is likely to differ between men and women, to rise with improved fitness and to fall with both inactivity and increasing age. An essential point is that the level of 'modest' activity – the first target for sedentary people – may rise over time if fitness levels improve. Similarly, required workloads at all levels need to increase as fitness improves in order to ensure further progress. This is often referred to as 'progression' in exercise training. There are also indications that after an athlete withdraws from competition, it is very important that he or she maintains an exercise programme to avoid health disturbances due to a sudden alteration (reduction) in activity levels. It is not uncommon for health disorders found in former athletes to be attributed to 'damage' caused by their former tough training schedule. However, a more plausible reason is the sudden change in physical activity level leading to a condition of relative hypokinaesia. However, this is currently merely a hypothesis that requires further testing. Further studies are also necessary to establish the quantitative relationships between fitness level and the minimum level of activity required to avoid 'relative hypokinaesia'. A schematic representation of the inter-relationships between the above concepts is shown in Figure 11.4.

There have been a number of recommendations for the amount of physical activity needed to enhance health (Cooper, 1968; ACCM, 1990; Blair *et al.*, 1992; Paffenbarger & Olson, 1996; US Department of Health and Human Services, 1996). The most recent of these (US Department of Health and Human Services, 1996) recommends that to avoid the condition of hypokinaesia, currently sedentary adults need to become moderately active for at least 30 minutes a day. In other words, they need to accumulate the equivalent of two miles walking at a moderate pace. Haskell *et al.* (1992) have suggested that in order to reduce the risk of coronary heart disease, endurance training at 65–80 per cent of functional capacity for 25 minutes or longer (expenditure of at least 300 kcal) for three or more sessions weekly is necessary. It seems that the protective effect is observed after a training programme of 16 weeks or longer. In his meta-analysis, Williams (2001) examined the contribution of both physical activity and fitness with respect to reduction of risk of cardiovascular disease. In this analysis the contribution of physical activity was 15 per cent and that of fitness was 20 per cent.

It seems obvious that there are different levels at which individuals can exercise and obtain health-promoting effects. The general guidelines given above are at a relatively low level and this is an excellent strategy because it renders them achievable by large numbers of people. Nevertheless, there are likely to be individuals who wish to progress beyond this level in order to achieve

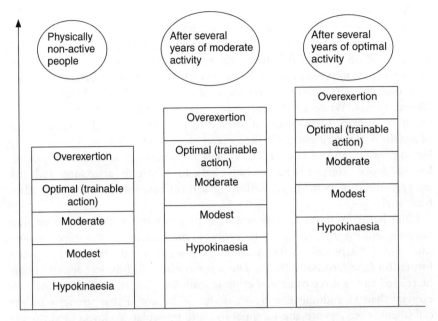

Figure 11.4   Energy expenditure for muscular activity

further improvements in both adaptivity and general fitness. For them, higher levels are obviously needed. Exercising five or more times weekly with a minimum duration of 20 minutes is considered the threshold for training effects to occur providing workloads are of a sufficient intensity to induce effective adaptive protein synthesis. For resistance exercise, the minimum effective dose is considered to be two sessions a week using one set of 8–12 repetitions of 8–10 exercises that condition the major muscle groups (ACSM, 1990). However, it seems obvious that there is an infinite number of possible exercise 'prescriptions', the effects of which will vary markedly between individuals. Nevertheless, it is important to gain a level of understanding of the differential effects of different levels of physical activity and exercise.

Effects of different types of physical activity

The changes that occur in the body as a result of physical activity and exercise depend on the type, volume, frequency, intensity and duration of performed exercises (Viru, 1995). A certain minimum level of energy expenditure is probably essential to avoid the condition of hypokinaesia. Paffenbarger and collaborators (Paffenbarger *et al.*, 1986; Paffenbarger & Olson, 1996) indicated that this minimum level of energy expenditure is within the range of 500–2000 kcal a week. While this has been widely accepted, less attention has been paid to the specific nature of physical activity, which may be equally significant.

There is general agreement that improvements in aerobic working capacity, cardiovascular function, energy stores, oxidative processes, lipoprotein profile and endocrine function are induced by aerobic endurance exercises (see Table 11.2). In 1968 Cooper originally recommended these exercises as the main tool for health improvement (Cooper, 1968). Since then, endurance exercises have been widely recommended for health (ACSM, 1990; Paffenbarger & Olson, 1996). While this 'prescription' has undoubtedly been accepted as being of primary importance, it should not be forgotten that other forms of activity – for example, resistance exercises, may improve insulin sensitivity, blood pressure and increase HDL-cholesterol levels in the blood. In particular, resistance exercises that include light-to-moderate resistance and that are performed with many repetitions and short rest intervals are particularly beneficial.

Callisthenic exercises are important, as they can support or stimulate brain function and mental activities. The probable mechanism for this effect involves stimuli from the proprioceptors in contracting muscles to the brain stem reticular formation (the 'arousal' effect). The arousal effect of physical activity could be related to the force of muscle contractions, which is stronger in callisthenic exercise than in endurance exercise. It should be noted that strength and/or callisthenic exercises are also essential to avoid muscular weakness (and thereby the loss of support to the joints) in elderly people. In older individuals, efficient muscular function brings independence in daily activities and can improve quality of life.

Aerobic dance and aerobic rhythmic gymnastics are attempts to combine the positive effects of both endurance and gymnastic exercises. Indeed, the marked increases in $\dot{V}O_2$max and HDL cholesterol levels seen with this sort of exercise (Jürimäe *et al.*, 1985; Williford *et al.*, 1989) are evidence of the improvement of aerobic working capacity together with a metabolic antisclerotic effect. This form of exercise can also maintain or improve flexibility, demonstrating the wide-ranging beneficial effects of these forms of exercise. However, it should always be remembered that all modes and levels of exercise are seen differently by sedentary individuals. Where exercises are seen as too challenging – despite a knowledge of how beneficial they are – they are unlikely to be adopted by any but a small number of individuals.

The phenomenon of too much exercise

As discussed previously, over-exertion or over-training phenomena may occur in individuals who perform too much exercise. Over-exertion phenomena are consequences of exercise(s) that exceeds the functional capacity of any of the body's systems, and the signs and symptoms of over-exertion are variable, depending on the exercise performed and on the individual characteristics of the subjects. Specific manifestations are probably related to genotypic peculiarities as well as to phenotypic changes in the body. These include previous experience in regard to the type of exercise, pre-existing diseases (particularly chronic sub-clinical syndromes), and lifestyles that influence adaptivity. The human body is actually well defended against over-exertion by several defence mechanisms – most notably *fatigue* – that guard against attempts to perform too much exercise. However, over-exertion is possible when a transitory decrease in adaptivity takes place but the exercise level remains high. The decrease in adaptivity may occur because of malnutrition, disease, drug taking, adverse climatic conditions, or dehydration. In some cases this form of imbalance may simply be the result of ageing. Fatal over-exertion cases have occurred when a person who is ill has successfully treated the symptoms of the disease with medications and then undertaken high-level physical exertion. Similar dangers exist in individuals who exercise under the influence of stimulatory drugs.

The over-training effect is, therefore, a phenomenon of chronic over-exertion. In athletes, it is often related to the desire to increase performance capacity beyond that which is actually possible. However, this level of motivation does not normally exist in health-related exercisers. Nevertheless, in health-related physical activity there is always the possibility of chronic overstraining of certain structures (for example, the knee joint, leg muscles, tendons and ligaments). There are no formal guidelines or recommendations on this and common sense and an appreciation of the need for slow, progressive adaptation of the body to an exercise programme currently guide the exerciser.

It is interesting to note that a feeling of 'staleness', similar to an overtraining effect in athletes, can be experienced in recreational exercises. However, this is not likely to be related to a decline in body adaptivity. The reasons for staleness may be too-frequent exercise sessions or sessions that lack variety and become monotonous. In this case, the reasons may be as much psychological as physiological. It should be noted that these effects are normally fairly minor, although there is no doubt that they can constitute a barrier to further progress and could even be a reason for giving up exercise. In this vein, Åstrand (1987) has commented that exercising is undoubtedly associated with a certain level of risk of experiencing adverse effects. However, the risk of health impairment due to hypokinaesia is 100 per cent for all those who remain lying on the couch!

Conclusion

Regular physical activity and exercise induces many changes in the body essential for health enhancement. The positive outcomes of exercising are founded on (1) removal of the harmful consequences of hypokinaesia, (2) specific preventive effects with relation to various pathological processes, and (3) enhanced adaptivity in parallel with improvements in fitness. For avoidance of the harmful effects of hypokinaesia, increased energy expenditure through muscular activity is required. Critical thresholds are likely to exist for (a) a general preventive effect, and (b) enhanced body adaptivity. Most of the physiological changes that confer improved health status are related to the process of adaptive protein synthesis. The accumulation of metabolites during physical activity specifically determines the adaptive synthesis of structural and enzyme proteins for the most active cellular structures. Hormonal changes, induced by exercise sessions, amplify this effect.

References

Abbott, R.D., Rodriguez, B.L., Burchfield, C.M. & Curb, J.D. (1994) Physical activity in older middle-aged men and reduced risk of stroke: the Honolulu heart program. *American Journal of Epidemiology*, **139**: 881–893.

American College of Sports Medicine (ACSM) (1990) Position Stand. The recommended quantity and quality of exercise for developing and maintaining cardiorespiratory and muscular fitness in healthy adults. *Medicine and Science in Sports and Exercise*, **22**: 265–274.

Andrew, G.M., Guzman, C.A. & Becklake, M.R. (1966) Effect of athletic training on exercise cardiac output. *Journal of Applied Physiology*, **21**: 603–608.

Arraiz, G.A., Wigle, D.T. & Mao, Y. (1992) Risk assessment of physical activity and physical fitness in the Canada health survey follow-up study. *Journal of Clinical Epidemiology*, **45**: 419–428.

Åstrand, P.-O. (1987) Exercise physiology and its role in disease prevention and in rehabilitation. *Archives of Physical Medicine and Rehabilitation*, **68**: 305–309.

Åstrand, P.-O. & Rodahl, K. (1986) *Textbook of Work Physiology. Physiological basis of exercise*. 3rd ed. New York: McGraw Hill.

Åstrand, P.-O., Cuddy, T.E., Saltin, B. & Stenberg, J. (1964) Cardiac output during submaximal and maximal work. *Journal of Applied Physiology*, **19**: 268–274.

Bailey, D.A. & Martin, A.I. (1994) Physical activity and skeletal health in adolescents. *Pediatric Exercise Science*, **6**: 330–347.

Barnard, R.J. (1975) Long-term effects of exercise on cardiac function. *Exercise and Sport Sciences Reviews*, **3**: 113–133.

Barnard, R.T., Jung, T. & Ikles, S.B. (1994) Diet and exercise in the treatment of NIDDM: the need for early emphasis. *Diabetic Care*, **17**: 1469–1472.

Berg, A., Frey, I., Baumstart, M.W., Halle, M. & Keul, J. (1994) Physical activity and lipoprotein disorders. *Sports Medicine*, **17**: 6–21.

Biddle, S. (1995) Exercise and psychological health. *Research Quarterly for Exercise and Sport*, **66**: 292–297.

Biering-Sörensen, F., Bendix, T., Jorgensen, K., Manniche, G. & Nielsen, H. (1994) Physical activity, fitness and back pain. In: Bouchard, C., Shephard, R.J. & Stephens, T. (eds) *Physical Activity, Fitness and Health*, Champaign, Il: Human Kinetics, pp. 737–748.

Blair, C.N., Kohl, H.W., Gordon, N.F. & Paffenbarger, R.S. (1992) How much physical activity is good for health? *Annual Review of Public Health*, **13**: 99–126.

Blair, H.R., Goodyear, N.N., Gibbons, L.W. & Cooper, K.H. (1984) Physical fitness and indices of hypertension in healthy normotensive men and women. *Journal of American Medical Association*, **252**: 487–490.

Blair, S.N., Horton, E., Leon, A.S., Lee, I.M., Drinkwater, B.L., Dishman, R.K., Mackey, M. & Kienholz, M.L. (1996) Physical activity, nutrition and chronic disease. *Medicine and Science in Sports and Exercise*, **28**: 335–349.

Blair, S.N., Kohl, H.W., Paffenbarger, R.S., Clark, D.G., Cooper, K.H. & Gibbson, L.W. (1989) Physical fitness and all-cause mortality: a prospective study of healthy men and women. *Journal of American Medical Association*, **262**: 2395–2401.

Bloomfield, S.A. & Coyle, E.F. (1993) Bed rest, detraining, and retention of training-induced adaptation: In: Durstine, J.L., King, A.C., Painter, P.L., Roitman, J.L. & Zkiren, L.D. (eds) *ACSM's Resource Manual for Guidelines for Exercise Testing and Prescription*. 2nd edn. Philadelphia: Lea and Febiger, pp. 115–128.

Booth, F.W. & Gould, E.W. (1975) Effects of training and disuse on connective tissue. *Exercise and Sport Sciences Reviews*, **3**: 83–112.

Booth, F.W. & Thomason, D.B. (1991) Molecular and cellular adaptation of muscle in response to exercise: perspectives of various models. *Physiological Reviews*, 71: 541–585.

Bouchard, C., Shephard, R.J. & Stephans, T. (eds) (1994) *Physical Activity, Fitness and Health*. Champaign IL: Human Kinetics.

Brill, P.A., Macera, C.A., Davis, D.R., Blair, S.N. & Gordon, N. (2000) Muscular strength and physical function. *Medicine and Science in Sports and Exercise*, 32: 412–416.

Brown, M. & Holloszy, J.O. (1993) Effects of walking, jogging, and cycling on strength, flexibility, speed and balance in 60- to 72-year-olds. *Ageing*, 5: 427–434.

Buettinger, G.R. (1993) The peaking order of free radicals and antioxidants: lipid peroxidation, alpha-tocopherol, and ascorbate. *Archives of Biochemistry and Biophysics*, 300: 535–543.

Caro, J.F., Sinha, M.K., Kolaczynski, J.W., Zhang, P.L. & Considine, P.A. (1996) Leptin: a tale of an obesity gene. *Diabetes*, 45: 1455–1462.

Chilibeck, P.D., Sale, D.G. & Webber, C.E. (1995) Exercise and bone mineral density. *Sports Medicine*, 19: 103–122.

Cooper, K.H. (1968) *Aerobics*. New York, Evans & Co.

Coyle, E.F. & Conzález-Alonso, J. (2001) Cardiovascular dift during prolonged exercise: new perspectives. *Exercise and Sports Science Reviews*, 29: 88–92.

Craig, B.W., Hammons, G.T., Garthwaite, S.M., Jarett, L. & Holloszy, J.O. (1981) Adaptation of fat cells to exercise: response of glucose uptake and oxidation to insulin. *Journal of Applied Physiology*, 51: 1500–1506.

Dempsey, J.A. (1986) Is the lung built for exercise? *Medicine and Science in Sports and Exercise*, 18: 143–55.

Després, J.-P., Trembley, A., Nadeau, A. & Bouchard, C. (1988) Physical training and changes in regional adipose tissue distribution. *Acta Medica Scandinavica*, 723: (Suppl.) 205–212.

Dohm, G.L., Sinha, M.K. & J.F. (1987) Insulin receptor binding and protein kinase activity in muscles of trained rats. *American Journal of Physiology*, 252: E170–E175.

Ducimetiere, P., Eschwege, E., Papoz, L., Richard, J.L., Claude, J.R. & Rosselin, G. (1980) Relationship of plasma insulin levels to the incidence of myocardial infraction and coronary heart disease morality in a middle-aged population. *Diabetologia*, 19: 205–210.

Dunn, A.L. & Dishman, R.K. (1991) Exercise and neurobiology of depression. *Exercise and Sport Sciences Reviews*, 19: 41–98.

Ekblom, B. (1970) Effect of physical training on circulation during prolonged severe exercise. *Acta Physiologica Scandinavica*, 78: 145–158.

Ekblom, B., Åstrand, P.-O., Saltin, B., Stenberg, J. & Wallström, B. (1968) Effect of training on circulatory response to exercise. *Journal of Applied Physiology*, 24: 518–528.

Ekelund, L., Haskell, W.L., Johnson, J.L., Whaley, F.S., Criqui, M.H. & Shops, D.S. (1988) Physical fitness as a predictor of cardiovascular mortality in asymptomatic North American Man: the lipid research clinics mortality follow-up study. *New England Journal of Medicine*, 319: 1379–1384.

Eskola, J., Ruuskanen, O., Soppi, E., Viljanen, M.K., Järvinen, M., Toivonen, H. & Kokalainen, K. (1978) Effect of sport stress on lymphocyte transformation and antibody formation. *Clinical and Experimental Immunology*, 32: 339–345.

Galbo, H. (1983) *Hormonal and Metabolic Adaptation to Exercise*. Stuttgart, New York: Thieme.

Gledhill, N., Cox, D. & Jammik, R. (1994) Endurance athletes stroke volume does not plateau: major advantage is diastolic function. *Medicine and Science in Sports and Exercise*, 26: 1116–1121.

Goodyear, L.J. & Kahn, B.B. (1998) Exercise, glucose transport, and insulin sensitivity, *Ann Rev Med*, 49: 235–261.

Gotovtseva, E.P., Surkina, I.D. & Uchakin, P.N. (1998) Potential interventions to prevent immune suppression during training. In: R.B. Kreider, A.C. Fry and M.L. O'Toole (eds) *Overtraining in Sport*. Champaign Ill: Human Kinetics, 243–272.

Green, H.J., Jones, L.L. & Painter, D.C. (1990) Effects of short-term training on cardiac function during prolonged exercise. *Medicine and Science in Sports and Exercise*, 22: 488–493.

Grimston, S.K., Willows, N.D. & Hanley, D.A. (1993) Mechanical loading regime and its relationship to bone mineral density in children. *Medicine and Science in Sports and Exercise*, 25: 1203–1210.

Hargreaves, M. (ed.) (1995) *Exercise Metabolism.* Champaign: Human Kinetics.

Harris, M.I., Hadden, W.C., Knowler, W.C. & Bennett, P.H. (1987) Prevalence of diabetes and impaired glucose tolerance and plasma glucose levels in U.S. population aged 20–74 ys. *Diabetes,* **36**: 523–534.

Haskell, W.L., Leon, A.S., Caspersen, C.J., Froelicher, V.F., Hagberg, J.M., Harlan, V.F., Holloszy, J.O., Regensteiner, J.G., Thomson, P.D., Washburn, R.D. & Wilson, P.W.F. (1992) Cardiovascular benefits and assessment of physical activity and physical fitness in adults. *Medicine and Science in Sports and Medicine,* **24**: (Suppl.) S201–S219.

Hebbelnick, M. & Casier, H. (1966) Effect of muscular exercise on the metabolism of 4-C^{14} labelled cholesterol in mice. *Internationale Zeitschriff für die angewante Physiologie,* **22**: 185–189.

Helmrich, S.P., Ragland, D.R., Leung, R.W. & Paffenbarger, R.S. (1991) Physical activity and reduced occurrence of non-insulin-dependent diabetes mellitus. *New England Journal of Medicine,* **325**: 147–152.

Ho, K.W., Roy, R.R., Taylor, J.F., Heusner, W.W. & Van Huss W.D. (1983) Differential effects of running and weight-lifting on the coronary arterial tree. *Medicine and Science in Sports and Exercise,* **15**: 472–477.

Holloszy, J.O., Schultz, J., Kusnierkiewicz, J., Hagberg, J.M. & Ehsani, A.A. (1987) Effects of exercise on glucose tolerance and insulin resistance. *Acta Medica Scandinavica,* **711**: (Suppl.) 55–65.

Inal, M., Akyüz, F., Turgut, A. & Getsfried, W.M. (2001) Effect of aerobic and anaerobic metabolism on free radical generation swimmers. *Medicine and Science in Sports and Exercise,* **33**: 564–567.

Jakovlev, N.N. (1977) *Sportbiochemie.* Leipzig, Barth.

Jürimäe, T., Neissaar, I. & Viru, A. (1985) The effect of similar aerobic gymnastics and running programs on physical working capacity and blood lipids and lipoproteins in female university students. *Hungarian Review of Sports Medicine,* **26**: 251–255.

Kaneley, J.A., Andersen-Reid, M.L., Oenning, L., Kottke, B.A. & Jensen, M.D. (1993) Differential health benefits of weight loss in upper-body and lower-body obese women. *American Journal of Clinical Nutrition,* **57**: 20–26.

Kannus, P., Jozsa, L., Renström, P., Järvinen, M., Kvist, M., Lehto, M., Oja, P. & Vuori, I. (1992) The effects of training, immobilization and remobilization on musculoskeletal tissue. 1. Training and immobilization. *Scandinavian Journal of Medicine and Science in Sports,* **2**: 100–118.

Keiser, A., Poortmans, J. & Bunnik, S.J. (1980) Influence of physical exercise on sex hormone metabolism. *Journal of Applied Physiology,* **48**: 765–769.

Keul, J., Dickhuth, H.-H., Lehmann, M. & Staiger, J. (1982) The athlete's heart – haemodynamics and structure. *International Journal of Sports Medicine,* **3**: (Suppl. 1) 33–43.

King, D.S., Staten, M.A., Kohrt, W.M., Dalsky, D., Elahi, D. & Holloszy, J.O. (1990) Insulin secretory capacity in endurance-trained and untrained young men. *American Journal of Physiology,* **259**: E155–E181.

Kirchner, E.M., Lewis, R.D. & O'Conner, P.J. (1996) Effect of past gymnastics participation on adult bone mass. *Journal of Applied Physiology,* **80**: 225–232.

Kjaer, M. (1992) Regulation of hormonal and metabolic responses during exercise in humans. *Exercise and Sport Sciences Reviews,* **20**: 161–184.

Kjaer, M., Christensen, N.J., Sonne B., Richter, E.A. & Galbott (1985) Effect of exercise on epinephrine turnover in trained and untrained male subjects. *Journal of Applied Physiology,* **59**: 1061–1067.

Koerner, J.E. & Terjung, R.L. (1982) Effects of physical training on coronary collateral circulation of the rat. *Journal of Applied Physiology,* **52**: 376–387.

Kovanen, V. & Suominen, H. (1989) Age- and training-related changes in the collagen metabolism of rat skeletal muscle. *European Journal of Applied Physiology,* **58**: 765–751.

Komadell, L., Barth, E. & Konavec, M. (1968) *Physiological Enlargement of the Heart.* Bratislava: Slovak Academy of Sciences.

Krølner, B., Toft, B., Pors Nielsen, S. & Tøndevold, E. (1983) Physical exercise as prophylaxis against involutional vertebral bone loss: a controlled trial. *Clinical Science,* **64**: 541–546.

Laughlin, M.H. (1994) Effects of exercise training on coronary circulation: introduction. *Medicine and Science in Sports and Exercise*, 26: 1226–1229.

Laughlin, M.H. & Tomanek, R.J. (1987) Myocardial capillarity and maximal capillarity diffusions in exercise-trained dogs. *Journal of Applied Physiology*, 63: 1481–1486.

Layon, L.E. (1996) Using functional loading to influence bone mass and architecture: objectives, mechanisms and relationship with estrogen of the mechanically adaptive progress in bone. *Bone*, 18: (Suppl. 1) S37–S43.

Lee, I.-M. (1995) Exercise and physical health: Cancer and immune function. *Research Quarterly for Exercise and Sport*, 66: 286–291.

Lehmann, M., Foster, C., Gastmann, U., Keizer, H. & Steinacker, J.M. (1999) Definition, types, symptoms, findings, underlying mechanisms, and frequency of overtraining and overtraining syndrome. In: Lehmann, M., Foster, C., Gastmann, U., Keizer, H. & Steinaker, J.M. (eds) *Overload, Performance Incompetence and Regeneration in Sport*. New York: Klükver Academic/ Plenum Publication.

Levando, V.A., Suzdalnitski, R.S., Pershin, B.B. & Zykov, M.P. (1988) Study of secretory and antiviral immunity in sportsmen. *Sports Training Medicine and Rehabilitation*, 1: 49–52.

Lindgårde, F. & Saltin, B. (1981) Daily physical activity, work capacity, and glucose tolerance in lean and obese normoglycaemic middle-aged men. *Diabetologia*, 20: 134–138.

Lipman, R.L., Raskin, P., Love, T., Triebwasser, J., Lecocq, F.R. & Schnure, J.J. (1972) Glucose intolerance during decreased physical activity in man. *Diabetes*, 21: 101–107.

Mackinnon, L. (2000) Chronic training effects on immune function. *Medicine and Science in Sports and Exercise*, 32: (Suppl.) S369–S376.

Mackinnon, L.T. & Hooper, S.L. (2000) Overtraining and overreaching: causes, effects, and prevention. In: Garrett, W.E. & Kirkendall, D.T. (eds) *Exercise and Sport Science*. Philadelphia: Lippincott Williams & Wilkins, pp. 487–498.

Malhorta, A., Penpargkul, S., Schaibe, T. & Scheuer, J. (1981) Contractile proteins and sarcoplasmic reticulum in physiologic cardiac hypertrophy. *American Journal of Physiology*, 241: H263–H267.

Marks, R. (1992) The effects of ageing and strength training on skeletal muscle. *Australian Journal of Physiotherapy*, 38: 9–19.

Meerson, F.Z. (1965) Intensity of function of structures of the differentiated cell as a determinant of activity of its genetic apparatus. *Nature*, 206: 483–484.

Mellerowicz, H. (1956) Vergleichende Untersuchungen über das ökonomieprinzip des trainierten Kreislauf und seine Bedeutung für die präventive und rehabilitive Medizin. *Archiv für der Kreislaufforsuchungen*, 24: 70–176.

Mole, P.A. (1978) Increased contractile potential of papillary muscles from exercise trained rat hearts. *American Journal of Physiology*, 234: H421–H425.

Moore, R.L. & Gollnick, P.D. (1982) Response of ventilatory muscles of the rat to endurance training. *Pflügers Archiv für die gesammte Physiologie*, 392: 268–271.

Musshoff, K., Reindell, H. & Klepzig, U. (1959) Stroke volume, arteriovenous difference, cardiac output and physical working capacity and their relationship to heart volume. *Acta Cardiologica*, 14: 427–452.

Nieman, D.C. (1994) Exercise, upper respiratory tract infection, and the immune system. *Medicine and Science in Sports and Exercise*, 26: 128–139.

Nieman, D.C. (1997) Exercise immunology: Practical applications. *International Journal of Sports Medicine*, 18: (Suppl. 1) 91–100.

Nieman, D.C. (2000) Exercise, the immune system and infections diseases. In: Garrett, W.E. & Kirkendall, D.T. (eds) *Exercise and Sports Science*. Philadelphia: Lippincott Williams & Wilkins, pp. 177–190.

Nieman, D.C., Nehlsen-Cassarella, S.L. & Markoff, P.A. (1990) The effect of moderate exercise training on natural killer cells and acute respiratory infection. *International Journal of Sports Medicine*, 11: 467–473.

Noakes, T.D., Higginson, L. & Opie, L.H. (1983) Physical training increases ventricular fibrillation threshold of isolated rat hearts during normoxia, hypoxia, and regional ischemia. *Circulation*, 67: 24–30.

O'Conner, G.T., Buring, J.E., Yusuf, S., Goldhaber, S.Z., Olmstead, E.M. & Paffenbarger, R.S. (1989) An overview of randomized trials of rehabilitation with exercise after myocardial infraction. *Circulation*, **80**: 234–244.

Paffenbarger, R.S. & Olson, E. (1996) *Life Fit*. Champaign: Human Kinetics.

Paffenbarger, R.S., Hyde, R.T., Wing, A.L. & Hsieh, C. (1986) Physical activity, all-cause mortality, and longevity of college alumni. *New England Journal of Medicine*, **314**: 605–613.

Paffenbarger, R.S., Jung, D.L., Leung, R.W. & Hyde, R.T. (1991) Physical activity and hypertension: an epidemiological view. *Annals of Medicine*, **23**: 319–327.

Pedersen, B.K. & Bruumsgaard, H. (1995) How physical exercises influences the establishment of infections. *Sports Medicine*, **19**: 393–400.

Pedersen, B.K. & Ullum, H. (1994) Natural killer cell response to physical activity: Possible mechanism of action. *Medicine and Science in Sports and Exercise*, **26**: 140–146.

Penpargkul, S., Repke, D.I., Katz, A.M. & Scheuer, J. (1977) Effect of physical training on calcium transport by rat cardiac sarcoplasmic reticulum. *Circulation Research*, **40**: 134–138.

Pershin, B.B., Kuzmin, S.N., Suzdalnitski, R.S. & Levando, V.A. (1988) Reserve potential of immunity. *Sports Training, Medicine and Rehabilitation*, **1**: 53–60.

Petruzzello, S., Landers, D., Hatfield, B., Kubitz, K. & Salazar, W. (1991) A meta-analyzis on the anxiety-reducing effects of acute and chronic exercise: Outcomes and mechanisms. *Sports Medicine*, **11**: 143–182.

Plough, T., Galbo, H., Vinten, J., Jørgenser, R. & Richter, E.A. (1987) Kinetics of glucose transport in rat muscle: Effects of insulin and contraction. *American Journal of Physiology*, **253**: E12–E20.

Powers, S.K., Ji, L. & Leeuwenburgh, C. (1999) Exercise training-induced alterations in skeletal muscle antioxidant capacity: a brief review. *Medicine and Science in Sports and Exercise*, **31**: 987–997.

Raab, W. (1970) *Preventive Myocardiology. Fundamentals and Targets*. Springfield, C.C. Thomas.

Rauramaa, R. (1986) Physical activity and prostanoids. *Acta Medica Scandinavica*, **711**: (Suppl.) 37–42.

Rauramaa, R., Salonen, J.T., Seppanen, K., Salonen, R., Venalainen, J.M., Ihanainen, M. & Rissanen, V. (1986) Inhibition of platelet aggregability by moderate-intensity physical exercise: a randomized clinical trial in overweight men. *Circulation*, **74**: 939–944.

Reindell, H., Klepzig, H. & Stein, H. (1957) *Die Sportliche Herz- und Kreislaufberatung*. Bern: Wander A/G.

Rost, R. (1989) The frontiers between physiology and pathology in the athlete's heart: to what limits can it enlarge and beat slowly? In: Lubich, T., Venerando, A. & Zeppilini, P. (eds) *Sports Cardiology*. Vol. 2. Bologna: Auto Gaggi Publisher, 187–198.

Rowell, L.B. (1986) *Human Circulation Regulation During Physical Stress*. New York: Oxford University Press.

Rönnemaa, T., Matila, K., Lehtonen, A. & Kalbo, V. (1986) A controlled randomized study on the effect of long-term physical exercise on the metabolic control in type 2 diabetic patients. *Acta Medica Scandinavica*, **220**: 219–224.

Sale, D.G. (1992) Neural adaptation to strength training. In: Komi, P.V. (ed.) *Strength and Power in Sports*. London: Blackwell Scientific, pp. 249–265.

Saltin, B. & Gollnick, P.D. (1983) Skeletal muscle adaptability. Significance for metabolism and performance. In: Peachy, L.D., Adrian, R.H. & Geiger, S.R. (eds) *Handbook of Physiology*, sect. 10: skeletal muscle. Baltimore: Williams & Wilkins, pp. 555–637.

Saltin, B., Blomqvist, G., Mitchell, J.H., Johnson, R.L., Wildenthal, K. & Champman, C.B. (1968) Response to exercise after bed rest and after training: a longitudinal study of adaptive changes in oxygen transport and body composition. *Circulation*, **38**: (Suppl. 7) 1–78.

Sawka, M.N., Convertino, E.R., Eichner, E.R., Schneider, S.M. & Young, A.J. (2000) Blood volume: importance and adaptation to exercise, and trauma/sickness (review). *Medicine and Science in Sports and Exercise*, **32**: 332–348.

Scheuer, J. & Tipton, C.M. (1977) Cardiovascular adaptation to physical training. *Annual Reviews of Physiology*, **39**: 221–251.

Seals, D.R., Hagberg, J.M., Spina, R.J., Rogers, M.A., Schechtman, K.B. & Ehsami, A.A. (1994) Enhanced left ventricular performance in endurance trained older man. *Circulation*, **89**: 198–205.

Sen, C.A. (2001) Antioxidant and redox regulation of cellular signaling: introduction. *Medicine and Science in Sports and Exercise*, **33**: 368–370.

Sorock, G.S., Bush, T.L., Golden, A.L., Fried, L.P., Breuer, B. & Hale, W.E. (1988) Physical activity and fracture risk in a free living elderly cohort. *Journal of Gerontology: Medical Sciences*, **43**: M134–M139.

Stratton, J.R., Chander, N.L. & Schwartz, R.S. (1991) Effects of physical conditioning on fibrinolytic variables and fibrinogen in young and old healthy adults. *Circulation*, **83**: 1692–1697.

Suominen, H. (1993) Bone mineral density and long term exercise. *Sports Medicine*, **16**: 316–330.

Szygula, Z. (1990) Erythrocytic system under the influence of physical exercise and training. *Sports Medicine*, **10**: 181–197.

Talmage, R.V., Stinnett, S.S., Landwehr, J.T., Vincent, L.M. & McCartney, W.H. (1986) Age-related loss of bone mineral density in non-athletic and athletic women. *Bone and Mineral*, **1**: 115–125.

Tepperman, J. & Pearlman, D. (1961) Effects of exercise and anemia of coronary arteries of small animals as revealed by the sion-cast technique. *Circulatory Research*, **9**: 576–584.

Tharp, G.D. & Wagner, C.T. (1982) Chronic exercise and cardiac vascularization. *European Journal of Applied Physiology*, **48**: 97–104.

Tibbits, G., Koziol, B.J., Roberts, N.K., Baldwin, K.M. & Barnard, D.J. (1978) Adaptation of the rat myocardium to endurance training. *Journal of Applied Physiology*, **44**: 85–89.

Tinetti, M.E., Baker, D.I., McAvay, G., Claus, E.B., Garrett, P. & Gottschalk, M. (1994) A multifactorial intervention to reduce the risk of falling among elderly people living in the community. *New England Journal of Medicine*, **319**: 1701–1707.

Tipton, C.M., Schild, R.J. & Tomanek, R.J. (1967) Influence of physical activity on the strength of knee ligaments in rats. *American Journal of Physiology*, **212**: 783–787.

US Department of Health and Human Services. *Physical Activity and Health. A Report of the Surgeon General*. The President Council on Physical Fitness and Sports, Pittsburgh, PA 1996.

Viru, A. (1992) Mechanism of general adaptation. *Medical Hypothesis*, **38**: 296–300.

Viru, A. (1994) Molecular cellular mechanisms of training effects. *Journal of Sports Medicine and Physical Fitness*, **34**: 309–322.

Viru, A. (1995) *Adaptation in Sports Training*. Boca Raton: CRC Press.

Viru, A. & Seene, T. (1985) Peculiarities of adjustments in the adrenal cortex to various training regimes. *Biology of Sport*, **2**: 91–99.

Viru, A. & Smirnova, T. (1995) Health promotion and exercise training. *Sports Medicine*, **19**: 123–136.

Viru, A. & Tendzegolskis, Z. (1995) Plasma endorphin species during dynamic exercise in humans. *Clinical Physiology*, **15**: 73–79.

Vranic, M. & Wasserman, D. (1990) Exercise, fitness and diabetes. In: Bouchard, C., Shephard, J.R., Stephens, T., Sutton, J. & McPherson, B. (eds) *Exercise, Fitness and Health. A Consensus of Current Knowledge*. Champaign IL: Human Kinetics, pp. 467–490.

Vuori, I. (1995) Exercise and physical health: Musculoskeletal health and functional capabilities. *Research Quarterly for Exercise and Sport*, **66**: 276–285.

Wahrenberg, H., Bolinder, J. & Arner, P. (1991) Adrenergic regulation of lipolysis in human fat cells during exercise. *European Journal of Clinical Investigation*, **21**: 534–541.

Wareham, R.W. & Jakes, N.J. (this volume) – See Chapter 3.

Whyte, G.P., George, K., Sharma, S., Lumbey, S., Gates, P., Prasad, K. & McKenna, W.J. (2000) Cardiac fatigue following prolonged endurance exercise of differing distances. *Medicine and Science in Sports and Exercise*, **32**: 1067–1072.

Williams, P.T. (2001) Physical fitness and activity as separate heart disease risk factors: a meta-analysis. *Medicine and Science in Sports and Exercise*, **23**: 754–761.

Williford, H.N., Scharff-Olson, M. & Blessing, D.I. (1989) The physiological effects of aerobic dance: a review. *Sports Medicine*, **8**: 335–345.

Wilmore, J.H., Stanforth, P.R., Gagnon, J., Rice, T., Mandel, S., Leon, A.S., Rao, D.C., Skinner, J.S. & Bouchard, C. (2001) Cardiac output and stroke volume changes with endurance training: The HERITANCE Family Study. *Medicine and Science in Sports and Exercise*, **33**: 99–106.

Wolfe, R.R., Nadel, E.R., Shaw, J.H.E., Stephansen, L.A. & Wolfe, M.H. (1986) Role of changes in insulin and glucose homeostasis in exercise. *Journal of Clinical Investigation*, **77**: 900–907.

Yu, B. (1994) Cellular defences against damage from reactive oxygen species. *Physiological Reviews*, **74**: 139–162.

Zhimkin, N.V. (1961) Stress in physical exercises and the state of unspecifically enhanced resistance of the body. *Sechenov Physiological Journal of the USSR*, **47**: 741–751.

CHAPTER 12

The Anthropology of Physical Activity

CATHERINE PANTER-BRICK

Introduction

It is often said that the activity patterns and energy requirements of modern humans were significantly shaped by evolution in the 'Stone Age'. Claims that we are 'designed as a species for physical activity' result from observing the lifestyles of hunter-gatherers (foragers), for whom food procurement depends directly upon energy expenditure, and projections onto ancestral foragers. The high physical activity, strength and endurance required for the pursuit of subsistence during 99 per cent of our evolutionary history are then contrasted with present-day low levels of physical activity. It is argued that an evolutionary understanding of activity patterns helps to understand both the human-specific physical capabilities and limitations, and the links between optimal physical activity and health. Cordain *et al.* (1998: 328) put it this way: 'the model for human physical activity patterns was established not in gymnasia,

263

athletic fields, or exercise physiology laboratories, but by natural selection acting over eons of evolutionary experience'.

Anthropological approaches take an essentially *comparative* perspective on physical activity levels in different societies, and an interest in evolutionary interpretations of the past and present. Anthropologists might ask themselves, 'How do levels of physical activity vary across different societies' for men, women and children, and, furthermore, 'How may we reconstruct ancestral activity profiles as daily life demands changed?' These are all-important questions which lead to a more informed discussion of the links between physical activity and health. Indeed, anthropologists are asked to comment not only on the transition between high to low physical activity, but also on the 'health transition' across hunter-gatherer, agriculturalist and modern industrial groups, to post-industrial (office) workers, which translates into different life expectancies and risk factors for specific diseases.

This chapter will review past and present activity patterns, presenting both evolutionary arguments regarding human-specific levels of energy expenditure and the best data available to date. As we shall see, descriptions of hunter-gatherer life – whether ancestral or modern – all too often promote over-simplified portrayals of levels of physical activity. There are few studies that do not lump together men and women, that portray the activities of children as well as adults, or that appraise variability in daily activity patterns. The net result is a stereotypical view of levels of activity to characterise the activity of humans. This is not helpful given current interest on the links between life-style activity and health, and efforts to uncover such links in children.

'Stone agers in the fast lane': an evolutionary discordance

In a series of papers, Eaton & Eaton (1999) outlined what our diet and exercise should be, in the present day, if we wanted to prevent the major degenerative diseases that are currently responsible for 75 per cent of deaths in Western countries. The evolutionary argument they espouse is powerful, yet simple. They argue that 'our biology is designed for a different era' (Eaton & Eaton, 1999: 455), such that there is now a 'discordance' between our genes, selected for a Paleolithic existence, and our present lifestyles, in terms of characteristic patterns of both diet and exercise. Essentially, present-day humans are 'Stone agers in the fast lane' (Eaton *et al.*, 1988a).

It is worth quoting their argument.

> *From a genetic standpoint, humans living today are Stone Age hunter-gatherers displaced through time to a world that differs from that for which our genetic constitution was selected.... Although our genes have hardly changed, our culture has been transformed almost beyond recognition during the past 10 000 years, especially since the Industrial Revolution. There is increasing evidence that the mismatch fosters 'diseases*

of civilization' that together cause 75 per cent of all deaths in Western nations, but that are rare among persons whose lifeways reflect those of our preagricultural ancestors (Eaton et al., 1988a: 739).

The discordance is not, strictly speaking, an evolutionary 'maladaptation', since it does not affect pre-reproductive changes in fertility or mortality through the action of natural selection. Nonetheless, it is a 'potent promoter of chronic illnesses: atherosclerosis, essential hypertension, many cancers, diabetes mellitus, and obesity among others' (*op. cit.* 1988a: 739).

This perspective sets the scene for this chapter. The links between 'lifestyle' and 'health' are situated within a broad and intuitively attractive evolutionary model, evidence for which requires careful examination of activity and health outcomes across populations.

An evolutionary model provides no proof of the health benefits of an active lifestyle (as might be obtained from prospective epidemiological studies), but it is a powerful and useful perspective. We turn to examine actual data on physical activity patterns that will help evaluate this evolutionary scenario. All data reviewed are based on direct measurements of time and energy expenditure, not self-completed activity questionnaires.

Chapter 3 (Epidemiology) describes the relationships between physical activity and health. Chapter 5 (Measurement) shows the importance of accurate and specific measurement of physical activity.

Levels of physical activity, past and present

How active were our ancestors? How great a gap exists, in terms of energy expenditure, between contemporary Western office workers and ancestral hunter-gatherers, or between modern-day fitness enthusiasts and our ancestors? And how do these various groups compare to our closest living relative, the chimpanzee, a forager sharing 98 per cent of our genetic material?

To answer these questions, Figure 12.1 allows comparison of data for modern-day urban groups, modern-day foragers, ancestral foragers, and non-human foragers (ancestral profiles are based on extrapolations from living human and non-human foragers). Comparisons between activity levels are usually expressed as total energy expenditure (TEE) and/or physical activity levels (PAL, defined as TEE/resting or basal metabolic rate, which corrects for variation in body size; see Table 12.1). Importantly, this information should be disaggregated by gender to reflect different life styles and practices. PALs are graded following the FAO/WHO/UNU (1985) thresholds of light, moderate and heavy activity (with the addition, for the purposes of comparisons in this chapter, of a 'very light' and a 'very heavy' category).

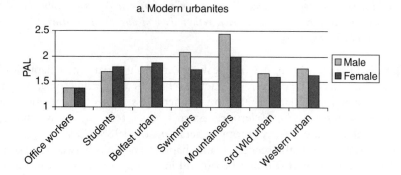

a. Modern urbanites

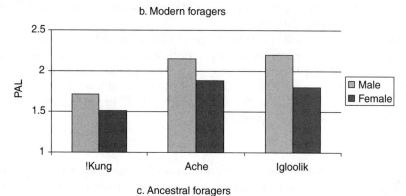

b. Modern foragers

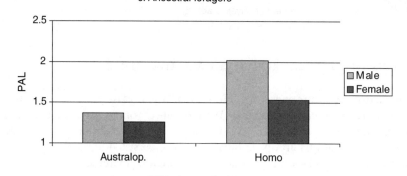

c. Ancestral foragers

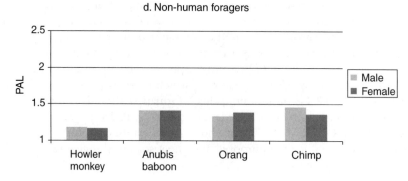

d. Non-human foragers

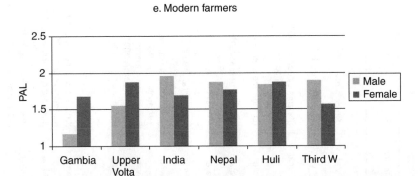

Figure 12.1 Physical activity levels (PAL) for men and women for (a) modern urbanites, (b) modern foragers, (c) ancestral foragers, (d) non-human primate foragers, and (e) modern farmers (Data from Table 12.1). Mean values are shown (measures of dispersion are not readily available in the literature)

Maximum and average activity levels in modern-day urban groups

The PAL of present-day Western office workers are 'very light' (see Figure 12.1a and Table 12.1). For both males and females, Cordain *et al.* (1998) published values equivalent to only 1.37 times resting expenditure from the Recommended Daily Allowances from the National Research Council (1989). Other authors (Chen, 1999) opted for even lower PAL values to describe the modern sedentary office worker, namely 1.18 times resting expenditure.

Scottish students and Belfast urbanites are relatively more active (PAL are moderate for males and heavy for women; Table 12.1). Unsurprisingly, swimmers in training, Everest mountaineers and Nordic skiers achieve heavy to very heavy PAL (data from doubly labelled water measurements). Maximum activity levels for humans are about five times the basal metabolic rate: $4.47 \times BMR$ for male Arctic explorers, or $4.69 \times BMR$ for male cyclists in the Tour de France pedalling up and down 34 mountains over 3800 km (Black *et al.*, 1996; Hammond & Diamond, 1997). Such extremely heavy exercise, however, is probably not sustainable as habitual energy expenditure. The upper range for 'sustainable lifestyles' – day in and day out activity – appears to be reached at a PAL of 2.5 (Black *et al.*, 1996).

An 'average' PAL for urban Western populations was calculated by Ferro-Luzzi & Martino (1996) and Yamauchi *et al.* (2001) on the basis of 55 studies selected for methodological reliability. The 'Western' PAL of 1.77 for men and 1.64 for women indicate a moderate energy expenditure. Surprisingly, this is similar to 'average' PAL for urban groups in the Third World (1.68 for men and 1.61 for women) and, unsurprisingly, much lower than the PAL for elite athletes (Table 12.1).

Table 12.1 A comparison of daily physical activity levels across populations

Population group	Sex	Weight Kg	RMR MJ	TEE MJ	PAL mean	Grade	M/F PAL ratio	Day range km	Nature of data	Sources
Modern day groups										
Western office workers	M	70	6.9	9.4	1.37	vL	1.00	–	Derived	(Cordain et al., 1998)
	F	58	5.6	7.7	1.37	vL				
Fitness enthusiast[1]	M	70	6.9	12.6	1.84	M	–	12	Derived	(Cordain et al., 1998)
	F	–			–					
Scottish students	M	65	–	12.26	1.7	M	0.94	–	Factorial	(Katzmarzyk et al., 1994; Durnin & Passmore, 1967)
	F	55	–	9.59	1.8	H				
Belfast urbanites	M	?	?	–	1.88	M	1.06	–	Dlwater	(Livingstone et al., 1992)
	F	?	?	–	1.77	H				
Swimmers in training	M	?	8.0	16.7	2.08	H	1.19	–	Dlwater	(Jones & Leitch, 1993; Black et al., 1996)
	F	?	6.2	10.9	1.75	H				
Everest mountaineers	M	?	6.0	14.7	2.44	H	1.22	–	Dlwater	(Westerterp et al., 1992; Black et al., 1996)
	F	?	6.0	12.0	2.00	H				
Nordic skiers	M	?	8.7	30.3	3.47	vH	1.23	–	Dlwater	(Sodin et al., 1994; Black et al., 1996)
	F	?	6.6	18.3	2.81	vH				
Western urban (mean)	M	76	–	–	1.77	M	1.08	–	Derived	(Ferro-Luzzi & Martino, 1996; Yamauchi et al., 2001)
	F	68	–	–	1.64	M				
Third World urban (mean)	M	56	–	–	1.68	L-M	1.04	–	Derived	Ferro-Luzzi & Martino, 1996; Yamauchi et al., 2001)
	F	51	–	–	1.61	M				
Elite athletes	M	73	–	–	2.27	vH	1.16	–	Derived	(Ferro-Luzzi & Martino, 1996)
	F	59	–	–	1.96	vH				
Modern day foragers										
Bostwana !Kung San	M	46	5.3	9.1	1.71	M	1.13	15	Factorial	(Leonard & Robertson, 1992; Katzmarzyk et al., 1994)
	F	41	4.9	7.4	1.51	L		9		
Paraguay Ache	M	60	6.5	13.9	2.15	H	1.14	19	Factorial	(Leonard & Robertson, 1992; Katzmarzyk et al., 1994)
	F	52	5.8	11.0	1.88	H		9		
Igloolik Eskimo[2]	M	65	7.0	15.4	2.19	H	1.22	?	Factorial	(Godin & Shepard, 1973; Katzmarzyk et al., 1994)
	F	55	5.5	9.8	1.8	H		?		

Ancestral foragers[3]

Homo sapiens	M	65	6.7	13.6	2.02	H	1.32	—	Simulation	(Leonard & Robertson, 1997)
	F	54	5.8	8.9	1.54	L		—		
erectus	M	63	6.6	13.2	2.02	H	1.32	—	Simulation	(Leonard & Robertson, 1997)
	F	52	5.7	8.7	1.53	L		—		
Australopithecine robustus/africanus	M	40	4.7	6.4	1.37	vL	1.09	—	Simulation	(Leonard & Robertson, 1997)
	F	31	3.9	5.0	1.28	vL		—		
afarensis	M	45	5.1	7.0	1.37	vL	1.09	—	Simulation	(Leonard & Robertson, 1997)
	F	29	3.7	4.7	1.28	vL		—		
Non-human foragers										
P. troglodytes (chimpanzee)	M	39.5	4.3	6.3	1.46	—	1.07	5	Factorial	(Leonard & Robertson, 1992)
	F	29.8	3.5	4.8	1.36					
P. pygmaeus (orang-utang)	M	83.6	8.2	10.9	1.33	—	0.96	3	Factorial	(Leonard & Robertson, 1992)
	F	37.8	4.5	6.3	1.39			0.3		
P. anubis (baboon)	M	29.3	4.0	5.4	1.41	—	1.00	5	Factorial	(Leonard & Robertson, 1992)
	F	13.0	2.2	2.9	1.41			4		
A. palliata (howler monkey)	M	8.5	1.5	1.8	1.18	—	1.01	0.4	Factorial	(Leonard & Robertson, 1992)
	F	6.4	1.2	1.4	1.17			0.3		
Modern-day farmers										
Gambia (dry season)	M			7.6	1.17	vL	0.70	—	Factorial	(Lawrence & Whitehead, 1988)
	F			12.5	1.68	M		—		
Upper Volta (dry season)	M			10.1	1.55	L	0.82	—	Factorial	(Bleiberg et al., 1980; Brun et al., 1981)
	F			9.7	1.88	H		—		

Table 12.1 (*Cont'd*)

Population group	Sex	Weight Kg	RMR MJ	TEE MJ	PAL mean	Grade	PAL ratio	Day range km	Nature of data	Sources
India (4 seasons)	M			12.0	1.96	M-H	1.16	–	Factorial	(Gillespie & McNeill, 1992)
	F			8.3	1.69	M		–		
Nepal (winter)	M			11.8	1.88	M	1.06	–	Factorial	(Panter-Brick, 1996)
	F			9.1	1.77	M		–		
THW rural (mean)	M	56	–	–	1.90	M	1.21	–	Derived	(Ferro-Luzzi & Martino, 1996; Yamauchi *et al.*, 2001)
	F	50	–	–	1.57	L		–		

RMR, resting metabolic rate (or BMR, basal metabolic rate, in some studies)
TEE, Total energy expenditure
PAL, physical activity level (TEE/RMR or BMR). Grades of PAL are light (L), moderate (M) and heavy (H) following FAO/WHO/UNU (1985) international recommendations, whereby thresholds are 1.55, 1.78 and 2.1 for men, respectively, and 1.56, 1.64 and 1.82 for women, respectively. The grades very light (vL) and very heavy (vH) are Panter-Brick's own.

[1] Fitness enthusiast exercising equivalent of running 7.5 mph 60 min/day (from Cordain *et al.*, 1998).
[2] Data for the Igloolik are for hunter men and for married/single women, after Godin & Shepard, 1973.
[3] From Leonard & Robertson (1997), Table 6, where activity for Australopithecine is modelled after chimpanzee and that of *Homo* is modelled after (male Ache?) foragers.

Are Western groups less active than modern foragers?

How do modern foragers compare (see Figure 12.1a and b)? There are only three groups of foragers for whom PAL have been derived from quantitative data, based on direct measurements of time allocation and energy expenditure, for both men and women (Table 12.1). PAL values for other forager groups (Jenike, 2001: 219) are based on less reliable data for dietary intakes and are composite for both men and women. For the !Kung San of Botswana, PAL are moderate for men (1.71) and light for women (1.51). For the Ache of Paraguay and the Igloolik of Canada, PAL are heavy for men (2.2) and for women (1.8). In brief, activity levels range from light to heavy.

!Kung San activity patterns are the most widely used to illustrate the kind of activity entailed in foraging subsistence. Women walk 2400 km annually (about 6.6 km a day) while carrying equipment, 7–10 kg of gathered food, and a child (Lee, 1979: 310–312; Bentley, 1985). Men go on hunting trips for up to four days a week, and travel 15 km or more on each trip. Yet the !Kung are demonstrably a model for low-energy hunting and gathering, associated with small body size and slow reproduction rates, when compared to the Ache, who live in a richer forest environment and who achieve higher levels of energy expenditure and intake, larger body sizes, as well as a higher reproductive rate (Jenike, 2001). There is significant cross-population variability in PAL, and it is likely that there would also be significant seasonal variation in energy expenditure (Jenike, 2001: 221). Understanding differences in foraging subsistence strategies and their consequences for health and biology is the remit of the field of evolutionary ecology (see review in Panter-Brick, 2002).

Cordain *et al.* (1998) makes the comparison between modern-day office workers and foragers in this way: 'the TEE/kg/d of typical contemporary humans is about 65 per cent that of late Paleolithic Stone Agers (assuming their TEE/kg/d was similar to that of recent foragers; 134 kJ/kg/d for contemporary humans compared to the average of 206 kJ/kg/d for !Kung and Ache)...For typical Americans to approximate the TEE/kg/d of recently-studied gatherers-hunters it would require adding (...) the equivalent of a 19 km (12 mile) walk for a 70 kg man, to each day's current activity level!'

However, the calculation of an 'average' TEE for recent foragers masks considerable cross-population variation, evident between the desert-living !Kung and the forest-living Ache. There are several different templates for forager-activity patterns, and the use of an 'average' TEE across forager (or Western) groups risks promoting an inadequate portrayal of levels of energy expenditure. In truth, some Western groups are less active, some more active, than Ache or !Kung foragers.

Are Western groups less active than human ancestors or wild chimpanzees?

What about ancestral foragers (Figure 12.1c)? Leonard and Robertson (1992, 1997) first estimated PAL values for species of ancestral Homo (who lived

2–0.5 million years ago) and Australopithecine (3.5–3 million years ago). In one simulation model (in Table 12.1), they derived TEE and PAL values for Homo (sapiens and erectus) from fossil body sizes and the activity patterns of modern foragers (Ache, men only), and values for Australopithecines from fossil body sizes and the activity patterns of living chimpanzee. The assumption was, of course, that ancestral Homo would compare more closely to hunter-gatherers such as the Ache while a more appropriate model for Australopithecines was the wild chimpanzee.

PAL values for chimpanzee, based on detailed activity budgets, are 1.46 for males and 1.36 for females. The other non-human primates align themselves with or below these values (Figure 12.1d). If graded as for humans, these values indicate very light PAL for both sexes.

It is therefore apparent that contemporary Western office workers are about as 'active' as chimpanzees in the wild. They are also (given the above assumptions) just about as active as Australopithecines, but much less active than ancestral Homo. Of course, absolute TEE is far greater for office workers than for chimpanzee, but this is because of their greater resting energy expenditure (linked to body weight) rather than because of physical activity. By contrast, the PAL of Western students and urbanites, fitness enthusiast, swimmers and mountaineers fall well within the range observed for modern foragers (and ancestral Homo).

In sum, there is a great deal of variability among foragers, Western urban groups, and also farmers (Figure 12.1e), which afford a plurality of models for patterns of energy expenditure in the past and present day. It is only when Western groups are contrasted with foragers such as the very active Ache that a clear decline in PAL for Western urban groups can be argued.

How do men and women compare?

Among foragers, the sexual division of labour – encapsulated in the memorable phrase 'Man the Hunter, Woman the Gatherer' – is an ubiquitous feature of subsistence activities (reviewed in Panter-Brick, 2002). Although the portrayal of subsistence activities whereby men hunt for meat and women gather vegetable matter has hardened into a stereotypical view of daily activities, it is still a consistent feature of the way in which men and women organise work responsibilities. How does this division of labour affect overall PAL? And did subsistence intensification and urbanisation bring about a significant change in relative male/female activity?

A common evolutionary scenario holds that PAL increased with the advent of agriculture (then fell to an all-time low with industrialisation) and that activities were more sharply differentiated in hunter-gatherers relative to farmers. Paleontologists look for evidence of this in the bones of prehistoric

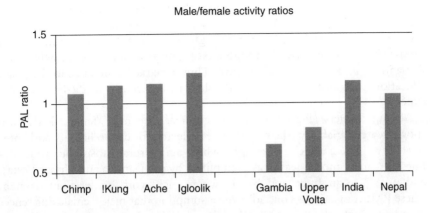

Figure 12.2 Male/female physical activity level (PAL) ratio (Data from Table 12.1)

foragers and farmers. According to Ruff (1987), bones help to appraise both overall levels of activity (affecting bone density) and types of habitual activity (affecting bone shape or geometry). A decrease in the sexual dimorphism of bone density accompanying a subsistence shift away from hunting and gathering is usually taken to reflect a decline in male long-distance hunting and an increase in sedentary activities for both sexes (Larsen, 1995: 203). Ruff argued that the shift to agriculture in the late Pleistocene led to a decline in sex differences in mobility, given that the greatest sexual dimorphism in bone shape showed a strong decline from modern hunter-gatherers to agricultural and again to industrial populations. For his part, Larsen (1995) maintains that there was no 'uniform' biological transition with the shift to agriculture, with respect to either activity patterns or consequences for health (as evidenced in bones or teeth).

In the present day, how do men and women compare in foraging, farming and urban populations? Figure 12.2 illustrates a simple way of comparing male/female levels of physical activity across groups, using a male/female PAL ratio. The PAL ratio approximates unity if males and females are equally physically active, and drops to below one if females are more active than males. The use of a simple *ratio* circumvents the problem of relying on absolute values to grade workload intensity: an absolute value can be graded differently according to sex (a PAL of 1.8 is 'moderate' for men but 'heavy' for women), given that the thresholds for moderate and heavy activity (FAO/WHO/ UNU, 1985) are sex-discrepant (Panter-Brick, 2002).

Among foragers (the !Kung, Ache and Igloolik, as well as the chimpanzee), differences between male and female overall activity levels are actually quite small (PAL ratios in Table 12.1). This does not support the common expectation that a hunter-gathering division of labour should imply a marked difference in male/female energy expenditure. Among traditional Igloolik, for instance, the PAL ratio is only 1.2, even though men were 'hunters' and women 'housewives' (women had the tough job of processing animal skins, which was demanding in both time and energy). Thus a marked difference in daily task allocation does not necessarily extrapolate to differences in 24-hour energy expenditure.

Among farmers (Figure 12.2), by contrast, the male/female PAL ratio show greater variability (the examples are selected for data reliability and comparability). There are clear examples where agricultural subsistence strategies burden women more greatly (as exemplified by the Gambia and Upper Volta), and others, as in India and Nepal, where men work harder than women. These PAL comparisons contradict the assumption that male/female differences in overall workloads were necessarily reduced during the transition from hunting and gathering to agriculture. Instead, male/female workloads show substantial variability across ecological contexts.

What data do we have to illustrate changes with 'urbanisation'? 'Average' data for Third World populations (Ferro-Luzzi & Martino, 1996; Yamauchi, 2001) indicate both a decline in PAL from rural to urban settings (Figure 12.3a) and a decrease in male/female PAL ratio (Figure 12.3b), with greater workload equality in urban settings. Yamauchi *et al.* (2001) do not provide measures of dispersion attached to 'average' PAL. From the above discussion, however, one would expect significant variability in this overall pattern (the Huli and Igloolik provide two contrasting examples in Figure 12.3b).

Among the Huli of Papua New Guinea, rural and urban populations differ significantly in time-allocation, physical exertion, and levels of energy expenditure (evaluated from heart-rate monitoring; Yamauchi *et al.*, 2001). The Huli are farmers in the highland and also have migrated to towns where they engage in a cash economy. The time-allocation data revealed a marked sex inequality between men and women in rural contexts, which is absent in urban contexts. From PAL data (Figure 12.3), Yamauchi *et al.* (2001) concluded that urbanisation for the Huli is associated with reduced physical activity, especially for females. They also drew attention to the fact that the precursors of chronic degenerative disease are in evidence in urban Papua New Guinea, and likely to be associated with reduced levels of physical activity.

Among the Igloolik Eskimo in Canada, the effects of sedentarisation were examined for men who traditionally hunted, engaged in wage labour, and settled in towns (Godin & Shepard, 1973; PAL in Katzmarzyk *et al.*, 1994). In line with expectations of declining activity levels from foraging to urban lifestyles, PAL fall from 2.2 for hunters to 2.0 for labourers and 1.5 for sedentarised men (PAL are 1.8 for women, described as 'housewives' for all groups). Thus male/female PAL ratios fall from 1.2 to 1.1 and 0.8 respectively for hunter, labourer and sedentarised groups. In this case, sedentarisation

a. Physical activity levels

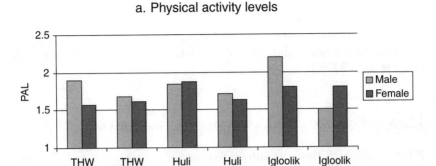

b. Male/female activity ratios

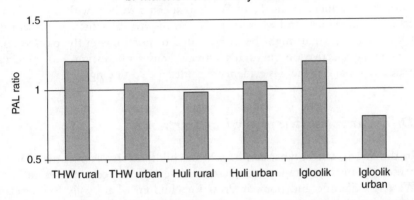

Figure 12.3 Rural to urban transition in (a) physical activity levels (PAL) and (b) male/female physical activity level ratio (Data from Table 12.1)

reversed the relative male/female differences in levels of physical activity (men were less active than women in an urban setting). The original study went on to examine the relative profile of each group in terms of specific health indicators.

There are many other studies of groups undergoing 'modernisation', 'urbanisation' or 'sedentarisation' either *in situ* or as a result of local or international migration. Such studies are designed to evaluate changes in the levels of risk for specific diseases accompanying the health transition, but they rarely provide quantitative data on physical activity patterns, expressed as PAL, which would facilitate cross-population comparison. Furthermore, studies of modernisation have been criticised for assuming either explicitly or implicitly that traditional groups follow a uniform path of development (towards resembling Western industrial societies), with a set of expected consequences (such as increased body weight, reduced daily physical activity, increased blood pressure). Current research models more carefully the energetic and psychosocial aspects of modernisation, and with respect to risks for cardiovascular health, and their differential impact on men and women (McGarvey, 1999).

How active are children in non-Western contexts?

What of the activities of children? We might expect a marked decrease of habitual levels of activity for children in urban Western countries relative to children in non-Western contexts. Surely there could be no greater contrast between Western children, enrolled in school in the week-day, and children of subsistence farmers in the Third World, expected to help with domestic and economic activities. And what are the levels of physical activity in present-day forager children that might be extrapolated to hominids in the past? A comparative perspective on children's activities raises interesting and important issues, especially as there is evidence for unexpected findings.

Different intensities of physical exertion

In the first instance, what can be said of children's involvement in vigorous exercise? This is an important question, given the concern expressed in the Western scientific and popular Press for children's habitually low levels of physical activity, involving few periods of high-intensity exercise. Recent reviews of the literature have called for a more careful examination of the assumptions that vigorous exercise in childhood confers cardiovascular fitness and that benefits to health will track into adulthood (Livingstone *et al.*, 1992: 351; Riddoch & Boreham, 1995; Riddoch & Boreham, 2000). However, the overwhelming majority of studies are done in Western contexts, with very few data on children in developing countries (Panter-Brick, 1998).

A small cluster of studies in the developing world concludes that the lifestyle of rural children actually involves very few periods of vigorous activity (Table 12.2). These studies are based on heart-rate monitoring, a non-invasive and fairly reliable method which is particularly well suited to cross-cultural comparisons of 10–15-years-old in free-living situations. Periods of 'vigorous' activity were defined as heart-rate elevations above 139 beats/minute. In British and Irish contexts, as expected, school-children engaged in vigorous activity for a very small proportion of the day (3–6 per cent of observation time). Perhaps unexpectedly, Senegalese children in a rural-subsistence community, engaged in farming activities, spent only 2–4 per cent of their day

Table 12.2 Vigorous physical activity among children: percentage time at heart rates above 140 beats per minute (selected studies, boys only)

	Age yr	Observed time	N boys	Vigorous activity % time (SD)
British school[1]	11–16	12 hr	103	6.2 NA
Irish school[2]	12–15	<16 hr	8	3.1 (1.9)
Senegal farmers[3]	11–16	NA	37	1.7 (0.7)
Senegal farmers[4]	10–12	6 hr	17	4.1 (4.2)
	12–14	6 hr	28	2.6 (3.0)
Nepal 4 groups[5]	10–13	10 hr	67	4 (5)

[1] Armstrong *et al.*, 1990 (HR > 139 bpm, roughly 70% of the maximal HR).
[2] Livingstone *et al.*, 1992 (HR > 50% of peak oxygen uptake for 'moderate vigorous physical activity', corresponding to HR > 147 bpm).
[3] Diaham & Prentice, 1993 (HR > 140 bpm for 'intense' activity).
[4] Benefice, 1992 (HR > 140 bpm).
[5] Panter-Brick *et al.*, 1996 (HR > 139 bpm for 'vigorous activity' among rural, urban slum-dwelling, homeless, and school children).

vigorously active. In Nepal, also, various groups of children selected for a marked contrast in lifestyles (to include middle-class urban school-children, slum-dwelling squatter children, homeless street-children, and rural villagers) all spent only 4 per cent of the day vigorously active.

Such low levels of vigorous physical activity undoubtedly reflect a common-sense behavioural strategy, namely a preference for children to spend more time working at a moderate rather than vigorous pace, in order to avoid physical exhaustion and to be able to sustain their activities throughout the working day. Rural Nepali boys, for instance, were 'active' for 73 per cent of daylight hours, moderately active for 33 per cent, and vigorously active for just 5 per cent of the day, as evidenced from 24-hour heart-rate monitoring and different intensities of physical exertion (measured from increasing thresholds of heart rate elevations; Panter-Brick *et al.*, 1996).

Children's activities across cultures

An evaluation of children's physical activity must include detailed studies of time-allocation to document what children actually do. Subsistence and domestic responsibilities are clearly the main tasks of pre-adolescents in many Third World communities. Super and Harkness (1986: 554) concluded from systematic observations of rural Kipsigis in Kenya that: 'in contrast to the middle-class Western emphasis on play as central to young children's development, work was clearly the main task of childhood' for the Kipsigis. In turn, Cain (1977) documented that Bangladeshi children began economically productive tasks at age six years, and worked a nine-hour day by age 13, with boys becoming net economic producers by age 12. Work responsibilities can be strongly gender-dependent. In Kerala, India, both boys and girls aged 5–15 years spent a total seven hours a day working in domestic, waged and unwaged work, but girls were co-opted more often to work in housekeeping and childcare, which increasingly bound them to the home environment (Nieuwenhuys, 1994). One study in Senegal reported that girls in early adolescence assumed a high level of physical activity, in both rural and rural-to-urban migrant contexts (Garnier & Benefice, 2001), compared to adolescents in North America (Benefice & Cames, 1999).

 Chapter 9 (Schools) identifies how physical activity may be encouraged among children using school-based interventions. Chapter 5 (Measurement) shows the importance of using validated devices to measure physical activity.

Do forager children work much less than children in farming contexts? Systematic spot-check observations of the !Kung San led Draper (1976: 213) to conclude that children 'do amazingly little work'! But here too one must caution against a simple portrayal of childhood among foragers, past and present. In direct contrast to San children, who seldom help adults forage for food, Hadza children (in neighbouring Tanzania) routinely walk a 10 km round trip to collect food from berry groves. Thus two well-known groups of modern foragers, the Hadza and the !Kung San, show very different involvement of children in subsistence activities. Such differences in children's 'activity' reflect behavioural strategies that relate to the ecological and social environments in which children are raised (Blurton Jones *et al.*, 1994). To model such differences in children's activities has already proven a complex exercise; to appraise health consequences is also a challenging task.

Types of activity and levels of fitness

Finally, let us examine the impact of habitual lifestyles on levels of physical fitness. To pursue a comparative and evolutionary perspective, what data do we have for modern foragers and what extrapolations are made for ancestral hominids? Eaton & Eaton (1999: 454) have argued boldly that: 'Hunter-gatherers are more like decathlon athletes than like either power lifters or ultra-marathoners. Their lifestyle generates both strength and endurance.' In their view, present-day fitness programmes should be directed towards these same goals.

Strength and stamina are characteristic of hunter-gatherers of both sexes at all ages (Eaton *et al.*, 1988: 24). Estimation of strength (muscularity) can be made from the skeletal remains of ancestral foragers: they were robust – as Eaton *et al.* (1988) would argue, more robust than their descendants who shifted to agriculture, and more robust than the average person in the industrialised West. The capacity for endurance (stamina) is, as Carrier (1984) argued, evidenced in our 'sweaty nakedness' – humans evolved sweat glands and hairlessness to provide for efficient heat dissipation, especially important for exercise activities such as running.

Where measurements of aerobic fitness have been made (largely for men), foragers demonstrate superior values relative to industrialised Westerners. Thus maximal oxygen uptake averages 56.4 ml/kg/min for 29-year-old Canadian Igloolik Eskimos and 47.1 ml/kg/min for young !Kung San men, as compared with a $\dot{V}O_2$max of 40.8 ml/kg/min for 20–29-year-old Canadian Caucasians (Eaton *et al.*, 1998: 24). These data indicate that age-matched physical fitness 'averages fully one-third higher for hunter-gatherers than for North Americans' (Eaton & Eaton, 1999: 450).

Aerobic fitness is primarily achieved from endurance-demanding activities. By contrast, high PAL can primarily result from working long hours on repetitive tasks demanding relatively low energy, rather than bursts of intense activity. Recent studies of contemporary farmers and agro-pastoralists, for instance, have shown that the bulk of high workloads (PAL) comes from working long hours rather than from espousing intense exercise (Panter-Brick, in press). This also has implications for modelling the types of activity 'suitable' for our species: in non-Western groups, women in particular achieve high levels of activity from a regimen of moderately demanding, regular exercise rather than high intensities of physical exertion.

Chapter 11 (Biology) describes how the body responds to different levels of physical activity and exercise.

The health transition

Do hunter-gatherers, then, enjoy better health than Western counterparts? Far from it. They have lower life expectancy and higher rates of infant mortality (two of the best indicators of the health of a population). Indeed, Eaton *et al.* (1988) were careful to acknowledge that in Western nations today, life expectancy is over 70 years – double what it was in pre-industrial times. 'Such vital statistics certify that the health of current populations, at least in the affluent nations, is superior to that of any prior group of humans' (1988: 739), resulting largely from declining rates of infection and trauma, 'the chief causes of mortality in the Paleolithic era'. However, the authors stick to their argument that our genetic make-up 'is poorly designed for modern life': the 'discordance' between genetic make-up and fast environmental change is expressed in increased risks of chronic degenerative diseases.

Chapter 2 (Lifespan) details the role of genetic factors in the growth and lifecourse development.

It is not the goal of this chapter to review the epidemiological transition and its association with physical activity (see Wareham & Jakes, this volume). But some important evidence in support of the evolutionary argument can be summarised here. Eaton *et al.* (1988: 740) argued that 'we have crossed an epidemiologic boundary...in which certain diseases...have become common, but were rare among traditional foragers'. Importantly, this is not because foragers die before old age, as they do *not* show the precursors of degenerative diseases in middle age. Thus Eaton *et al.* (1988: 743–745) have contrasted the slenderness of 'traditional' populations to the prevalent obesity in Western groups, the prevalence of diabetes in traditional settings (0.0–2.0 per cent) and Western populations (3–10 per cent), and serum cholesterol values (125 mg/dl in foragers versus 220 mg/dl in Sweden; in Eaton & Eaton, 1999: 452). They famously developed (Eaton *et al.*, 1998) a 'Paleolithic prescription' for health, based on the lifestyle of modern foragers: diet, exercise, and avoidance of noxious substances such as alcohol and tobacco. With respect to exercise, four simple recommendations were offered, in line with the probable features (aerobic exercise and resistance training) of lifestyle in the Late Paleolithic. These were: high levels of physical exertion starting in childhood and lasting until old age; daily life activities promoting both aerobic endurance and muscular strength; an exercise pattern alternating days of exertion with days of relative rest; variation of specific forms of exercise, according to the seasons (*op. cit.*, pp. 196–197).

The fact that risks of chronic ill-health are preventable was well illustrated by a simple intervention study among sedentarised Australian Aborigines, for whom non-insulin dependent diabetes mellitus (NIDDM) is a serious problem (affecting as many as 25 per cent of Aborigines, compared with only 3 per cent of Australians of European descent; Pain, 1988). One group of diabetic Aborigines was persuaded to revert to a hunter-gatherer lifestyle for seven weeks (adopting a diet lower in carbohydrates, lower in saturated fat, with quality protein, as well as increasing energy expenditure with the pursuit of food). The results were promising in that blood-glucose levels fell – suggesting that even though diabetes mellitus takes years to develop, the condition may be partly reversible.

Froment (2001), however, tempered the tendency to portray health among foragers in glowing terms, by showing that modern foragers suffer multiple infections and uncertain survival. In his view, we cannot contrast 'healthy' foraging ways of life with 'diseases of civilization', since foragers are far from healthy, albeit with fewer chronic degenerative conditions. Importantly, both Froment (2001) and Jenike (2001) argue that foraging populations do not constitute a 'biological entity' with health characteristics and morphological profiles that are invariably different from farmers or industrialist populations.

Another approach has been to search for evidence of epidemiologically relevant thresholds of physical activity. For instance, Ferro-Luzzi & Martino (1996), in their review of links between physical activity and obesity, looked for a 'critical threshold level of energy expenditure' (p. 216) to stave off the risks of obesity. Their analysis of 55 studies across the world identified a 'critical' or 'desirable' PAL of 1.80, below which the risks of becoming overweight (a $BMI > 25 \, kg \cdot m^2$) were increased sevenfold. They then explored some simple changes (regarding the nature, duration, timing of weekday/weekend) in 'active leisure' required to raise the activity levels of a fairly sedentary (PAL 1.58) Western male.

Conclusion

The model of 'discordance' between the past and present day (between our genetic constitution and modern habits of diet and exercise) is largely based on contrasting 'average' levels of physical activity for Westerners and modern foragers. The 'Paleolithic prescription' for a programme of diet and exercise that would forestall disorders such as obesity, diabetes, hypertension and certain cancers stems from a simple recommendation to bring specific aspects of our lifestyle more closely in line with those of our hunter-gathering ancestors.

We might like to conclude that Western office workers are about as active as wild chimpanzees, that dedicated Western sportsmen and women approximate the heavy levels of physical activity espoused by the Ache foragers in Paraguay, and that students typically average intermediate activity profiles (Figure 12.1). We might like, for the sake of simplicity, to say that our ancestors had activity levels (shown as PAL values) similar to modern-day foragers such as the Ache, or half-way between that of the !Kung San, adopting a figure undifferentiated for men and women. We could then argue that we were 'designed', as a species, for this particular level of physical activity, and associate critical thresholds of energy expenditures with specific health outcomes (such as obesity). This approach is but a simplistic approximation of the links between health and physical activity, one which overlooks actual variation in human activity behaviour, and extrapolates activity from socio-economic, cultural or ecological context.

There is now good evidence for considerable variability in activity levels for men, women, and children across population groups. We still need a more fine-grained understanding and portrayal of physical activity – its amount, nature, intensity, and timing – as well as a sophisticated understanding of what constrains or facilitates activity across ecological and social environments. In particular, we lack data on children, who constitute an important and interesting group. Our aim for future studies should be to grasp the opportunity to espouse a range of models for human-specific levels of physical activity, as illustrated in the range of activity profiles among modern-day foraging, farming, and urban populations.

Some findings regarding PAL variation across population groups are counter-intuitive. Some apparently obvious expectations regarding PAL differences across populations are not supported by the evidence. Thus, Ferro-Luzzi & Martino (1996) reported no systematic differences in levels of habitual activity between Western (PAL of 1.74 for men, 1.64 for women) and Third World countries

(1.84 for men and 1.65 for women). In their words, 'this conclusion is difficult to reconcile with the profound differences in terms of mechanization of labour and home activities between Third World and industrial societies, and with the widespread belief that daily life in less-developed countries demands a vastly superior physical effort. It seems counter-intuitive that a Third World woman, who spends 30–150 minutes every day of her life simply fetching water (...), or walks while attending to her daily chores for up to 1.5 hours (...), should have a PAL value that is not dissimilar from that of a Western housewife who just turns a tap to get water and drives to the shops' (p. 213). Perhaps Third World women spare as much energy as possible by spending non-work time in low-intensity activities.

Similarly, studies of children have unexpectedly found low levels of 'vigorous' physical activity in non-Western contexts, and these probably reflect the same commonsense strategy to accomplish a demanding workload by pacing one's activity. In cross-population comparisons of habitual lifestyles, a more sophisticated evaluation of physical activity, in terms of the intensity and the pace of habitual tasks, remains a challenge for future studies.

References

Armstrong, N., Balding, J., Gentle, P. & Kirby, B. (1990) Patterns of physical activity among 11 to 16 year-old British children. *British Medical Journal*, **301**: 203–205.

Benefice, E. (1992) Physical activity and anthropometric and functional characteristics of mildly malnourished Senegalese children. *Annals of Tropical Paediatrics*, **12**: 55–66.

Benefice, E. & Cames, C. (1999) Physical activity patterns of rural Senegalese adolescent girls during the dry and rainy seasons measured by movement registration and direct observation methods. *European Journal of Clinical Nutrition*, **53**: 636–643.

Bentley, G.R. (1985) Hunter-Gatherer Energetics and Fertility: A Reassessment of the !Kung San. *Human Ecology*, **13(1)**: 79–109.

Black, A.E., Coward, W.A., Cole, T.J. & Prentice, A.M. (1996) Human energy expenditure in affluent societies: an analysis of 574 doubly-labelled water measurements. *European Journal of Clinical Nutrition*, **50**: 72–92.

Blurton Jones, N., Hawkes, K. & Draper, P. (1994) Foraging patterns of !Kung adults and children: why didn't !Kung children forage? *Journal of Anthropological Research*, **50**: 217–248.

Cain, M. (1977) The economic activities of children in a village in Bangladesh. *Population and Development Review*, **3(3)**: 201–227.

Carrier, D.R. (1984) The energetic paradox of human running and hominid evolution. *Current Anthropology*, **25**: 483–495.

Chen, J. di (1999) Evolutionary aspects of exercise. In: Simopoulos, A.P. (ed.) *Evolutionary Aspects of Nutrition and Health, Diet, Exercise, Genetics and Chronic Disease*. World Rev. Nutr. Diet, Basel: Karger, **84**: 106–117.

Cordain, L., Gotshall, R.W., Eaton, S.B. & Eaton, III S.B. (1998) Physical activity, energy expenditure and fitness: An evolutionary perspective. *International Journal of Sports Medicine*, **19**: 328–335.

Diaham, B. & Prentice, A. (1993) Are modern British children too inactive? *British Medical Journal*, **306**: 998–999.

Draper, P. (1976) Social and economic constraints on child life among the !Kung. In: Lee, R. & Devore, I. (eds) *Kalahari Hunter-Gatherers*. Cambridge, MA: Harvard University Press, pp. 199–217.

Durnin, J.V.G.A. & Passmore, R. (1967) *Energy, work and leisure*. London: Heinemann.

Eaton, S.B. and Eaton, III S.B. (1999) Hunter-gatherers and human health. In: Lee, R.B. & Daly, R. (eds) *The Cambridge Encyclopedia of Hunters and Gatherers.* Cambridge: Cambridge University Press, pp. 449–456.

Eaton, S.B., Konner, M. & Shostak, M. (1988) Stone agers in the fast lane: Chronic degenerative diseases in evolutionary perspective. *The American Journal of Medicine*, **84**: 739–749.

Eaton, S.B., Shostak, M. & Konner, M. (1988) *The Paleolithic Prescription: A program of diet & exercise and a design for living.* New York: Harper & Row.

FAO/WHO/UNU Expert Consultation (1985) *Energy and Protein Requirements.* Technical Report Series 724, World Health Organization, Geneva.

Ferro-Luzzi, A. & Martino, L. (1996) Obesity and physical activity. In: *The origin and consequences of obesity* (Ciba Foundation Symposium 201), Wiley: Chichester, pp. 207–227 and 259–266 (Appendix).

Froment, A. (2001) Evolutionary biology and health of hunter-gatherer populations. In: Panter-Brick, C., Layton, R. & Rowley-Conwy, P.A. (eds) *Hunter-Gatherers – An Interdisciplinary Perspective.* Cambridge: Cambridge University Press, pp. 239–266.

Garnier, D. & Benefice, E. (2001) Habitual physical activity of Senegalese adolescent girls under different working conditions, as assessed by a questionnaire and movement registration. *Annals of Human Biology*, **28**: 79–91.

Godin, G. & Shepard, R.J. (1973) Activity patterns of the Canadian Eskimo. In: Edolhm, O.G. & Gunderson, E.K.E. (eds) *Polar Human Biology.* London: Heinemann Medical, pp. 193–215.

Hammond, K.A. and Diamond, J. (1997) Maximal energy budgets in humans and animals. *Nature*, **386**: 457–462.

Jenike, M. (2001) Nutritional ecology: diet, physical activity, and body size. In: Panter-Brick, C., Layton, R. & Rowley-Conwy, P.A. (eds) *Hunter-Gatherers – An Interdisciplinary Perspective.* Cambridge: Cambridge University Press, pp. 205–238.

Katzmarzyk, P.T., Leonard, W.R., Crawford, M.H. & Sukernik, R.I. (1994) Resting Metabolic rate and daily energy expenditure among two indigenous Siberian populations. *American Journal of Human Biology*, **6(6)**: 719–730.

Larsen, C.S. (1995) Biological changes in human populations with agriculture. *Annual Review of Anthropology*, **24**: 185–213.

Lee, R.B. (1979) *The !Kung San: Men, Women and Work in a Foraging Society.* Cambridge: Cambridge University Press.

Leonard, W.R. & Robertson, M.L. (1992) Nutritional Requirements and Human Evolution: A Bioenergetics Model. *American Journal of Human Biology*, **4**: 179–195.

Leonard, W.R. & Robertson, M.L. (1997) Comparative Primate Energetics and Hominid Evolution. *American Journal of Physical Anthropology*, **102**: 265–281.

Livingstone, M.B.E., Coward, W.A., Prentice, A.M., Davies, P.S.W., Strain, J.J., McKenna, P.G., Mahoney, C.A., White, J.A., Stewart, C.M. & Kerr, M.J. (1992) Daily energy expenditure in free-living children: comparison of heart-rate monitoring with the doubly labelled water (^{2}H$_2$^{18}O) method. *The American Journal of Clinical Nutrition*, **56**: 343–352.

McGarvey, S.T.M. (1999) Modernization, psychological factors, insulin and cardiovascular health. In: Panter-Brick, C. & Worthman, C.M. (eds) *Hormones, Health and Behavior: A Socio-Ecological and Lifespan Perspective.* Cambridge: Cambridge University Press, pp. 244–280.

National Research Council: Diet and Health (1989) *Implications for Reducing Chronic Disease Risk.* Washington DC. National Academy Press, **142**: 52.

Nieuwenhuys, O. (1994) *Children's Lifeworlds – Gender, Welfare and Labour in the Developing World.* London: Routledge.

Pain (1988) The healthiest restaurant in Australia. *New Scientist* 18th August, pp. 42–47.

Panter-Brick, C. (1996) Seasonal and sex variation in physical activity levels among agro-pastoralists in Nepal. *American Journal of Physical Anthropology*, **100**: 7–21.

Panter-Brick, C. (1998) Biological anthropology and child health: context, process and outcome. In: Panter-Brick, C. (ed.) *Biosocial Perspectives on Children.* Cambridge: Cambridge University Press, pp. 66–101.

Panter-Brick, C. (2002) Sexual division of labor: energetics and evolutionary scenarios. *American Journal of Human Biology*, **14**.

Panter-Brick, C., Todd, B.A., Baker, R. & Worthman, C. (1996) Heart rate monitoring of physical activity among village, school and homeless Nepali boys. *American Journal of Human Biology*, **8**: 661–672.

Riddoch, C.J. & Boreham, C.A.G. (1995) The health-related physical activity of children. *Sports Med*, **19(2)**: 86–102.

Riddoch, C.J. & Boreham, C.A.G. (2000) Physical activity, physical fitness and children's health: current concepts. In: Armstrong, N. & van Mechelen, W. (eds) *Paediatric Exercise Science and Medicine*. Oxford: Oxford University Press, pp. 243–252.

Ruff, C. (1987) Sexual dimorphism in human lower limb bone structure: relationship to subsistence strategy and sexual division of labor. *Journal of Human Evolution*, **16**: 391–416.

Super, C.M. & Harkness, S. (1986) The developmental niche: a conceptualization at the interface of child and culture. *International Journal of Behavioral Development*, **9**: 545–569.

Yamauchi, T., Umezaki, M. & Ohtsuka, R. (2001) Physical activity and subsistence pattern of the Huli, a Papua New Guinea Highland Population. *American Journal of Physical Anthropology*, **114**: 258–268.

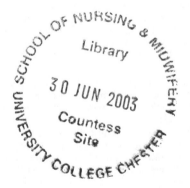

Index